bon appétit

THE FOOD LOVER'S CLEANSE

bon appétit
THE FOOD LOVER'S CLEANSE

140 Delicious, Nourishing Recipes
That Will Tempt You Back into Healthful Eating

SARA DICKERMAN

NUTRITIONAL ADVISER Marissa Lippert, MA, RD
FOREWORD BY Adam Rapoport
PHOTOGRAPHS BY Michael Graydon and Nikole Herriott

WM
WILLIAM MORROW
An Imprint of HarperCollins*Publishers*

This book is written as a source of information only. The information contained in this book should by no means be considered a substitute for the advice of a qualified medical professional, who should always be consulted before beginning any new diet, exercise, or other health program.

HarperCollins books may be purchased for educational, business, or sales promotional use. For information please e-mail the Special Markets Department at SPsales@harpercollins.com.

FIRST EDITION

Designed by MGMT. design
Photographs by Michael Graydon and Nikole Herriott

Library of Congress Cataloging-in-Publication Data has been applied for.

ISBN 978-0-06-239023-3

15 16 17 18 19   INDD/QGT   10 9 8 7 6 5 4 3 2 1

For Mary Dickerman, who taught me to cook and let me pore over all her copies of *Bon Appétit* when I was growing up.

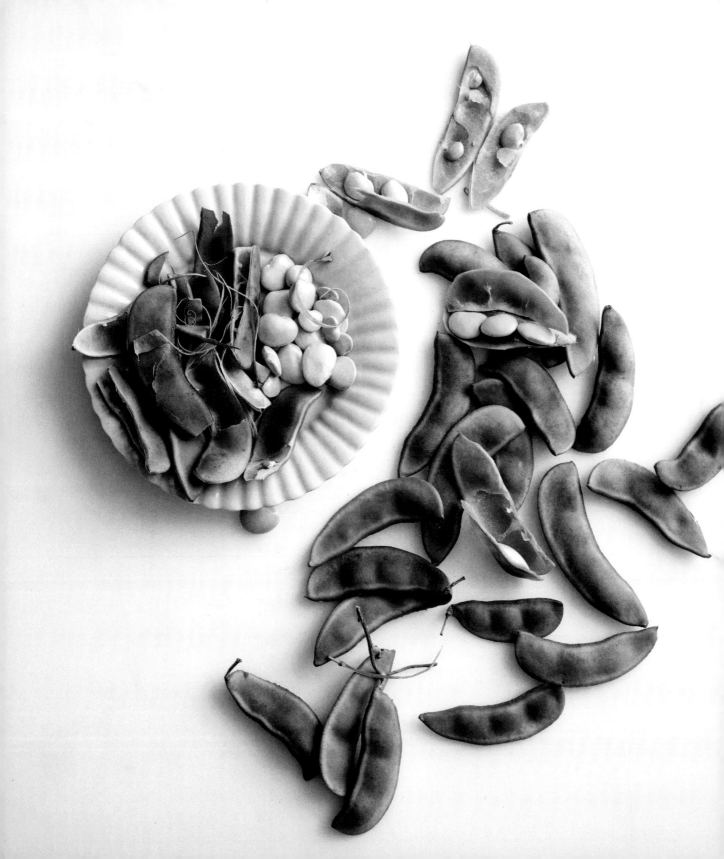

CONTENTS

FOREWORD

You know how every couple of years everyone goes nuts over some new diet? *Eat like a caveman! Eat like you live in South Beach! Don't eat, just drink juice!*

Well, at *Bon Appétit,* that's not how we roll. As a staff, we try to eat sensibly, but we also really, really love food. We've always felt it's possible to have it both ways. So when Sara Dickerman worked up the idea for The Food Lover's Cleanse, we listened up. Here was a "cleanse" that didn't *feel* like a cleanse. It was manageable, not monastic. When we read the cleanse guidelines in the pages of the magazine, we couldn't help but smile:

* "Avoid booze (mostly)." (I mean, c'mon—how awesome is the "mostly" part?)
* "Choose healthy fats." (Code for "avocados"; praise the Lord.)
* "Limit sugar." (Not abstain, *limit.*)

And it turns out that it's not only we who dig the cleanse; our readers and online users love it too. Sara and nutritionist Marissa Lippert tap into a desire that so many Americans share. After an indulgent holiday season, we want to recalibrate. And more than anything, Sara preaches doability. The cleanse is two weeks, not in perpetuity. She provides the user with detailed online shopping lists for the entire two-week run, and three recipes a day that mix and match ingredients. And all of the recipes can be repurposed thoughout the week.

Oh, and did I mention that the recipes are delicious? You'll find yourself serving them to friends and family even when you're not technically on a cleanse. When so many fad diets come and go, there's a reason The Food Lover's Cleanse has thrived for six years. Because it works.

And, hey, it's now a book, with a flavorful cleanse for each season! So go ahead and enjoy it. I can say that, because I know you will.

— Adam Rapaport

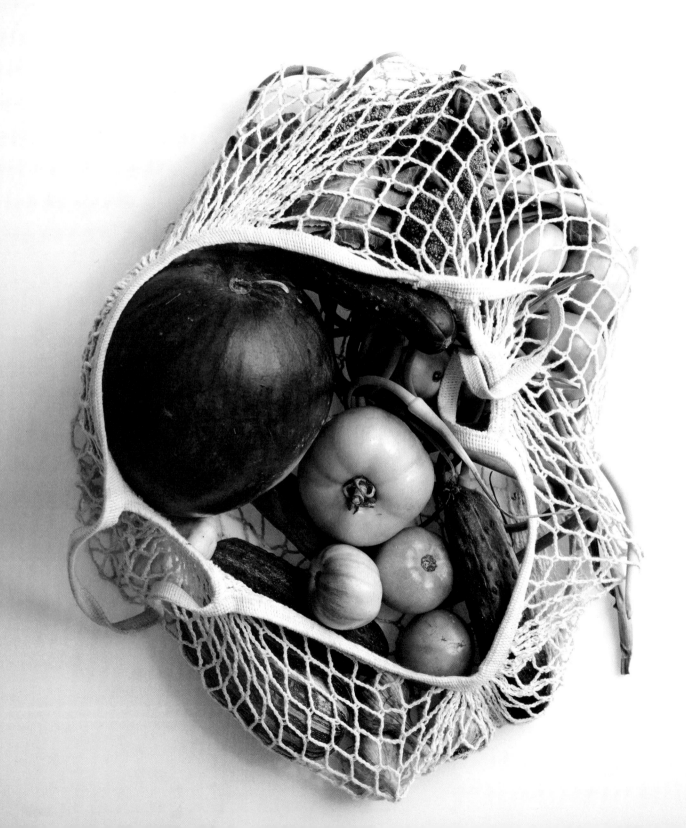

INTRODUCTION

It All Started Online . . .

Six years ago, at the suggestion of my editor, I set out to get bonappetit.com readers back into the kitchen after the holidays by designing a healthy and appealing two-week eating plan with Marissa Lippert, a registered dietician. The plan would put an emphasis on home cooking and whole foods, and the key rules in my mind were: no feelings of denial and absolutely no "diet-y" foods such as turkey bacon, artificially sweetened protein shakes, or egg-white omelets (for me, the only proper place for solo egg whites is in the meringue coating a baked Alaska). I wanted to show readers that flavor was the best way to coax ourselves into eating less of the super-refined stuff we all crave and more of the skin-on, whole-grain, lower-sugar food we could all use a little more of. I make a point of avoiding words like *detoxing* or *superfoods,* which are rooted more in media health hype than in science. If food can be the source of great temptation, why not harness the desire it creates by putting together healthier—or, as *Bon Appétit* editor in chief Adam Rapoport called it, "healthy-ish"—recipes that are full of big, seductive flavors?

And Evolved . . .

With each annual cleanse, we've tried to streamline for real-life logistics, while at the same time delving into exciting new flavor territory. We've all been astounded by the growing enthusiasm year after year. I have done the annual program along with readers, blogging about my cleanse successes and hunger-induced temper fits alike. The community response was a huge part of the appeal: readers were Instagramming their delicious meals and actively commenting on bonappetit.com (catching typos with incredible accuracy, I should add!). Just like me, readers were eager to take good cooking into their own hands and retool their kitchens for good taste and good health.

With Lots of Reader Input . . .

Some followers stuck to the exact specifications of the program, even the snacks. They would write in upset that they couldn't find some odd ingredient—say, the salad green mizuna—at the grocery store. Don't worry! Eat some spinach instead, I would write back. Many readers would just pick and choose recipes from the plan. That was fine too: if I could get people excited about one great recipe for quinoa, or black cod, or Brussels sprouts, it felt as if I was doing some good. And one of the most frequent comments from readers was: "Do more cleanses, for different times of year!"

And Now a Book!

It may have taken a while, but with the publication of this book, we're doing just that. We have a section for each season. If you want to do a full two-week cleanse, we have four schedules for you as well. If you'd rather use the book as a springboard for your own à la carte version of healthier eating, by all means do that. Just remember that at the heart of the book is a true desire on my part to let the pleasures of eating guide you toward healthy habits. Enjoy!

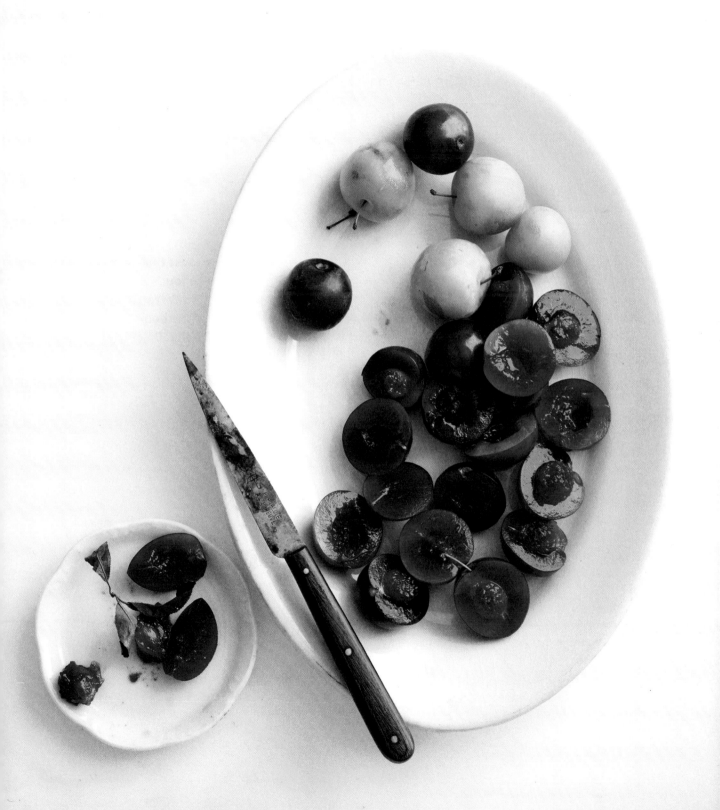

THE CONCEPT OF THE CLEANSE

I've been putting together The *Bon Appétit* Food Lover's Cleanse for six years now, and I have a confession to make: I have misgivings about the word *cleanse*. It's more appealing, I suppose, than *diet* or *regimen,* but using it is hard for me, because it suggests that the opposite of cleansing is getting dirty. And I'm pro-food. I don't think eating, no matter how indulgent, is a sullying experience.

IS THIS REALLY A CLEANSE?

There are plenty of cleanses, such as all-juice cleanses and lemon-water cleanses, that are far more radical than ours and are taken on as a kind of penance for the previous enjoyment of food. They promise, with little scientific evidence, to flush the body of toxins and give you a near-ecstatic energy boost. **The problem with these cleanses is that they tend to vilify food, treating it as the enemy of health rather than a key to it.** This kind of relationship to food is troubling to me and antithetical to a publication like *Bon Appétit,* which sets out to celebrate food and eating. Such withdrawal from typical eating patterns makes it too tempting to rebound from a program with defiant overeating. That said, I think there are moments when you can fine-tune the trajectory of your eating in a healthier direction.

A CLEANSE IS A PROMISE TO YOURSELF

What I do like about the idea of a cleanse is the idea of a resolution. If you set up a series of healthy rules and follow them for a limited time, **I think you can discover some key things about your own eating habits.** You might discover, as I have, that some of your most ingrained habits are more changeable than you think. Cravings for sugar or starchy snacks do get less pointed; you may find that you need far less meat in a meal to feel satisfied. You might realize that you have the strength to make a few small, meaningful tweaks to your diet for the long term. We don't promise weight loss (though it could happen!) or an extra five years on your life, but I do think that working with this book can help you find a new equilibrium in your eating.

RADICAL MODERATION

The parameters of "healthier food" are ever shifting, even treacherous. To make sure our suggestions are sound, I have worked together with Marissa Lippert, both a registered dietician and a card-carrying Food Lover (she owns the West Village cafe, Nourish Kitchen + Table), to create a set of guidelines for four two-week clean-eating plans.

The boundaries are more radical in their moderation than anything else: it's a program based more on saying yes than no. *Yes* to lots of vegetables; *yes* to whole grains; *yes* to healthy fats like avocado, nuts, and fish. *Yes* to cultured dairy that delivers protein and immune-supporting bacteria. Most important, **we want you to say *yes* to flavor**.

PLEASURE LEADS THE WAY TO BETTER HABITS

For me, the key to making these tweaks is in knowing that they can be even more pleasurable than the habits you had before you tried them. If plain steamed cauliflower makes you sad, you aren't likely to eat it once you're done with a diet. But if you love the way cauliflower tastes roasted and tossed with garlic, thyme, and olives, then you'll likely eat more of it. As I developed the recipes, **I looked to amplify flavor wherever I could**. Condiments are a signature of the cleanse, as is technique. Knowing how to cook a great pot of beans or quinoa makes it much more likely that whole grains and legumes can displace some of the white pasta or rice you may have leaned on.

Read on to discover more about our guidelines, and most important, dip into the straightforward and rewarding recipes we have developed for each season.

OVERVIEW FROM MARISSA LIPPERT, MS, RD

I teamed up with Sara six years ago to collaborate on The Food Lover's Cleanse, creating a cleanse that fused together nutritional balance, beautiful flavors, and simply vibrant, enticing food. From the first New York–to–Seattle phone call, I knew that Sara and I were well matched (I'm pretty sure that wine, chocolate, and cheese came up in the first three minutes of our conversation). Like her, I'm a food lover (and longtime *Bon Appétit* devotee). I love dining out, and I've been known to cook with a good bit of bacon and butter, but I also love sautéing a pan full of gorgeous leafy greens after a trip to the Greenmarket. Once we found our common enthusiasm, we dove into crafting a road map of pointers, portions, meals, and snacks that allow readers to start the cleanse with zeal and finish it with results: more energy, a sense of lightness, possibly fewer headaches or colds, sounder sleep, an overall feeling of better wellness, and maybe even a bumped-up sex drive.

For over 11 years, I've worked closely with hundreds of nutrition clients. That's a whole lot of experience in the patterns, frustrations, lifestyles, and schedules of people like you, Sara, and me, who are trying to feel better and eat better. **With that in mind, we chose not to overemphasize calories or nitty-gritty details around nutrients and health (too much information can get jumbled and take up unnecessary headspace).** I've found that for many people, setting small, strategic yet manageable goals is the golden key to long-term habit change. That change could be as simple as incorporating whole grains into your meals more frequently, or as broad as shifting your pantry and fridge to be more balanced year-round. Sara and I hope the program and recipes in this book provide you a foundation to reset yourself; to connect back to what your body is trying to tell you; to explore inherently healthful ingredients that are truly delicious; and **to create balanced, sustainable "default" eating routines that you can return to** long after doing a two-week round of the cleanse.

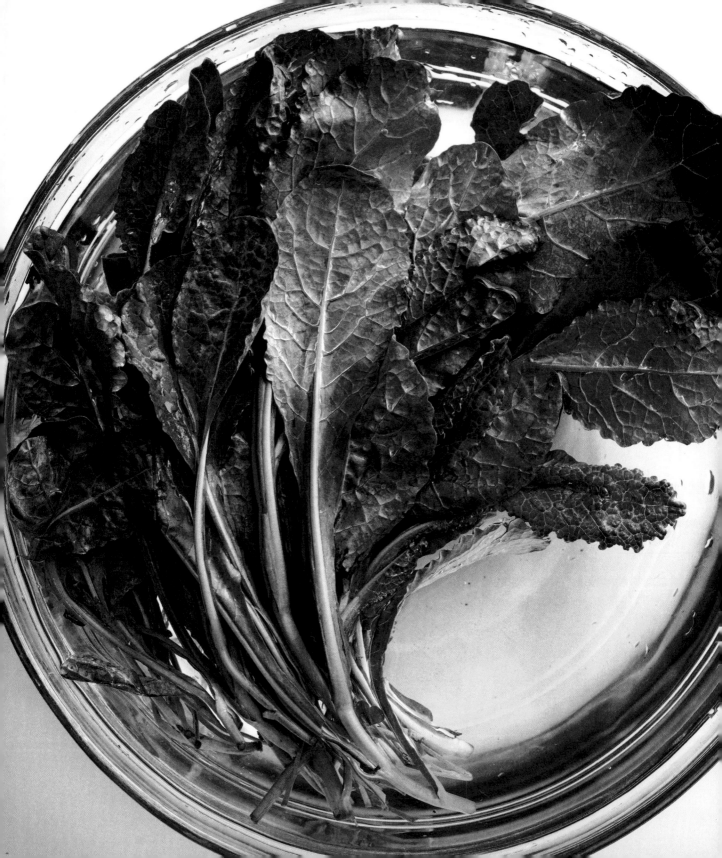

BASIC RULES*

EAT ON THE REGULAR

Don't skip meals, which tends to encourage binge eating later on: aim to eat every 3 to 4 hours to keep your metabolism on an even keel during the day. That said, once you're done with dinner and a modest dessert, stop eating for the night, ideally giving yourself 3 hours after dinner before getting to sleep.

RATCHET UP FLAVOR

If you want to reduce the amount of food you eat semiconsciously during the day, make sure the food you do eat tastes vibrant. Season your food thoughtfully with salt, and then let chiles, spices, herbs, citrus juice and zest, and flavor-boosting condiments make what you eat seem all the livelier.

KICK UP YOUR WATER TO 8 CUPS A DAY

There's no magic number for the amount of water an individual needs to drink in a given day. You should basically drink when you're thirsty. That said, drinking water conscientiously does a couple of things during the plan. It displaces other things you might be drinking (such as wine, diet soda, or cold-pressed green juice). It's also something to do when you'd rather be eating a handful of tortilla chips. And finally, drinking more water can help your body deal with the increased fiber that comes with eating more whole grains and vegetables.

CUT OUT THE WHITE STUFF

Get your complex carbs from a variety of whole grains, vegetables, and legumes instead. Whole grains give you more fiber per bite, which helps you feel more satisfied with your food, and the husks and skins of the grains also contain more diverse nutrients than bleached and polished grain products. I love white bread, pizza, and pasta, but it's good to know how delicious other whole options—such as quinoa, bulgur, and barley—can be.

*Please keep in mind that these are general rules for an adult of average health. If you have specific weight goals or health concerns, you may need to work with your doctor or a dietician to adapt our plans or recipes to your needs.

DIG INTO PRODUCE

The great thing about making a cleanse for each season is that we can incorporate fruits and vegetables that haven't been available in our winter cleanses. The principle is the same whether we're talking spring asparagus, summer green beans, or fall squash. See if you can get half your plate covered with produce.

EAT MORE YOGURT, LESS CHEDDAR

We cut way back on dairy, because it may give your digestive system a break. But we're very interested in keeping some live cultured foods in our program, so we include a fair amount of yogurt and some young fresh cheeses. Nondairy sources of calcium include almond milk and dark leafy greens.

CHOOSE QUALITY OVER QUANTITY WITH MEAT

Meat is less of a focus in FLC meals, and processed meat is excised altogether. Portions are pared back to 4 to 6 ounces per meal. If you're a meat eater, it's important to think about the context you're eating it in: a hamburger on a bun with fries tells a very different story from a grilled hanger steak served with homemade tomato relish and a quinoa salad with roasted figs and walnuts.

STOP THE SUGAR CREEP

Sugar isn't evil, but it can pile up in our daily diets, especially when we eat a lot of ready-made foods. For sweetness, there's a bit of honey, maple, fruit, and dark chocolate, but even those we keep moderate, since we're aiming to curb sugar cravings.

DRINK LESS

Limit your alcohol consumption to 4 drinks per week max. See more about drinking on page 22.

SAY YES TO THE AVOCADO (AND OTHER SOURCES OF HEALTHY FATS)

We incorporate plenty of foods that are rich in omega-3 fatty acids, such as nuts, salmon, of course avocados.

DIAL BACK THE LATTES

If you can't give up your morning coffee, we understand (and you're still getting a nice boost of antioxidants), but the results of cutting back can be interesting. One of the personal effects of this cleanse is that I discovered I sleep much, much better without a regular coffee habit. This isn't true for everyone, but it's a discovery I wouldn't have made without the FLC. Try to keep coffee to a single cup, low on the added milk and sugar. After that, swap it for unsweetened tea throughout the day: green, white, and herbal are generally lower in caffeine, are good sources of antioxidants, and can give you that nice afternoon lift you might be looking for.

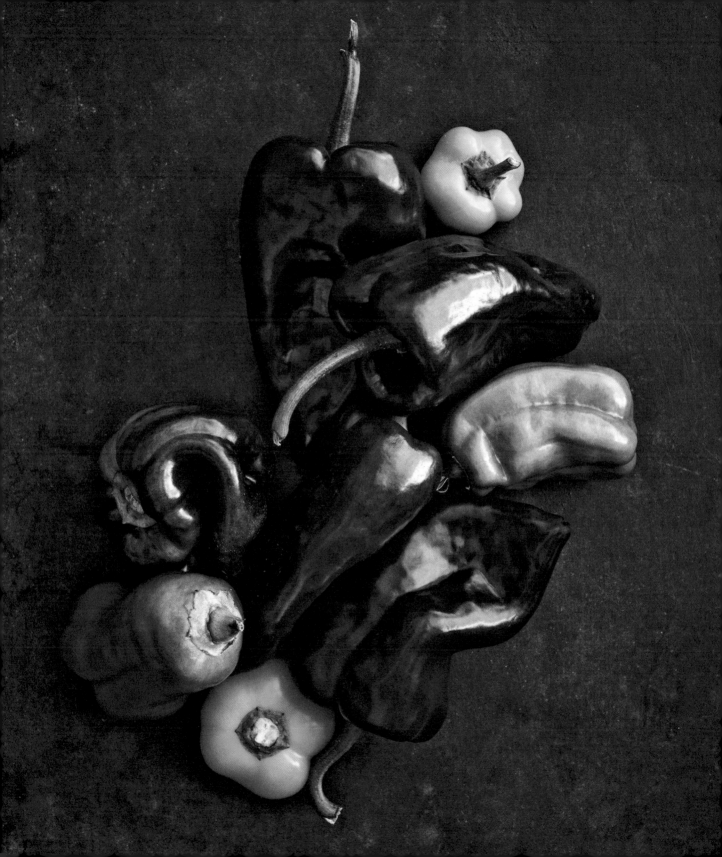

PORTIONS GUIDE

The Food Lover's Cleanse urges you to keep an eye on your portions. We want you to learn to observe your own hunger levels and adjust your eating to fit. Often, if you take a breather three-quarters of the way through a meal, you may decide you don't need to clean your plate—or at least you may calm your cravings for seconds. Thoughtfulness is one thing, but sometimes you need a way to visualize how much you should put on your plate. Here's a quick cheat sheet for portion sizes: take a look at your fist to get a good ballpark serving size for protein, and then double it for vegetables and salads! Here are guidelines for servings of other foods:

PROTEIN (MEAT, FISH, TOFU)
Size of your fist (3 to 4 ounces for women, 6 ounces for men).

GRAINS AND PASTA
Grains: ½ to 1½ cups cooked; pasta: 1 to 2 cups cooked. Go a little smaller if you're a petite female, a little larger if you're a guy or if you're extremely active.

POTATOES AND OTHER STARCHY VEGETABLES/WINTER SQUASHES
Size of your fist (yup, love that fist!).

VEGGIES AND SALADS
They should take up at least half of your plate most of the time.

TREATS AND DESSERTS
Keep them small—1 ounce maximum for chocolate or a piece of fruit. See page 16 for more details.

FRESH FRUIT
1 serving = 1 piece whole, or about 1 cup sliced.

DRIED FRUIT
¼ cup or less (2 or 3 dates, apricots, or figs).

NUTS
As a stand-alone snack, 1 good handful (about 20); for pistachios you can go up to 50.

YOGURT/KEFIR/BUTTERMILK
4 to 6 ounces per serving.

VINAIGRETTE/DRESSING
1 to 2 tablespoons per serving.

OLIVE OIL
Stick with moderate amounts for cooking/drizzling.

AVOCADO
¼ to ⅓ avocado is a serving for most women; ½ avocado is a serving for most men.

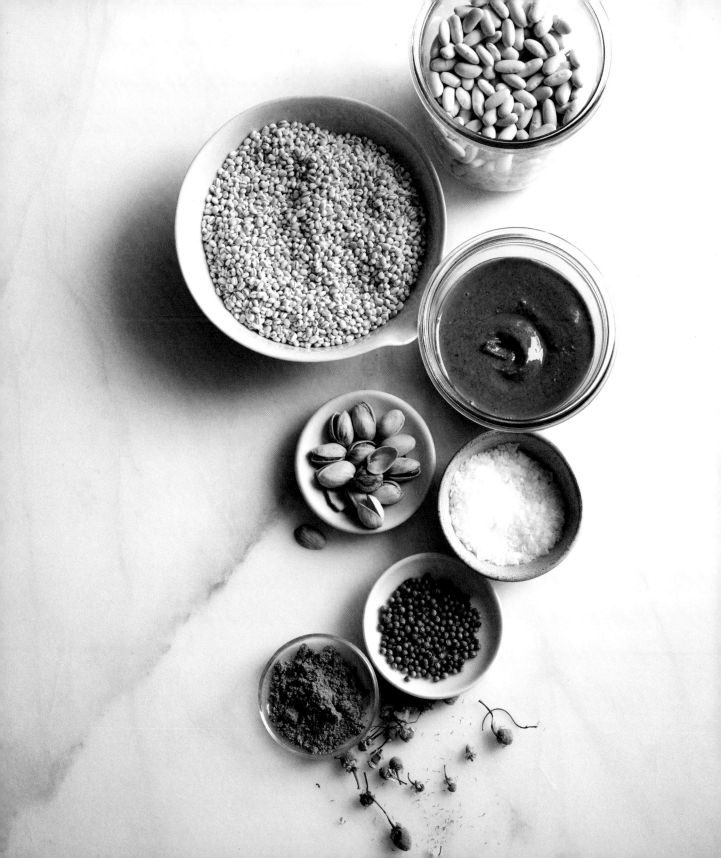

A DAY IN THE LIFE OF THE CLEANSE

Since we're trying to make healthier eating a (good) habit for you, we're setting up a regular pattern for meals; this will help you avoid weird dips in energy and keep you going at a steady pace all day long. Here's a look at the daily structure of The Food Lover's Cleanse.

BREAKFAST

A solid breakfast gets you going for the day and keeps you from lurching hungrily into midmorning snacks or lunchtime. It's even possible to resist office doughnuts if you start the day with a healthy, satisfying breakfast. But breakfast is a meal that should fulfill your most basic comforts, and you should feel free to repeat your favorite recipes more frequently or improvise your own meal that meets our guidelines. We're looking for a good bit of fiber and some protein in the morning, even enough fat (yay!) to keep you feeling sated until lunch. **If you like a whole-grain breakfast, look to eat ¾ to 1 cup cooked unsweetened oats or other porridge, mixing in about ½ cup fresh fruit or 2 tablespoons chopped dried fruit, plus about 1 tablespoon nuts or seeds or some almond milk for additional protein.** Try to limit honey or agave syrup to a teaspoon or so. **If you crave eggs, allot yourself 2 and feel free to stir herbs, vegetables, one of the pantry condiments, or a crumble of fresh chèvre into the mix.** If you like a smoothie, try to balance fruit and yogurt with some protein: nuts, silken tofu, or almond milk can all give you something to anchor the fruity sugars in the drink.

LUNCH-O-MATIC

You'll notice that we don't provide explicit lunch recipes in the book. Because everything in The Food Lover's Cleanse is so prescribed, over the years I've discovered that it's nice to let lunch be a place to improvise a bit. We encourage you to make your daily lunch a salad, which fills you up with the flavor and fiber of raw vegetables and also makes you *feel* energized and fresh. We want your salads to be significant, not insubstantial, and **we invite you to use them to reframe leftovers from the previous dinner.** We like this approach because it's a practical way to deal with extra food, and **it also gives you a little freedom to indulge flavor cravings that you might have.** Each seasonal schedule does have a suggested lunch combination based on leftovers from the previous dinner. But if you're at the neighborhood salad bar, or if you've ended up without those leftovers, don't worry. Just follow these guidelines.

BASIC LUNCH FORMULA

3 to 6 ounces protein	Leftover meat, seafood, or tofu from the previous dinner, hard-boiled egg, canned tuna, canned sardines, chickpeas, black-eyed peas, edamame, lentils, white beans, tempeh
3 to 4 cups greens or other green vegetables (frequently opt for dark greens, but it's okay to mix in lighter-hued lettuces and the like)	Kale, spinach, arugula, romaine, cabbage, radicchio, frisée, mâche, Belgian endive, mustard greens, tatsoi, mizuna, herbs, shaved asparagus, shaved fennel, shaved celery, shaved cucumber
½ cup to 1½ cups grains, starchy vegetables, beans, or fruit (choose the smaller amount for more rib-sticking foods like quinoa or barley)	Brown, black, or red rice, quinoa, barley, bulgur, roasted squash, roasted sweet potatoes, roasted beets, roasted celery root, apples, pears, plums, nectarines, orange slices
1 to 2 tablespoons dressing	At a salad bar, choose vinaigrettes over creamy dressings, or make your own: see pantry, page 310, for recipes.
1 to 2 tablespoons textural garnish	Chopped hazelnuts, walnuts, almonds, sesame seeds, pumpkin seeds, hemp seeds, flaxseeds, sunflower seeds, pine nuts, Chickpea and Hazelnut Dukkah (page 320), Spiced Pumpkin Seed and Cashew Crunch (page 318), chopped dried apricots, dried cherries, raisins, chopped avocados, olives

SNACKS

Snacks are critical to The Food Lover's Cleanse. In my experience, a well-planned snack makes the difference between a harried, cranky dinner prep and a relatively relaxed evening. In our plans, we've included snack suggestions for every day, and the pantry section of this book is loaded with dips and spreads that can be a part of your daily snacking. But we recommend you chart your own course with snacks; after all, they may be the most personal of all meals, and it's important that they be fundamentally satisfying to you, whether you seek crunch or a bit of sweetness, or something as substantive as a hard-boiled egg. **The key to an FLC snack is that it clocks in at around 150 calories or less, and that it has a good bit of fiber or protein (or both) in it to keep you feeling full enough to make it to dinner.**

- 2 to 3 tablespoons Roasted Beet and Tahini Dip (page 318) with 2 or 3 small carrots
- Hard-boiled egg with Smoked Salt Furikake (page 323) or chopped olives
- 1 apple with 1 tablespoon almond butter
- 2 to 3 tablespoons hummus or White Bean Dip (page 316) and 1 cup crudités, such as radishes, carrots, celery, or fennel
- 1 pear with a crumble of chèvre
- 1 nectarine with 1 tablespoon almonds
- Blanched cauliflower (see page 304) with Chickpea and Hazelnut Dukkah (see page 322) and 1 tablespoon olive oil
- Sliced peach with toasted coconut flakes
- All-rye crackers with ¼ avocado, lemon, salt, and chile flakes
- ½ cup plain Greek yogurt with Spiced Pumpkin Seed and Cashew Crunch (page 316)
- 1 cup of miso soup with tofu
- 1 cup of chicken stock (page 301) with green onions and ginger
- Herbed Yogurt Spread (page 321) with blanched green beans (see page 304)
- Fresh-pressed juice (12 ounces or less: you might end up with an extra bit for another time)
- Banana with 2 tablespoons Toasted Rye and Coconut Muesli with Apricots (page 30)
- 2 dates with 1 tablespoon Marcona almonds

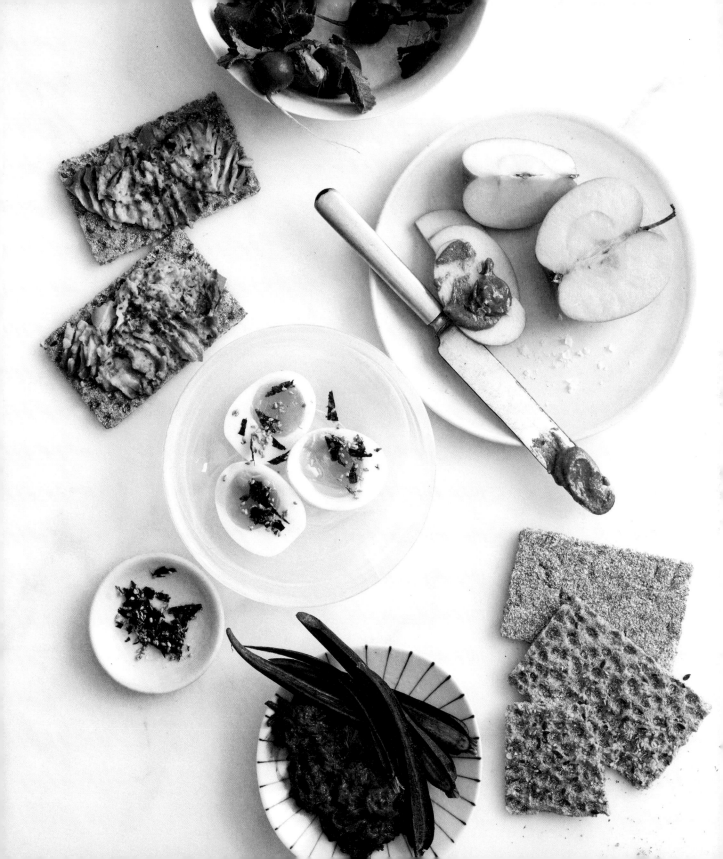

DINNERS

Dinners are less free-form, since we provide recipes for everything, but if you can't do the planned meal, once again, look to provide yourself with **4 to 6 ounces of meat, seafood, eggs, or tofu, plus ½ to 1½ cups vegetables and whole grains or legumes**. Also, slow down and take the time to appreciate your dinner: dine at a leisurely pace and enjoy the smells and the visual appeal of the food in front of you and conversation with your family or friends.

DESSERTS

While desserts can be problematic if they get to be too habitual, we know it's hard to end the day's eating without a touch of something sweet. If you're satisfied with your evening meal, you don't need to eat dessert. But we provide suggestions within each plan that alternate between a small portion of bittersweet chocolate bark and a lovely bit of fruit, perhaps dressed up with a morsel of fresh chèvre.

For portions, think 4 to 8 ounces fruit—such as a cup of berries or a single navel orange—with 1 tablespoon or less of higher-energy accompaniments, such as nuts or cheese.

Warm drinks are another way to extend conversation at the dinner table without a full-on dessert; herbal infusions, fresh mint tea, and steamed nut milks are soothing ways to end your day.

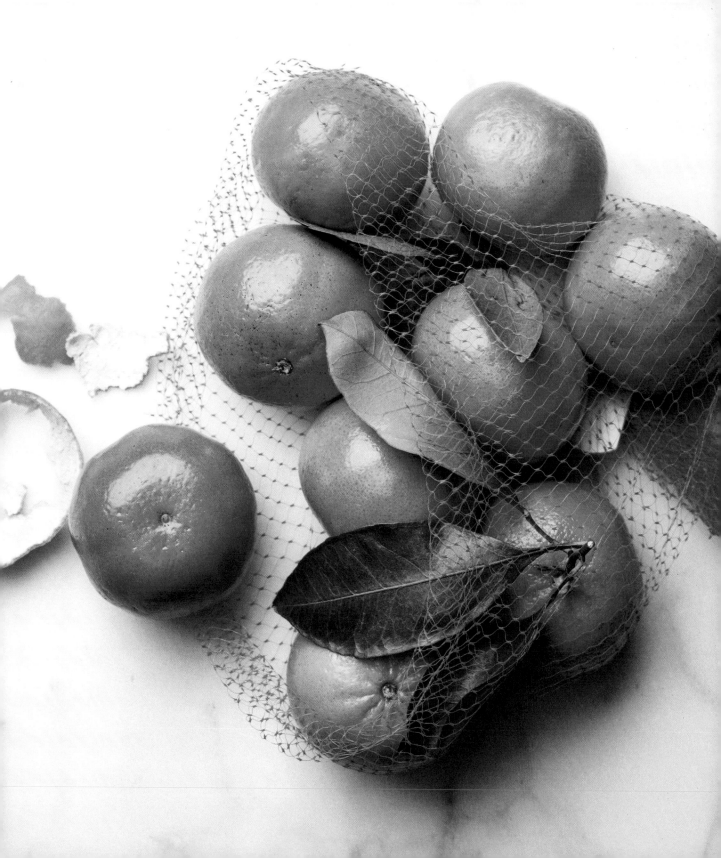

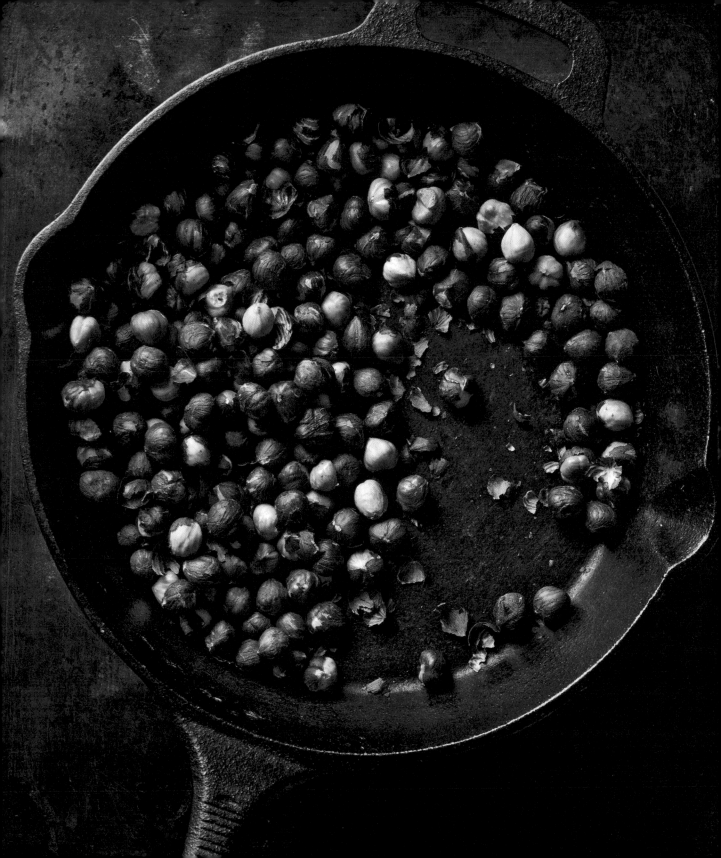

PREPPING FOR THE CLEANSE

If you're committing to the whole shebang, you should know that it will take you some time, as well as an investment in good ingredients. Your busy cleansing self will welcome as much prep work as you can do ahead of time.

CLEAN OUT YOUR FRIDGE AND CUPBOARDS

This will make space for items in your shopping list and also get rid of items that might cause you trouble when you're feeling crave-y, whether it's Nutella or tortilla chips.

GRAB SOME FOOD CONTAINERS

You're going to have a fair number of pantry items and leftovers to juggle: make sure you have enough containers on hand (with lids to match!) and plenty of zip-top bags to store salad greens or cooked grains.

SHOP THE BULK SECTION

A week or two in advance, you can knock out the shelf-stable pantry items on the seasonal shopping lists. Seek out a store with a diversely stocked bulk department for grains, nuts, spices, and dried fruit. You'll save money buying unpackaged goods, and you'll be able to buy just the right amount for your home. If you're diligent, label everything. (I am not that good.)

GET YOUR PERISHABLES

We break down the perishable part of the shopping lists into two separate weeks, so in theory you could get all you need for one week on the first trip and head out the next weekend for the second half. This works pretty well, but I would recommend saving any seafood purchases until no more than a day before you're going to prepare them.

WASH YOUR GREENS (AND OTHER PRODUCE)

This sounds like minor advice, but I find washing greens once I am in the middle of the cleanse to be one of the most soul-draining chores. It's easiest done in bulk before you start cooking in earnest every night. After your big shopping trip, scrub your sink, rinse it impeccably, and fill it up with water. Then wash each type of green one by one in the water (refilling if the water gets too murky). Dry the greens and store them in zip-top bags.

MIX, ROAST, AND TOAST

There are pantry items in every menu that can be done ahead, mostly vinaigrettes and condiments. You can also streamline your cooking by roasting vegetables for snacks or lunchtime salads, toasting nuts and seeds a few days ahead, cooking a big batch of morning porridge for the week, and hard-boiling a bunch of eggs to have on hand for snacking.

GET A BUDDY

One of the best things about doing the FLC has been having the online support of all the *BA* readers who are doing it along with me. If you're working from the book, you might not be able to coordinate on that scale, but get some friends to join in with you. You can trade off cooking dinners or just create an e-mail chain for support and questions. You could repeat the setup throughout the year.

MAKING THE CLEANSE WORK FOR YOU

As I put together the plans for each cleanse, I try to strike a balance, however tricky. Since these are plans for easily bored food lovers like me, I want to incorporate enough variety and novelty to make meals exciting. That means instead of asking you to make salads with spinach every day, I might suggest radicchio for one meal and frisée or kale for another. One dinner may call for a hot lick of harissa, the spicy North African condiment, while another leans on good soy sauce and fresh ginger. But I know you all live different lives, with preferences, allergies, budgets, and shopping scenarios. It's important that you feel as if you can make the right choices for your pleasure and your health. (After all, the FLC is just two weeks; you'll need to make good decisions later on anyway!) This section is dedicated to helping you adapt the plan for your own lifestyle.

SUBSTITUTIONS

SEAFOOD

We try to emphasize higher-oil fish in our recipes, so don't eat Dover sole at every meal, delicious as it can be. Still, specific fish can be hard to find in different markets. We provide alternatives for each of those recipes. Throughout the book, I've chosen fish that, at the time of writing, could be found on the Monterey Bay Aquarium's Seafood Watch list (seafoodwatch.org) as a "good-" or "best-" choice option. Keeping track can be confusing, but if we're to keep eating fish for its flavor and health benefits, it's in our interest as consumers to protect the ocean the best we can.

MEAT AND POULTRY

The amount of meat I eat from day to day has definitely gone down, but I still include it in my diet—and in this book. I hope this cleanse still has appeal for those of you who don't eat meat. In many preparations you can substitute a vegetarian option: beans are great in salads and soups in lieu of meat; on the grill, you can go for pressed tofu or tempeh (just make sure to give it a good coating of oil so that it doesn't stick). Almost any meal tastes good with a fried or soft- or hard-boiled egg on top of it. Or you can simply repeat some of the all-veggie meals that are presented in the book. That said, meat can do many good things as part of a well-rounded diet: It makes you full, it offers a protein boost, and it's delicious. If you're enjoying the meat and poultry recipes in this book, please look to choose quality over quantity. Organic meats and poultry let me relax my worries about excessive antibiotics in farm animals (and us!). Choose whatever meat you do eat with care.

GREENS

Almost any one green can be substituted for another. Darker greens, such as collards, kale, spinach, and mustard greens, have more nutritional mojo than light greens, including butter lettuce or frisée, but they're all a key part of the cleanse. Some greens, such as collards and chard, don't taste great raw, and others, such as spinach and arugula, lose almost all their volume when you cook them, so make sure to use more if you're substituting them in a recipe.

NUTS

Nuts and seeds are mostly interchangeable within the recipes.

VEGETABLES

Most vegetables can be exchanged, too, but try to keep textures in mind when swapping: root vegetables can be promiscuously switched for one another; fennel, celery, and onions all braise well; and winter squashes have different textures when roasted, but can basically be swapped freely.

WHOLE GRAINS AND OTHER SIDES

Whole grains can be switched in and out. In general, try to keep the size of the grains similar if you're substituting one for the other (barley and farro make a good swap, as do millet and quinoa).

LEGUMES

Lentils, beans, and peas are pretty interchangeable, too, but if you're cooking them dried, keep in mind that they often have different cooking times.

ON NOT DRINKING

Every January, it seems as if a majority of my friends resolve not to drink for (at least) a few weeks. Far fewer of them actually make it through the month. Because we're all about moderation at The Food Lover's Cleanse, we like to offer you a middle road. If you need to toast your friend's birthday or just a Tuesday, have a drink by all means. If you're not facing any specific health issues, drinking a moderate amount doesn't present serious problems. Still, it can be a space where habits are created (and calories pile up). So we ask you to limit your consumption to 4 drinks a week. It's a chance for you to see what life feels like without that automatic predinner drink, or what a night out feels like without more beers than you can count. Since I am a wine drinker, I sometimes find it hard to stop before my husband and I have finished a bottle, so I tend not to drink at all during the FLC. It's up to you, though. If you're going to have a few drinks during the plan, you might want to lean toward lighter-weight spritzers, Champagne, or low-alcohol cocktails like the lovely drink Marissa created a couple of years ago (at right).

WHAT TO DRINK WHEN YOU'RE NOT DRINKING

When I'm sticking to The Food Lover's Cleanse and snacking only at an appointed time, I find myself drinking a lot. Just not alcohol. Of course, I drink lots of water: I try to bring a quart bottle to my desk to keep me irrigated while I work. But a girl needs breaks, both from writing and from plain tap water. I start the day as Marissa suggests, with a glass of hot lemon water; she says it jump-starts digestion for the day, which it may do, but for me it's mostly a way to cool my jets about eating. It's soothing and slows me down, which helps me approach breakfast less like a snarling bear and more like a relatively domesticated human.

I also drink a lot of tea. During the program, I wean myself off the highly caffeinated black milky tea I tend to drink every morning and stick to oolongs and green, white, and herbal teas (or tisanes). Teas, in all their variety, provide a rich medium for the kind of geeking out I often reserve for wine or cheese. Oolongs are only somewhat fermented (compared with fully oxidized—and caffeinated—blacks), and they have really interesting floral and candied notes. Depending on the tea, they often get better with multiple steepings. Greens are a harder sell for me, since they can be a little stern and grassy; I tend to like fruitier Chinese green teas like Dragonwell. And after dinner, when I get an urge to snack in front of *The Americans* or whatever show I'm bingeing on at the time, I fix myself an herbal tisane: I like ones with fennel and licorice in them, such as Pukka—argh, I have to say it—Detox, which have a natural sweetness that feels right after dinner.

If I'm with friends who are drinking and I want something to clink glasses with, I turn to soda with a little bitters. As much as I like esoteric bitters made with celery and cardamom, I recommend starting with a classic, like Peychaud's, and putting a few drops in your bubbly water. It looks something like a sparkling rosé, and adds a little edge and elegance to yet another glass of water.

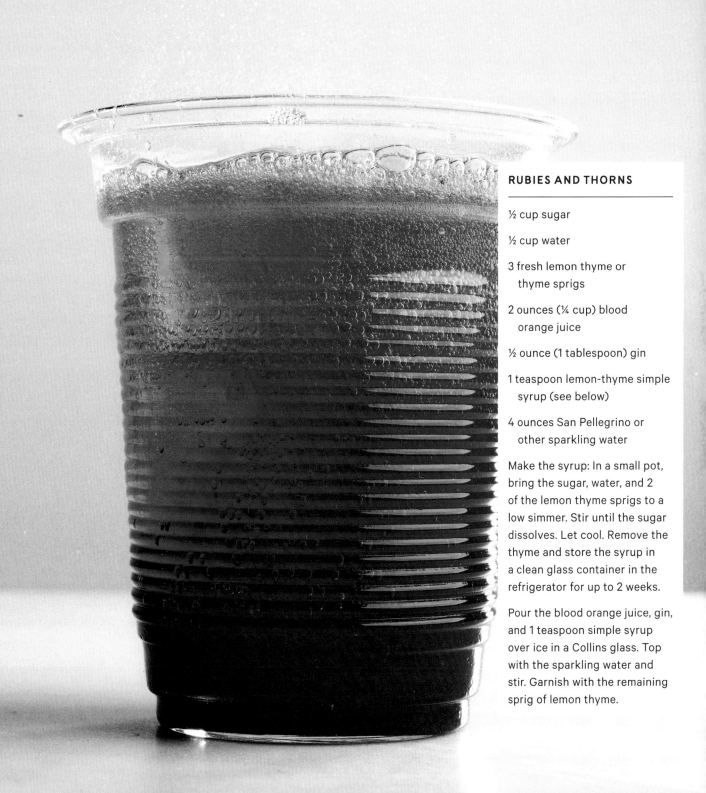

RUBIES AND THORNS

½ cup sugar

½ cup water

3 fresh lemon thyme or
thyme sprigs

2 ounces (¼ cup) blood
orange juice

½ ounce (1 tablespoon) gin

1 teaspoon lemon-thyme simple
syrup (see below)

4 ounces San Pellegrino or
other sparkling water

Make the syrup: In a small pot,
bring the sugar, water, and 2
of the lemon thyme sprigs to a
low simmer. Stir until the sugar
dissolves. Let cool. Remove the
thyme and store the syrup in
a clean glass container in the
refrigerator for up to 2 weeks.

Pour the blood orange juice, gin,
and 1 teaspoon simple syrup
over ice in a Collins glass. Top
with the sparkling water and
stir. Garnish with the remaining
sprig of lemon thyme.

CLEANSE BASICS

This book gives you recipes for four two-week cleanses, one for each season. If you want a fully mapped-out plan, we give you recipes and guidelines for every meal, even snacks. But just in case you want to find your own course, we include portion guides and broad guidelines. Feel free to improvise!

TROUBLESHOOTING

I'VE GOT A WORK TRIP. IS THERE ANY WAY I CAN STAY TRUE TO THE PLAN WHILE I'M AWAY?

Work travel can be the worst, because you're sequestered in offices and hotels where healthy food may not be readily available. Try to keep things as normal as possible. Order a balanced breakfast from room service the night before, before morning hunger (and a cinnamon roll) get the best of you. Evaluate menus for less-sauced protein, whole grains, and vegetables. Stock your carry-on with nuts and sturdier fruit to handle on-plane eating from boredom. And shove aside the minibar vodka to make room for some Greek yogurt or hummus for impromptu snacking.

I JUST REALIZED THAT MY FRIEND'S BIRTHDAY PARTY IS IN THE MIDDLE OF THE CLEANSE. WHAT TO DO?

Join in the fun. Offer to contribute one of the gorgeous dips at the back of the book, or a lovely salad, so that you'll know you'll have something good to eat. If you have some birthday cake or an extra margarita, don't beat yourself up; just get back to the plan the next day.

I'M TRAINING FOR A MARATHON (OR WORKING OUT REALLY HARD, OR BREAST-FEEDING); HOW SHOULD I ADAPT THE PLAN?

Keep eating on a regular schedule, and don't skip complex carbohydrates, such as roasted sweet potatoes, soba noodles, or quinoa. If you're feeling hungry, increase your portions at each meal only slightly: an ounce more protein here or ¼ to ½ cup more whole grains. If you need an extra snack, you can work one in. As Marissa says, "Learn what shuts the door on hunger for you; often that's hard-boiled eggs, avocado, smoked salmon, cottage cheese, or nut butters."

I'M FEELING GASSY. ANY ADVICE?

I've been there, and all I can say is that your body will likely adjust to the increase in fiber. Keep drinking lots of water, and perhaps add in a little more healthy fats and oils to your meals. (Avocado, anyone? Or fish oil . . . or a bit more olive oil . . .) They can help keep your suddenly unpredictable gut happy. Finish your meals with some peppermint or fennel tea, which is lovely and can help with that awkward gassiness.

PLEASE! I CAN'T HAVE ANOTHER SALAD FOR LUNCH!

We really like the idea of an abundant raw vegetable meal once a day to give you fiber and reinforce—through sheer crunchiness—that you are eating clean and fresh foods. That doesn't mean you can't rethink your salad a bit: Maybe it leans harder on roasted vegetables than raw. Maybe you mix in something irresistible, like avocado, dried cherries, or chèvre. Maybe you serve more of a whole-grain bowl with veggie garnishes. If you really need a break, you can also mix in something warm. Make a big batch of vegetable soup (such as the minestrone on page 278), and work a bowl of that into your lunch: you can up the protein by having a boiled egg alongside it.

IT'S JUST TWO OF US IN THE HOUSE, HOW SHOULD WE DEAL WITH LEFTOVERS?

We write dinner recipes to serve four people, generally with enough leftovers for the next day's lunch. But if you have a smaller household, you have two options: you can divide the recipes in half, or you can alternate days, serving your leftovers for a second dinner (and mixing other sources of protein into your lunch salads).

MY SPOUSE WON'T PLAY ALONG. WHAT SHOULD I DO?

If you're making and serving beautiful food, you might get more traction than you think: De-emphasize the healthy and emphasize the novelty and adventure. But you may also want to find a neighbor or friend who wants to do the cleanse with you (so you can trade prep with them as well). If your spouse wants more volume, you can serve something hearty alongside the cleanse meals, such as bread, cheese, sweet potatoes, or rice—if you're able to resist them.

HOW DO I HANDLE MY PICKY KIDS WHILE I'M ON THE CLEANSE?

I wish I could claim to have a couple of mussel- and harissa-loving kids who see food as a grand adventure. But no, they're as picky as any other kid. I compartmentalize for them a bit: pulling chicken out of the sauce it was cooked in, giving them plain quinoa before the garnishes are tossed in, and surrounding newer foods with old comforts, such as tortillas, or pasta, or plain raw veggies.

SPR

ING

Spring is supposed to be about rebirth, right? But sometimes that renewal can take an awfully long time to get going. Personally, I—and honestly most of the chefs I know—get some serious root-vegetable fatigue around March, when my mind starts pondering the green glories of summer but my garden is still in its earliest sprouting phase. That doesn't mean you can't seek renewal in your wholesome spring eating. Change the palette of your cooking toward the vivid greens of scallions, spinach, and asparagus (you can never eat too much asparagus, since it's at its best for such a short season). Switch from heavier braises to lighter, steamier techniques. Lighten up your broths a bit and brighten them with tender herbs. Grab those baby radishes at the first farmers' market of the year. Find a local cheesemaker and enjoy the new season of fresh chèvre. Eat some rosy lamb. These cues can give you a feeling of newness that will prime you for garden-fresh eating as the season becomes more abundant.

SPRING'S KEY INGREDIENTS

VEGETABLES

Baby turnips
Green garlic
Green onions
Morels
New lettuce
Peas and pea tendrils
Radishes

Tender herbs: dill, chives, mint, chervil
Watercress

FRUIT

Rhubarb
Strawberries

OTHER

Eggs
Fresh chèvre
Halibut
Lamb

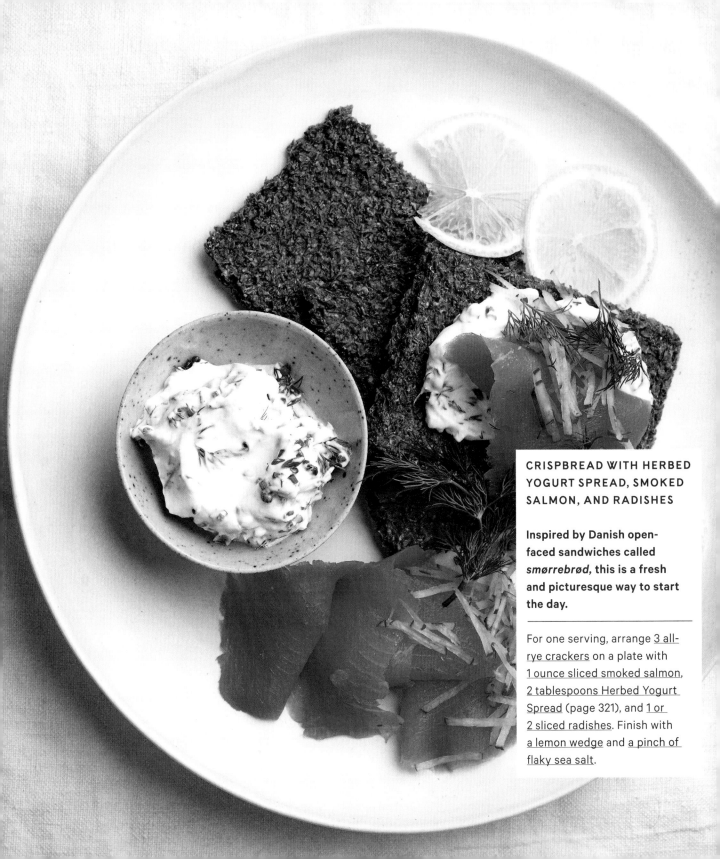

CRISPBREAD WITH HERBED YOGURT SPREAD, SMOKED SALMON, AND RADISHES

Inspired by Danish open-faced sandwiches called *smørrebrød*, this is a fresh and picturesque way to start the day.

For one serving, arrange 3 all-rye crackers on a plate with 1 ounce sliced smoked salmon, 2 tablespoons Herbed Yogurt Spread (page 321), and 1 or 2 sliced radishes. Finish with a lemon wedge and a pinch of flaky sea salt.

TOASTED RYE AND COCONUT MUESLI WITH APRICOTS

25 MINUTES (5 MINUTES ACTIVE)	MAKES 3 CUPS

- ½ cup chopped walnuts
- 2 cups rolled rye flakes or rolled oats
- ½ cup unsweetened flaked coconut (the wide kind, also known as coconut chips)
- ½ teaspoon fine sea salt
- 4½ teaspoons agave syrup
- 4½ teaspoons coconut oil, melted
- ½ cup dried apricots, cut into ¼-inch pieces
- Plain Greek yogurt or almond milk, for serving

Muesli has two faces: it can be a cold porridge, made with oats, fruit, and milk or yogurt, and soaked overnight for a hearty, soothing breakfast (page 102). It can also be a loose, less-sweet cousin to granola, as here. It serves as a nutty toasted fillip to add to your morning routine. Here I suggest rye flakes instead of oatmeal; they're thicker and chewier than oats, and are available at most health food stores or directly from Bob's Red Mill. Feel free to substitute old-fashioned oats if you can't get your hands on rye (or if you're avoiding gluten). Serve the muesli with almond milk or yogurt, and by all means, soak it overnight if you'd like something soft, comforting, and ready to go when you get up in the morning.

Preheat the oven to 300°F.

Stir together the walnuts, rye flakes, coconut, and salt. Pour in the agave syrup and coconut oil and toss to evenly distribute. Spread the mixture in a thin layer on a baking sheet. Toast in the oven until the coconut is lightly browned on the edges, about 20 minutes, rotating once halfway through the baking time.

Let the muesli cool, then toss in the apricots. Store in an airtight container in the pantry for up to 2 weeks (a serving is ⅓ cup with ½ cup plain Greek yogurt or almond milk).

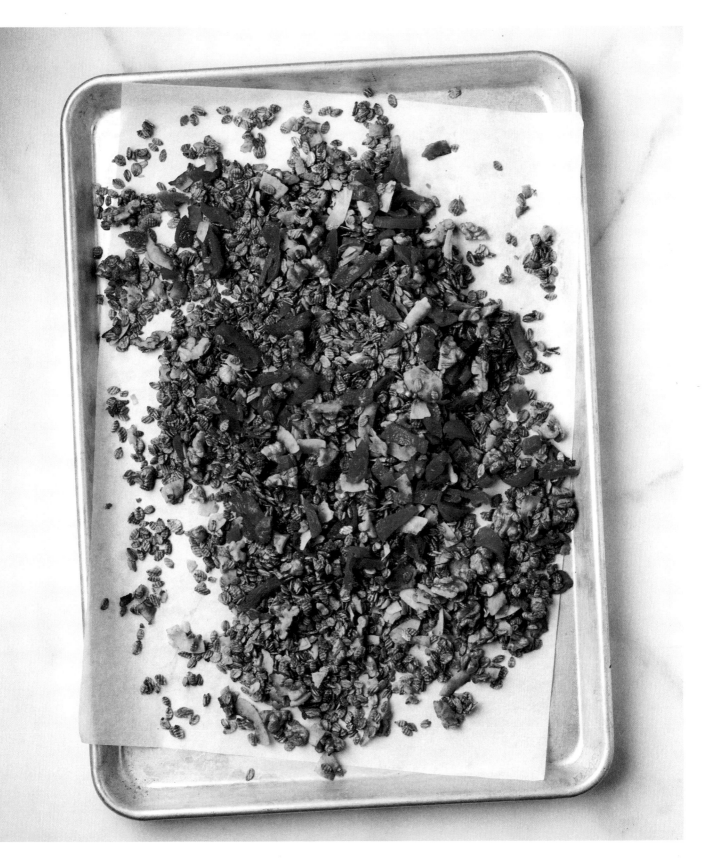

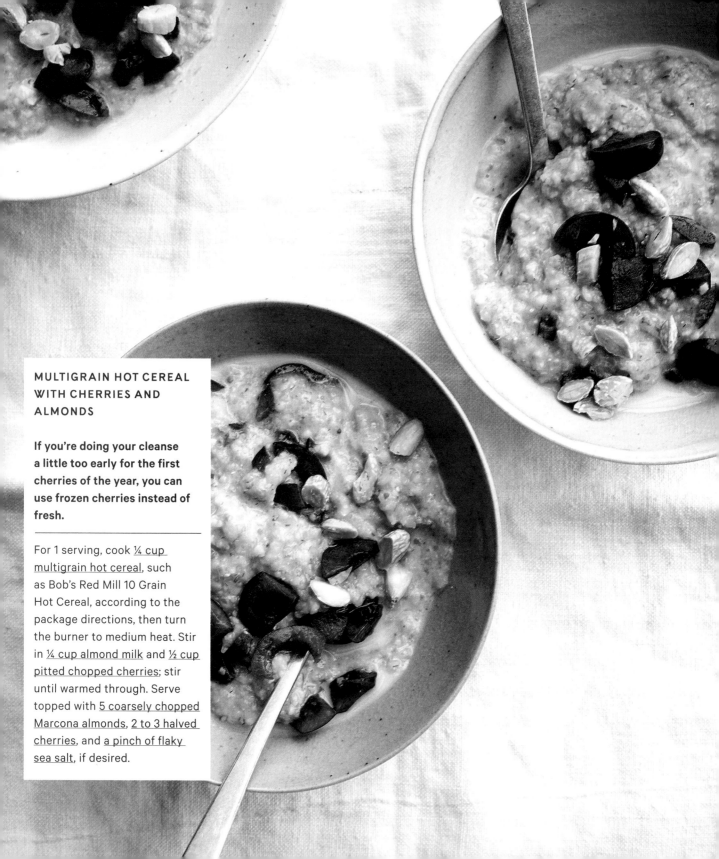

MULTIGRAIN HOT CEREAL WITH CHERRIES AND ALMONDS

If you're doing your cleanse a little too early for the first cherries of the year, you can use frozen cherries instead of fresh.

For 1 serving, cook ¼ cup multigrain hot cereal, such as Bob's Red Mill 10 Grain Hot Cereal, according to the package directions, then turn the burner to medium heat. Stir in ¼ cup almond milk and ½ cup pitted chopped cherries; stir until warmed through. Serve topped with 5 coarsely chopped Marcona almonds, 2 to 3 halved cherries, and a pinch of flaky sea salt, if desired.

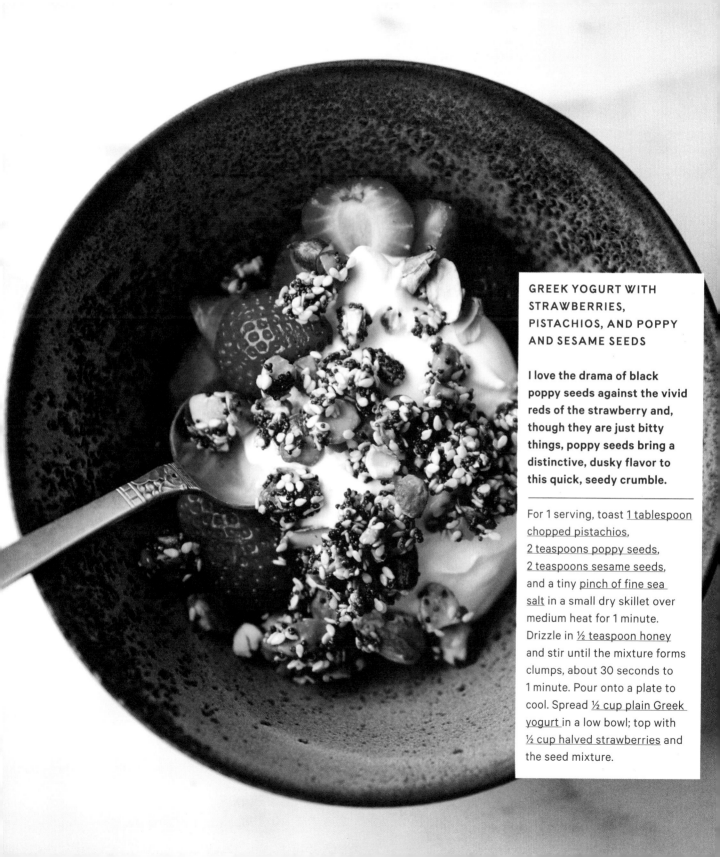

GREEK YOGURT WITH STRAWBERRIES, PISTACHIOS, AND POPPY AND SESAME SEEDS

I love the drama of black poppy seeds against the vivid reds of the strawberry and, though they are just bitty things, poppy seeds bring a distinctive, dusky flavor to this quick, seedy crumble.

For 1 serving, toast 1 tablespoon chopped pistachios, 2 teaspoons poppy seeds, 2 teaspoons sesame seeds, and a tiny pinch of fine sea salt in a small dry skillet over medium heat for 1 minute. Drizzle in ½ teaspoon honey and stir until the mixture forms clumps, about 30 seconds to 1 minute. Pour onto a plate to cool. Spread ½ cup plain Greek yogurt in a low bowl; top with ½ cup halved strawberries and the seed mixture.

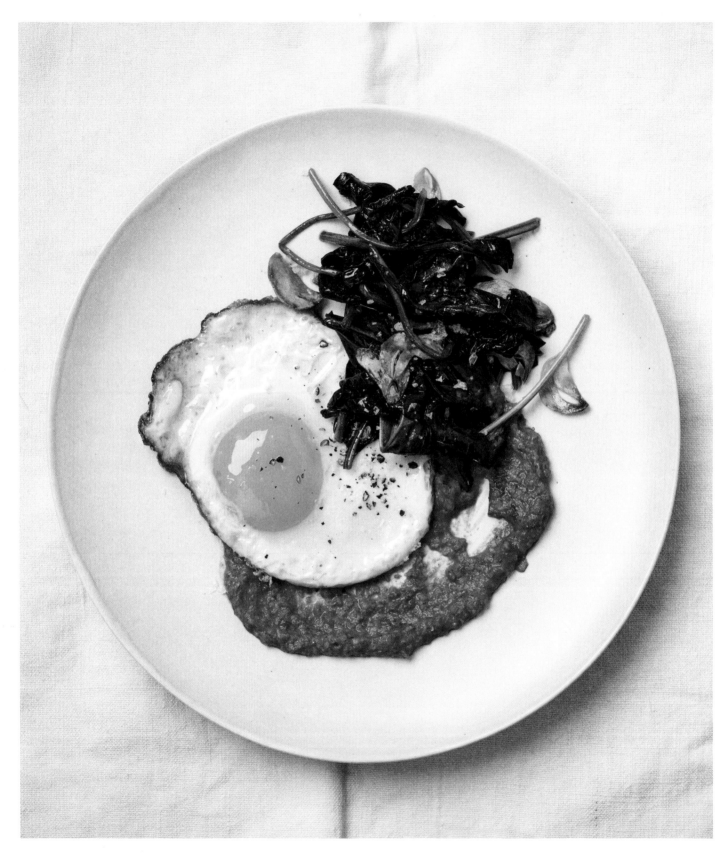

FRIED EGG WITH SPINACH, TOASTED GARLIC, AND PIQUILLO PEPPER ROMESCO

5 MINUTES	MAKES 1 SERVING

- 1 tablespoon olive oil
- ½ teaspoon thinly sliced garlic
- 2 cups well-washed spinach
- Fine sea salt to taste
- 1 or 2 large eggs, each in a small cup, bowl, or ramekin
- Flaky sea salt and freshly ground black pepper
- 1 rounded tablespoon Piquillo Romesco Sauce (page 53)

A fried egg offers so many textural delights: a crackly browned edge, a supple white, and a sinuous yolk. Here a bed of spinach gives that yolk a place to go when you're not eating toast: a softer-set yolk will coat the greens like a good salad dressing, and a bright red hit of piquillo pepper romesco gives you a bold dose of flavor to tie it all together.

Heat ½ tablespoon of the oil in a small nonstick skillet over medium heat. Add the garlic and cook until slightly browned, about 1½ minutes. Add the spinach and 1 tablespoon of water. Cover the skillet and cook until the spinach is wilted and bright green, about 1 minute. Season to taste with fine sea salt. Remove to a plate.

Wipe out the pan and heat the remaining ½ tablespoon of oil over medium-high heat. Pour in the egg(s), season with flaky salt and pepper, and let the eggs bubble and brown a bit at the edges. Using tongs or a slotted spoon, add the spinach back to the pan and cover the skillet. Cook the eggs to the desired doneness; you will get a well-set white and runny yolk with 1 minute of cooking. Serve with spinach and a spoonful of Romesco.

STEEL-CUT OATS WITH RHUBARB APPLESAUCE AND HAZELNUTS

5 MINUTES	MAKES 1 SERVING

- ¾ cup cooked steel-cut oats (see page 301 for the basic big-batch method)
- Pinch of fine sea salt (optional)
- ½ cup Rhubarb Applesauce for Spring Breakfasts and Snacks (recipe follows)
- 1 tablespoon chopped hazelnuts, toasted (see page 322)
- Flaky sea salt (optional)

Homemade applesauce goosed with a bit of tangy rhubarb makes oatmeal so much less ordinary, in no small part because of the chic blush tone of the fruit compote. Choose for yourself whether to warm up the applesauce in the microwave before dolloping it on top of the oatmeal; sometimes I like the cool contrast of chilly applesauce against my piping-hot oats.

Warm the oatmeal in a small saucepan with a splash of water. Season to taste with fine sea salt, if desired, and top with the applesauce, hazelnuts, and a few flakes of flaky sea salt, if desired.

RHUBARB APPLESAUCE FOR SPRING BREAKFASTS AND SNACKS

22 MINUTES (6 MINUTES ACTIVE)	MAKES 3 CUPS

- 4 large apples, such as Gala or Fuji
- 3 large rhubarb stalks, cut into 1-inch pieces (about 4 cups)
- ¼ cup honey
- Pinch of fine sea salt

Leaving the apple skin in the pot (you remove it after cooking) gives you a deeper flavor and imbues a lovely rosy tint.

Peel the apples, reserving the peel of 1 apple for cooking. Core the apples and cut them into 1-inch chunks. Place the apples, apple peel, rhubarb, honey, and salt in a nonreactive 3-quart saucepan. Cover the pan and cook the fruit over medium heat for 15 minutes, or until it has broken down into a chunky sauce, stirring frequently. Pluck out the apple peel and cool the applesauce before serving.

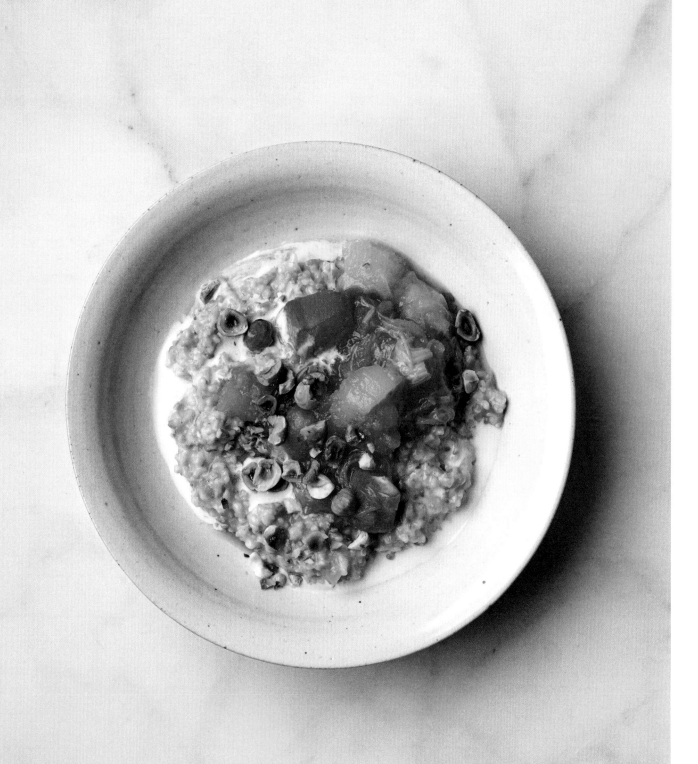

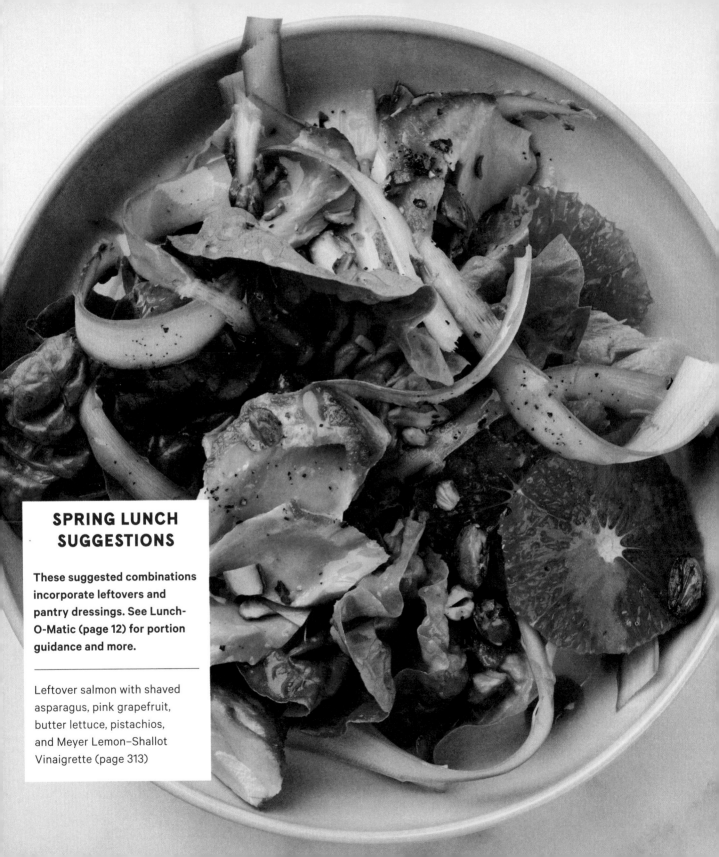

SPRING LUNCH SUGGESTIONS

These suggested combinations incorporate leftovers and pantry dressings. See Lunch-O-Matic (page 12) for portion guidance and more.

Leftover salmon with shaved asparagus, pink grapefruit, butter lettuce, pistachios, and Meyer Lemon–Shallot Vinaigrette (page 313)

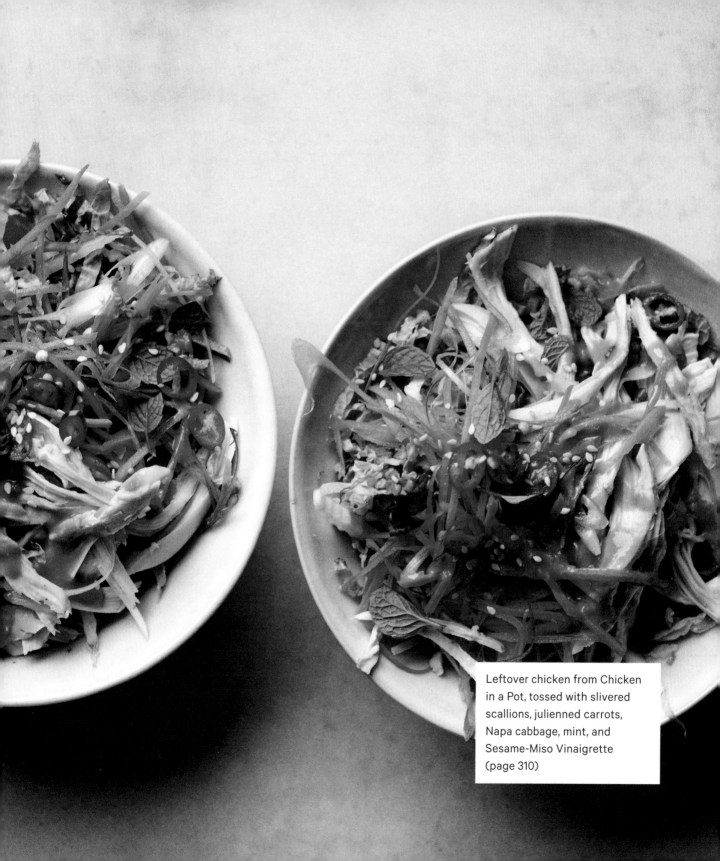

Leftover chicken from Chicken in a Pot, tossed with slivered scallions, julienned carrots, Napa cabbage, mint, and Sesame-Miso Vinaigrette (page 310)

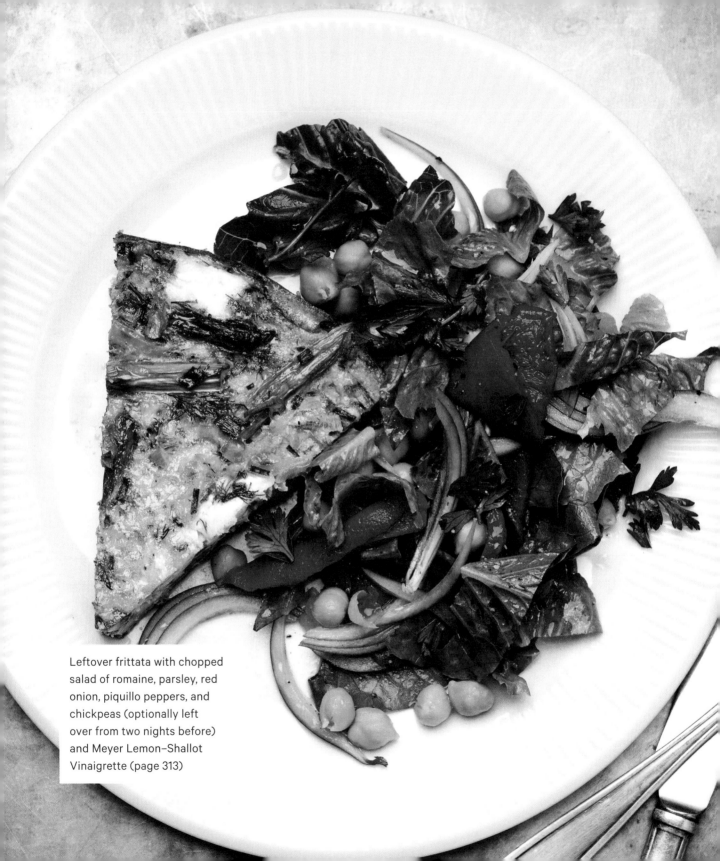

Leftover frittata with chopped salad of romaine, parsley, red onion, piquillo peppers, and chickpeas (optionally left over from two nights before) and Meyer Lemon–Shallot Vinaigrette (page 313)

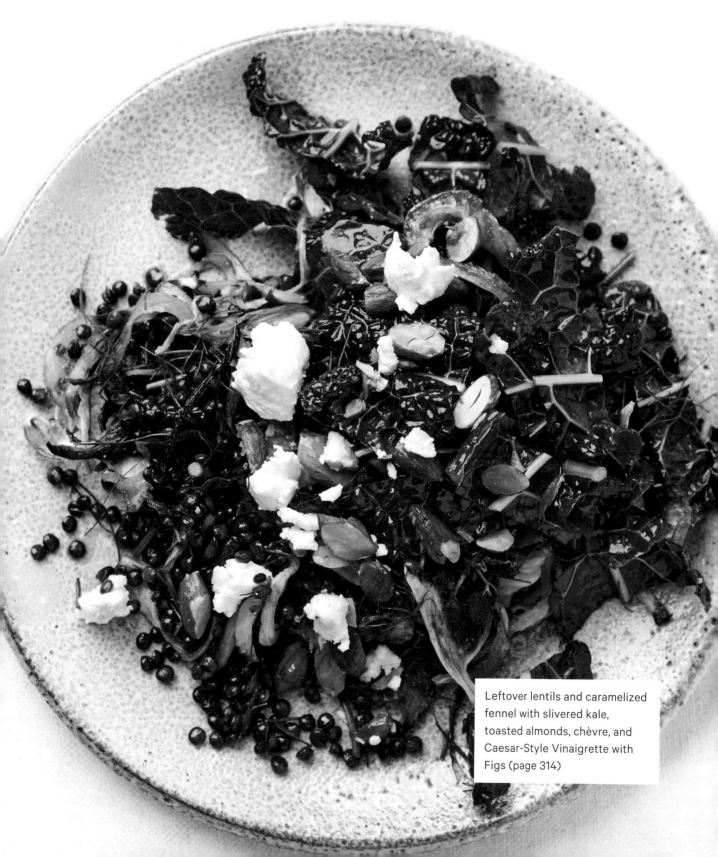

Leftover lentils and caramelized fennel with slivered kale, toasted almonds, chèvre, and Caesar-Style Vinaigrette with Figs (page 314)

CHARMOULA-RUBBED MAHI-MAHI

35 TO 40 MINUTES (10 ACTIVE)	4 SERVINGS

- ½ cup finely chopped fresh cilantro
- ¼ cup olive oil
- ½ teaspoon ground cumin
- ½ teaspoon sweet or smoked paprika
- Fine sea salt to taste
- Juice of 1 lime
- 1 small garlic clove, grated
- 4 (6-ounce) mahi-mahi fillets

Every region in the world has its green sauce, delivering deep flavor and antioxidant-rich herbs in one swoop. There is South American chimichurri, Italian pesto, Mexican salsa verde, and this one, North African charmoula. Though it tastes delicious raw, it's used most commonly as a marinade, and I love the deeper, musky herbal story it tells when broiled or grilled, especially with an extra squeeze of lime when the fish comes off the heat. Mahi-mahi is a solid, steaky fish; it is okay to substitute other rich, firm fish such as swordfish, ono, or mackerel, but feel free to play around, too. This marinade is also delicious with shrimp or squid.

In a medium bowl, stir together the cilantro, oil, cumin, paprika, salt, lime juice, garlic, and 1 tablespoon water (alternatively, pulse the ingredients in a food processor for a smoother texture and a slightly more intense herbal flavor). Rub the mixture onto the fish and chill for at least 15 minutes and up to 1 hour.

Preheat the oven to 425°F. Place the marinated fish on a rimmed baking sheet and roast until the fish is just opaque in the center, 10 to 15 minutes.

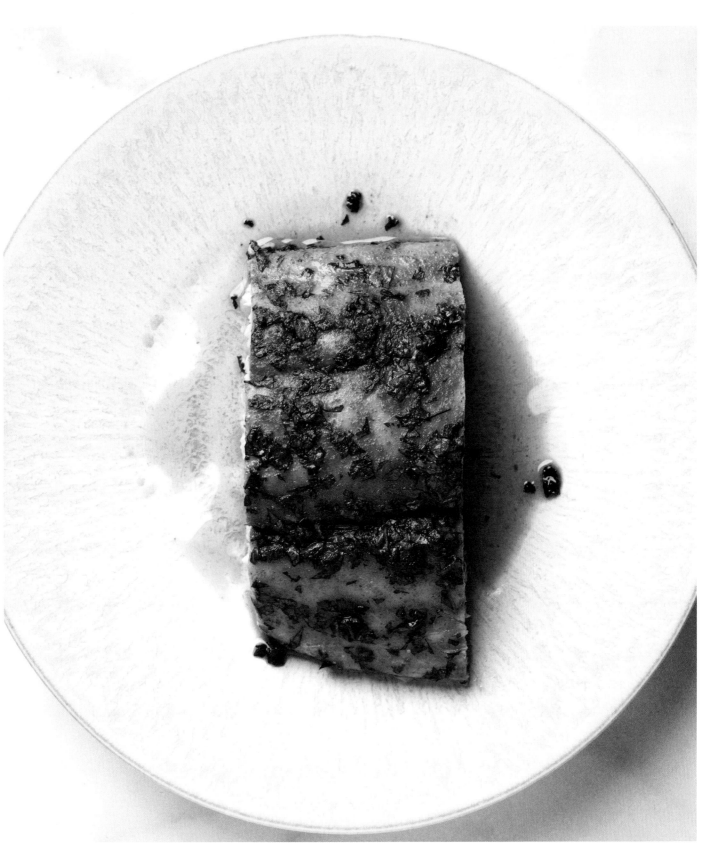

ROASTED ASPARAGUS WITH SHALLOTS, THYME, AND ALMONDS

10 MINUTES (5 ACTIVE)	4 SERVINGS AND 1 LUNCH THE NEXT DAY

- 2 pounds asparagus, tough stems snapped off
- 25 to 30 fresh thyme sprigs (1 small bunch)
- 2 shallots, sliced
- 2 tablespoons olive oil
- 2 teaspoons fine sea salt
- ¼ cup chopped almonds, toasted (see page 306)
- Flaky sea salt to finish

Here in Washington State, we get such a glut of good asparagus from the east side of the Cascades that in the midst of spring it can feel like a cliché. But I serve it all the time anyway, because the season is gone in a blink, and the fiber- and antioxidant-packed asparagus of spring is so vividly good. I shave it lengthwise to serve raw in salads, peel fat stems and blanch them until just tender, and, easiest of all, throw whole unpeeled asparagus into a screaming-hot oven to get a little crispy-caramelized contrast to the juicy interior of the stalks.

Preheat the oven to 450°F.

Toss together the asparagus, thyme, shallots, olive oil, and fine sea salt. Lay the asparagus mixture out in a single layer on 2 baking sheets and roast until the asparagus is tender and browned in spots but still crisp, about 5 minutes. Remove most of the thyme sprigs from the asparagus (though a few sprigs here and there look lovely).

Top with the almonds and season with flaky sea salt to taste.

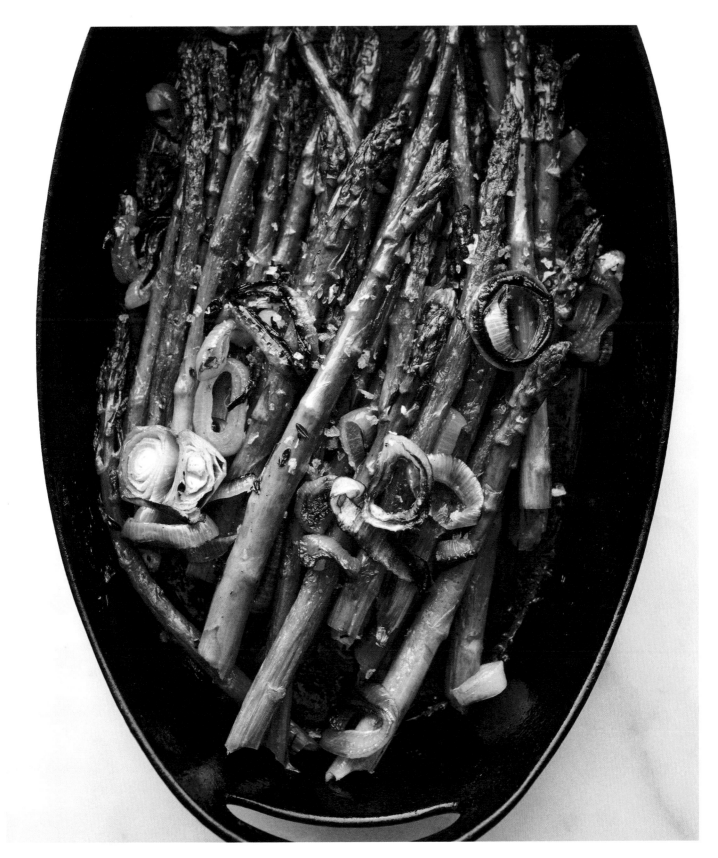

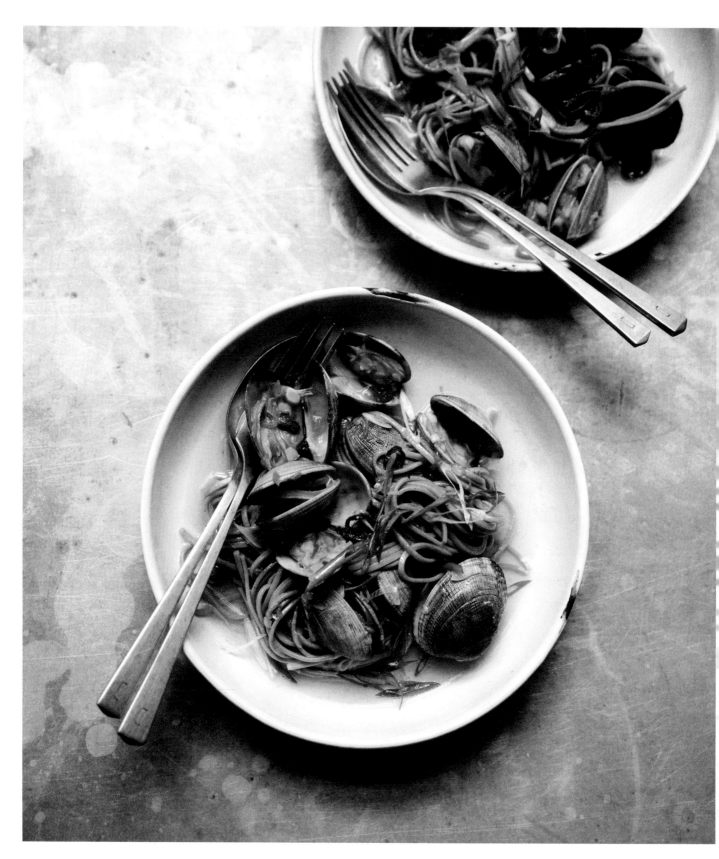

SAKE-STEAMED CLAMS WITH SOBA NOODLES

15 MINUTES (10 ACTIVE)	4 SERVINGS

- 8 ounces soba noodles (preferably all buckwheat; available at Asian markets and in many groceries and health food stores)
- Fine sea salt
- 1 tablespoon vegetable oil
- 1 bunch scallions, white and dark green parts separated, thinly sliced
- 1 jalapeño chile, seeded (unless you crave lots of heat) and sliced
- 1 (1-inch) piece of fresh ginger, peeled and sliced into 3 rounds
- 2½ pounds Manila clams, scrubbed
- ¾ cup dry sake

Clams are surprisingly high in protein, iron, and minerals such as potassium and zinc. But cook them for their bright, briny flavor; they're easier to prepare than you might think. When you cook clams in sake, they get a clean complexity that's amped up with ginger, chiles, and scallions. It takes a minute to prep clams before cooking: after rinsing them well in water, I gently squeeze each open clam to see if it clamps tightly shut. If not, I toss it, along with any broken shells. (I always buy a few more than necessary so that I can be rigorous with my culling.) Once sorted, clams are ready in a flash, and the soba noodles are perfect for sopping up the delicious clam broth.

Cook the soba noodles in a large pot of boiling salted water (try adding 1½ teaspoons salt per liter of water in the pan), stirring occasionally, until al dente. Drain and rinse in cold water.

Heat the oil in a large skillet over medium-high heat. Add the white parts of the scallions, the jalapeño, and ginger. Stir until aromatic, about 1 minute. Add the clams; stir to coat and cook for 1 minute, then pour in the sake. Cover and cook until the clams open, 4 to 6 minutes (discard any clams that don't open). Using a slotted spoon, transfer the clams to a bowl. Discard the ginger slices.

Transfer the noodles to the clam juices in the skillet and cook for 1 minute to warm them through. Divide the noodles among bowls. Toss the clams and scallion greens in the clam juices. Divide the clams and broth evenly among the bowls.

GREEN PEAS AND EDAMAME

8 MINUTES (6 ACTIVE)	4 OR 5 SERVINGS

- 2 tablespoons olive oil
- 4 garlic cloves, minced
- Small pinch of red pepper flakes, preferably Aleppo or Marash
- 2 cups frozen shelled edamame or green chickpeas (about 1 pound unshelled)
- Fine sea salt to taste
- 3 cups peas, either freshly shucked English peas or frozen petite peas
- Freshly ground black pepper to taste

Sweet, tender, and urgently green, this dish shoos away wintry cabin fever, even if I sometimes have to resort to frozen peas and edamame. I won't tell if you use frozen; I know plenty of chefs who prefer good frozen peas to starchy out-of-season "fresh" in-pod peas. In the meantime, you can adjust this dish easily to reflect the season as different items come into the markets. If you can get your hands on green garlic bulbs, they add a sharp green intensity. Sliver the whole bulb and then chop it finely; use about 2 teaspoons chopped in place of the mature garlic. Green garbanzos should hit many markets by March, too. Feel free to use them instead of edamame, shelling them first for a wonderfully nutty but herbaceous taste. And of course, the second you do get good English peas at the market, pounce on them and get shelling!

Heat the oil in a 2- or 3-quart saucepan over medium heat. Stir in the garlic and the red pepper flakes and cook for 30 seconds, then add the edamame. Cook for 1 minute and add ½ cup water and season with salt. Cook until the edamame is tender but still a bit al dente. Stir in the peas and cook until the peas are tender, 1 to 2 minutes. Drain the liquid and season with salt and black pepper.

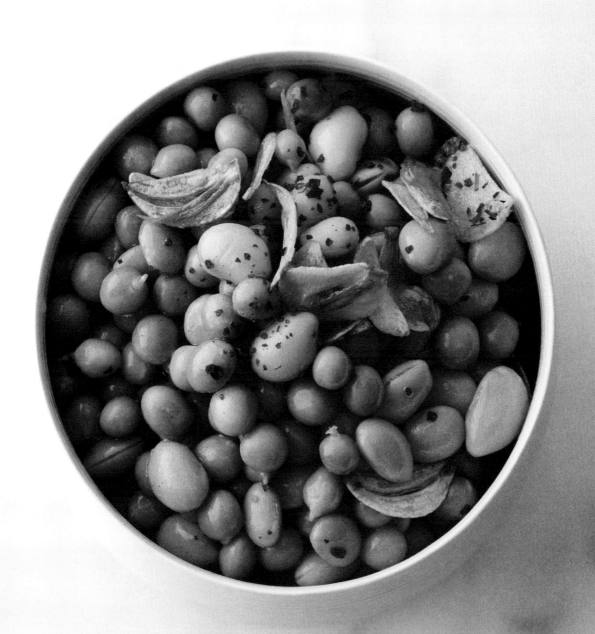

PORK RAGOUT WITH MORELS AND CELERY ROOT

2½ HOURS (15 MINUTES ACTIVE)	4 SERVINGS AND 1 LUNCH THE NEXT DAY

- 3 cups homemade chicken stock (see page 301) or low-sodium canned
- 1 ounce dried morels or porcini (about 1 cup)
- 4 teaspoons olive oil
- 1 pound pork shoulder, trimmed of excess external fat
- Fine sea salt and freshly ground black pepper to taste
- 1 medium onion, sliced
- 2 cups chopped peeled celery root (in 1-inch chunks)
- 1 garlic clove, sliced
- 1 tablespoon all-purpose flour or 2 teaspoons cornstarch
- 4 cups torn well-washed kale leaves, preferably lacinato (about 1 bunch)

The heart of this cleanse is context: here's a stew built around a rich cut of meat, pork shoulder. But there's a modest amount of it, and the rest of the stew is loaded with the flavors of kale and celery root, not to mention spring's best foraged ingredient: the morel. Though the recipe calls for dried morels, if you can get fresh, by all means use them. Just make sure to remove any grit by swishing them around and rinsing briefly in two or three changes of water.

Preheat the oven to 350°F.

Bring 1 cup of the stock to a boil. Soak the mushrooms in the hot stock for at least 20 minutes. Drain the mushrooms, reserving the stock. Pour the broth through a coffee filter to remove any grit, and add to the remaining chicken stock. Rinse the morels, trim away any tough stems, and slice on the bias into ½-inch rings.

In a large soup pot or Dutch oven, heat the oil over medium-high heat. Season the pork with salt and pepper and place in a single layer in the pot. Cook until the meat is browned, turning to get an even color on all sides, about 9 minutes. Remove the meat to a plate.

Place the onion and 1 teaspoon of salt in the pot and turn the heat down to medium. Scrape well to deglaze the bottom of the pot. Cook for 2 minutes, then add the celery root and garlic. Cook for 2 minutes, then add the morels and the flour. Stir well to keep the flour from sticking to the bottom of the pot, and then whisk in the stock. Use the whisk to scrape up any remaining browned bits from the bottom of the pot.

Return the pork to the pot, cover, and place the pot in the oven. Braise until the meat is fork tender and falls apart easily, about 2 hours. Let cook for another 15 minutes, uncovered.

Stir in the kale the last 5 minutes of cooking and adjust the seasoning with more salt if needed.

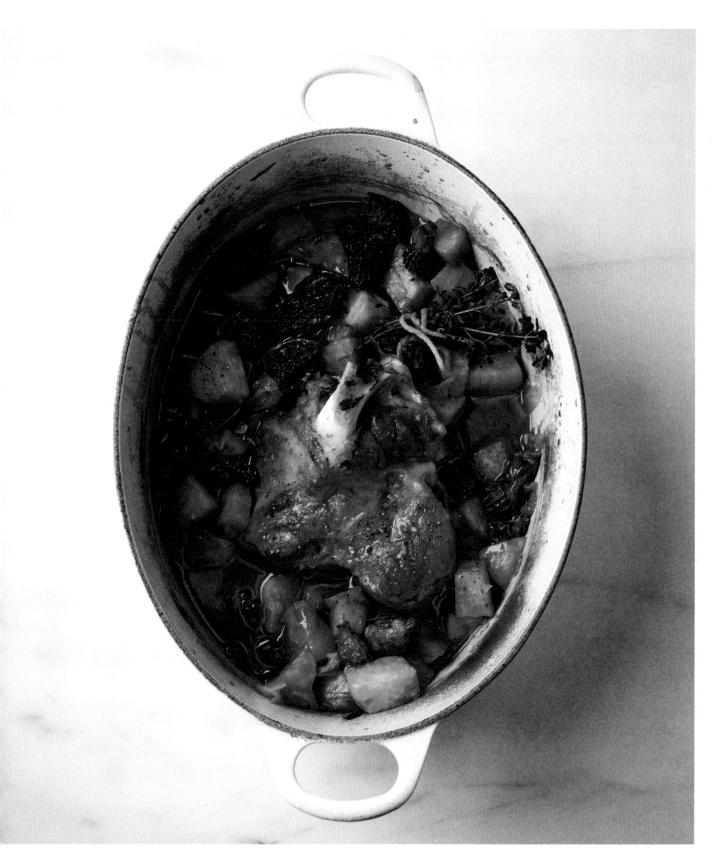

BUCKWHEAT POLENTA

Pictured on page 74

40 MINUTES (30 ACTIVE) | **4 TO 6 SERVINGS**

- ¼ cup kasha (roasted buckwheat groats)
- ¾ cup polenta (not quick-cooking)
- Fine sea salt
- 1 tablespoon olive oil
- 1 medium onion, finely minced
- 2 cups homemade chicken stock (see page 301), low-sodium canned, or water
- 1 ounce chèvre, crumbled
- Freshly ground black pepper to taste

Gluten free and protein rich, buckwheat isn't really a grain at all; it's more closely related to rhubarb than wheat. I use it whenever I want to rough up a dish a bit with some earthy flavor. Here, the addition of ground kasha (roasted buckwheat groats) gives mild mellow polenta a little more character. You can find kasha at your local health food store, or take a trip to an Eastern European imports store and look for it among the pickled mushrooms and sour cherry preserves.

Place the kasha in a blender or small food processor and whiz on high to grind the grains into a coarse powder. Pulse in the polenta and 1½ teaspoons salt to mix.

In a 3-quart saucepan or Dutch oven, heat the oil over medium-high heat. Stir in the onion, and cook, stirring occasionally, for 2 minutes, or until softened. Pour in 3 cups water and the stock and bring to a boil.

Vigorously whisk the buckwheat mixture into the liquid. Whisk for 1 minute, then turn down the heat to a very low simmer—a lazy bubble should burst onto the surface every other second or so. Cook, stirring frequently, until the polenta is soft, about 30 minutes. If it seems too thick and stodgy, add more water, ¼ cup at a time, to make a smooth porridge.

Stir in the chèvre and taste the porridge. Season with salt and pepper.

Notes on Saving:

If you're holding the polenta to serve the same evening, place a layer of plastic wrap across the top to prevent a skin from forming.

To save any leftover buckwheat polenta, pour the extra porridge into a lightly greased baking dish and chill overnight. Cover the surface of the polenta with plastic wrap. In the morning, cut it into rectangles and crisp it in a nonstick pan with a teaspoon or two of oil.

Polenta squares freeze well.

PIQUILLO ROMESCO SAUCE

Pictured on page 54

10 TO 12 MINUTES	MAKES 2 CUPS

- ¼ cup hazelnuts
- ¼ cup almonds
- 2 tablespoons plus ¼ cup olive oil
- 6 garlic cloves
- 2 medium tomatoes (about 10 ounces), cored and cut into large chunks
- Fine sea salt to taste
- ¼ cup piquillo peppers, drained
- White wine vinegar or sherry vinegar
- 1 teaspoon ancho chili powder

Piquillo peppers, the jarred, roasted, not-too-sweet Spanish peppers, are one of my favorite pantry shortcuts (if they're not in your local stores, look for them at spanishtable.com). They're delicious in salads, they can be stuffed with tuna or salt cod, and they can garnish your rice dishes. In this case, I use them as a tasty variation on bell peppers in Catalonian romesco sauce. The key to making romesco is browning the nuts and the garlic just a bit more than you might for other purposes; you want to teeter on the edge of bitterness without tumbling over it.

Preheat the oven to 325°F. Spread the hazelnuts and almonds on a baking sheet and toast the nuts until quite dark at the center, 10 to 12 minutes. Let cool and coarsely chop.

In a 2-quart saucepan, heat 2 tablespoons of the oil over medium-high heat. Place the garlic cloves in the pan and cook until they are nut brown on all sides, 3 minutes. Add the tomato chunks and about a teaspoon of salt: be careful, as the moist tomatoes may splutter. Cook as the tomatoes first their exude juices and then become thick and saucy, about 5 minutes.

In a food processor or a blender, combine the chopped nuts, tomato-garlic sauce, piquillo peppers, 1 teaspoon of vinegar, the chili powder, and the remaining ¼ cup oil. Puree until smooth, about 1 minute. Taste the sauce and add more salt or vinegar, if desired.

PAN-ROASTED CHICKEN WITH SAUTÉED PEA SHOOTS AND PIQUILLO PEPPER ROMESCO

24 MINUTES (6 ACTIVE)	4 SERVINGS AND 1 LUNCH THE NEXT DAY

- 4 bone-in, skin-on chicken breasts
- 1 garlic clove, grated
- Fine sea salt and freshly ground black pepper
- ½ teaspoon ground cumin
- 2 tablespoons olive oil
- 6 cups fresh pea shoots or vines, trimmed of tough stems, or spinach
- ¼ cup Piquillo Romesco Sauce (page 53)

Pan-roasted chicken breasts are a year-round weeknight staple for me. To make them seem special and springlike, serve them alongside quickly sautéed pea shoots. These young pea plants make an early payment on the promise of garden goodness to come. You can find pea shoots (or the more developed vines) at health food stores or Asian groceries. Then, for a bit of vibrant earthiness, add a dollop of romesco, a variation on the Catalonian condiment. While I prefer to cook the chicken with its skin on for flavor, when I'm doing The Food Lover's Cleanse, I usually pluck it off before eating. You decide.

Preheat the oven to 425°F.

Lift the skin of the chicken breasts and rub some of the garlic under the skin of each breast. Season the chicken, top and bottom, with salt and pepper and the cumin. Heat 1 tablespoon of the oil in an ovenproof skillet over medium-high heat. Place the chicken skin side down in the skillet and cook until the skin is golden brown, about 5 minutes. Turn the chicken skin side up and transfer the skillet to the oven. Roast until an instant-read thermometer inserted into the thickest part of the breast registers 165°F, 15 to 20 minutes.

In a large skillet, heat the remaining 1 tablespoon oil over medium-high heat. Add the pea shoots and season with salt. Toss the shoots frequently until they are bright green and glossy and have wilted just a bit, 1 to 2 minutes.

Serve the chicken with the sautéed pea shoots and piquillo romesco sauce.

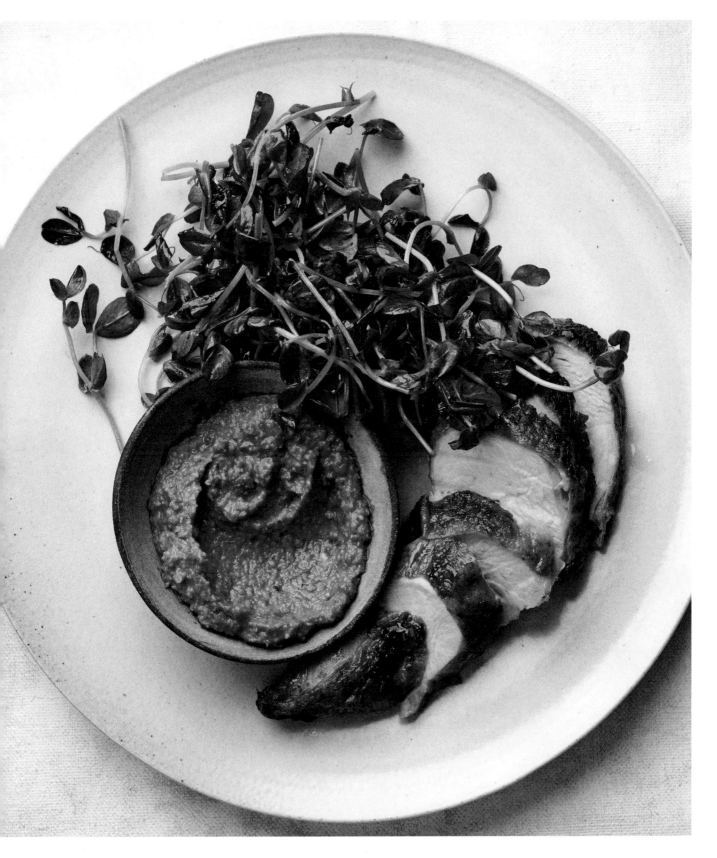

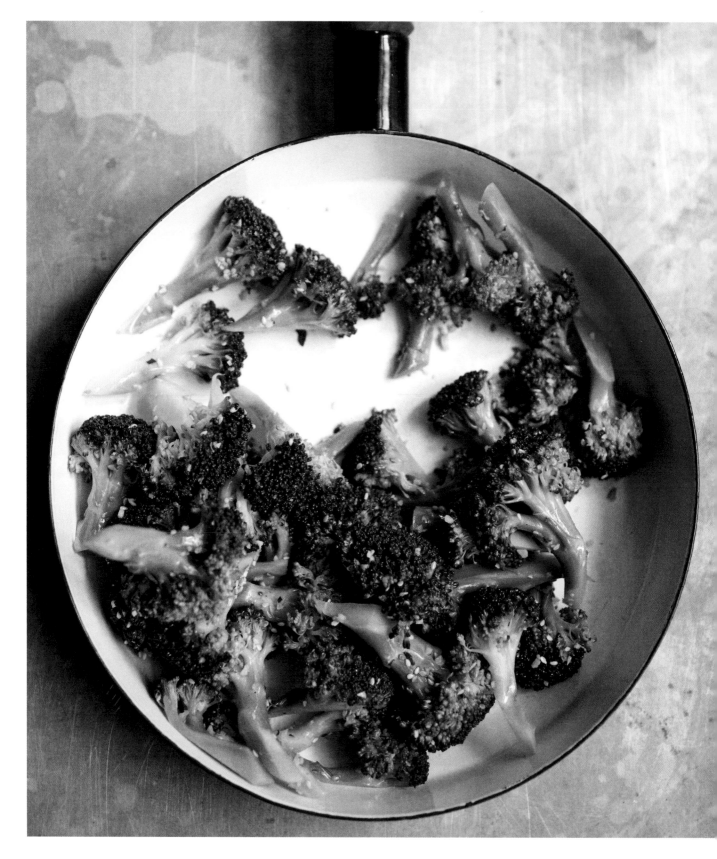

STEAM-SAUTÉED SESAME BROCCOLI

5 MINUTES	4 SERVINGS AND 1 LUNCH THE NEXT DAY

- 1 tablespoon sesame seeds
- 1 tablespoon canola oil
- 3 garlic cloves, chopped
- Pinch of red pepper flakes
- 2 small broccoli heads (about 2 pounds), cut into small 1-inch florets
- Fine sea salt to taste
- 2 teaspoons toasted sesame oil

I didn't think I needed a new approach to broccoli, but then I reread a 1970s classic, *The Key to Chinese Cooking,* by Irene Kuo, who introduced me to the idea of steam-sautéeing. Think hot pan, quick stir-fry, and almost instantly after that, a small amount of water plus a lid to cover the pan. The result is the brilliant green, crispy, yet fully cooked broccoli I always had in mind when I used to steam or blanch it. See what you think, and don't hesitate to use the (peeled) stems of the broccoli in there, too.

In a dry skillet, toast the sesame seeds over medium heat until fragrant and a shade darker, about 1 minute. Transfer the seeds to a small bowl and reserve.

In a wide skillet or wok, heat the canola oil over medium-high heat. Add the garlic, red pepper flakes, and broccoli and toss to combine. Add a good pinch of fine sea salt and ¼ cup water. Cover the pan and let the broccoli steam until it's cooked but still quite crisp, 1½ to 2 minutes. Turn off the heat, pour in the sesame seeds and sesame oil, and stir well. Taste the broccoli and season as needed with more salt.

LAMB LEG WITH GREENEST TAHINI AND SAUTÉED SWISS CHARD

20 TO 22 MINUTES (15 ACTIVE)	4 SERVINGS AND 1 LUNCH THE NEXT DAY

- 1½ pounds butterflied leg of lamb (about 2¼ pounds before boning and trimming)
- 3 tablespoons extra-virgin olive oil
- 1 garlic clove, minced
- 1 teaspoon finely minced fresh rosemary leaves
- Fine sea salt and freshly ground black pepper to taste
- 3 garlic cloves, thinly sliced
- Pinch of red pepper flakes
- 2 bunches Swiss chard, well washed, trimmed, and cut into 1-inch strips
- Flaky sea salt to taste
- Greenest Tahini Sauce (page 64)

Rosy lamb is the iconic roast of springtime, and here it's all the more lovely surrounded by vivid green tahini sauce and Swiss chard. Leg of lamb becomes a quick-cooking meat if you butterfly it first. This means cutting the round roast into one flat, even layer. You can give yourself a little butchery lesson (with the help of online videos like this one: bbcgoodfood.com/technique/how-butterfly-leg-lamb), or get your butcher to help you out.

Place an oven rack in the upper third of the oven and preheat the oven to 450°F.

Trim any large pieces of fat off the lamb. Mix 1 tablespoon of the oil with the minced garlic and the rosemary. Rub the meat with the oil mixture, then season it generously with fine sea salt and black pepper. Let the lamb sit at room temperature for at least 20 minutes before cooking.

In a large saucepan, heat 1 tablespoon of the oil over medium heat. Add the sliced garlic and red pepper flakes and stir for 30 seconds. Stir in the chard and cook until the greens are tender, about 3 minutes. Season with the flaky sea salt.

In a large ovenproof sauté pan, heat the remaining 1 tablespoon oil over medium-high heat. Brown the lamb on both sides, about 3 minutes per side. Remove from the heat, place in the oven, and cook to the desired temperature (remember, the temperature will rise slightly while the meat is resting): medium-rare is approximately 130°F, 6 to 8 minutes. Let the meat rest at least 10 minutes, then cut it into ½-inch slices.

Garnish the lamb with flaky sea salt and more black pepper, if desired. Serve with the tahini sauce and the sautéed chard.

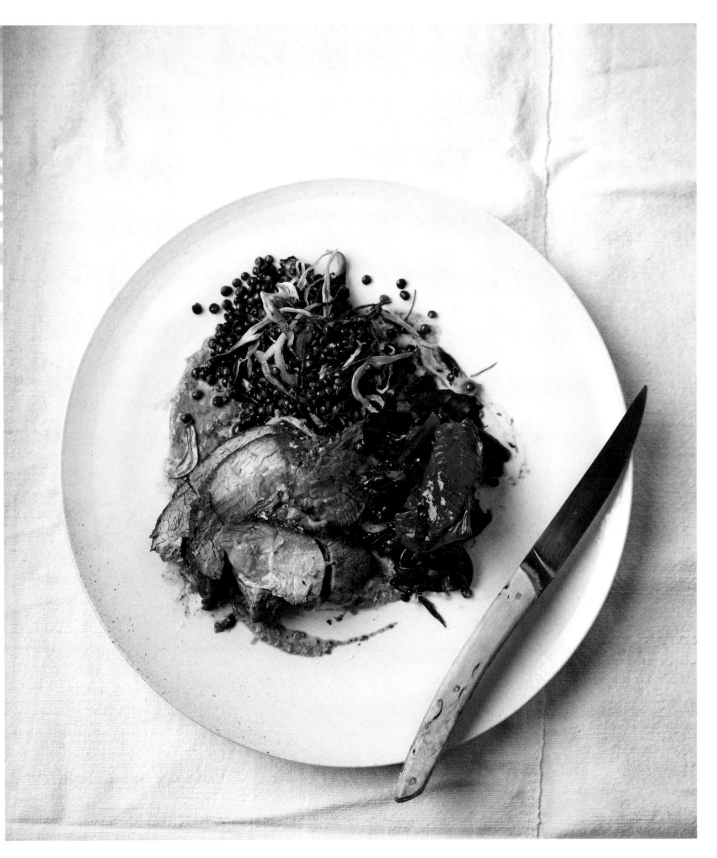

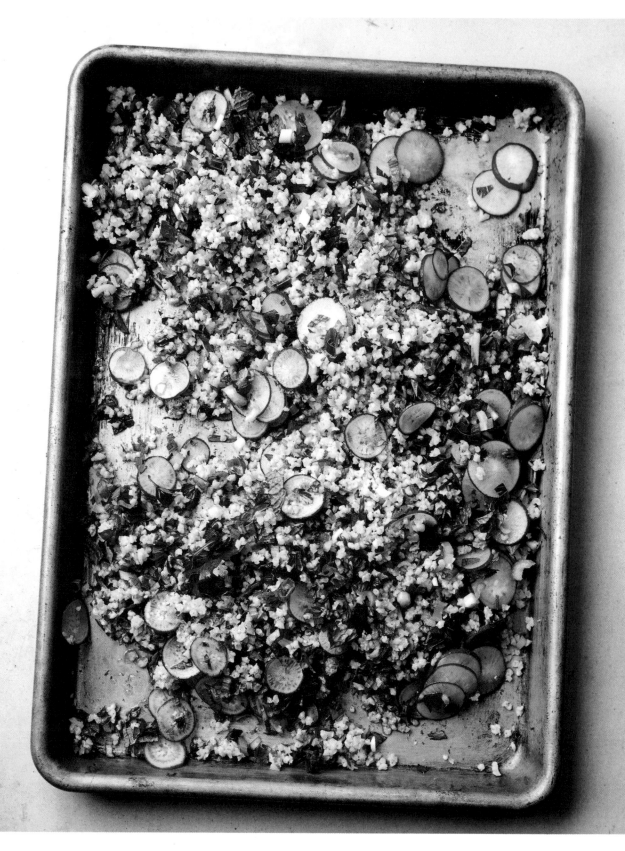

MILLET TABBOULEH

18 MINUTES (6 ACTIVE)	4 TO 6 SERVINGS

- Fine sea salt
- 1¼ cups millet
- 3 tablespoons extra-virgin olive oil
- ½ teaspoon ancho chili powder
- Freshly ground black pepper to taste
- 3 cups chopped fresh flat-leaf parsley leaves (from about 1 bunch)
- 1 cup chopped fresh mint leaves
- 4 scallions (white and light green parts), chopped
- 4 radishes, very thinly sliced
- 2 tablespoons freshly squeezed lemon juice, plus more to taste (from about 1 large lemon)

London's most celebrated champions of Mediterranean cuisine, Yottam Ottolenghi and Sami Tamimi, caution that tabbouleh, "not always understood in the West, is all about parsley. . . . This is essentially a parsley salad, not a bulgar salad." In my spring take on the concept, I've swapped the bulgur entirely and substituted golden seeds of millet, which give a nutty, cornlike taste to the salad. Instead of tomatoes, which are nowhere near ready in springtime, I add lovely slivers of radish. In the end, though, I'm with Ottolenghi: it's all about the green herbs. Feel free to add too many!

Bring a large pot of salted water to a boil. Pour in the millet and cook it until tender but still toothsome, stirring occasionally, about 15 minutes. Strain, then run cool water over the millet to rinse and cool.

Place the millet in a bowl and toss it with the oil, 1¼ teaspoons salt, the chili powder, and pepper. Stir in the parsley, mint, scallions, radishes, and lemon juice. Taste the salad and add more salt or lemon juice, if desired.

SALMON WITH THE GREENEST TAHINI SAUCE, SHAVED RADISHES, AND CUCUMBERS

10 TO 12 MINUTES (8 ACTIVE)	4 SERVINGS AND 1 LUNCH THE NEXT DAY

- 5 (4-ounce) salmon fillets, preferably wild-caught sockeye or king, skin on and pin bones removed
- Fine sea salt and freshly ground black pepper to taste
- 1 tablespoon neutral oil, such as canola or grapeseed
- 4 radishes, slivered
- 1 small cucumber, sliced thinly
- 1 tablespoon mint leaves
- 1 tablespoon chopped flat-leaf parsley
- 1 teaspoon lemon juice
- ¼ teaspoon lemon zest
- Flaky sea salt, for garnish
- 6 tablespoons Greenest Tahini Sauce (page 64)

Easy to find and full of good-for-your-heart omega-3 fatty acids, wild salmon is a staple for my household. Though king salmon gets the biggest hype for its ultra-silky flesh, I'm fond of sockeye, which is redder, firmer, and less meltingly rich. In the end, though, I pick whatever fish looks best in the market. In between salmon seasons, there's no shame in buying frozen-at-sea sockeye, though you could also substitute any oily fish here, such as albacore, wahoo, or bluefish for you lucky East Coasters. Here the lush fish gets necessary sharpness from the watercress in the sauce, the radishes, and the lemony herb salad.

Preheat the oven to 350°F. Season the fish with fine sea salt and pepper.

Heat the oil in a large ovenproof skillet over medium-high heat. Place the salmon in skin side down. Cook without moving until the salmon skin has crisped and browned, about 5 minutes. Transfer the skillet to the oven and roast until the salmon is just opaque at the center, 3 to 4 minutes for medium-rare.

Just before serving, in a medium bowl, toss together the radishes, cucumber, mint, parsley, lemon juice, and lemon zest. Season to taste with fine sea salt.

Season the salmon with flaky sea salt and serve skin side up with the tahini sauce and the radish and cucumber salad.

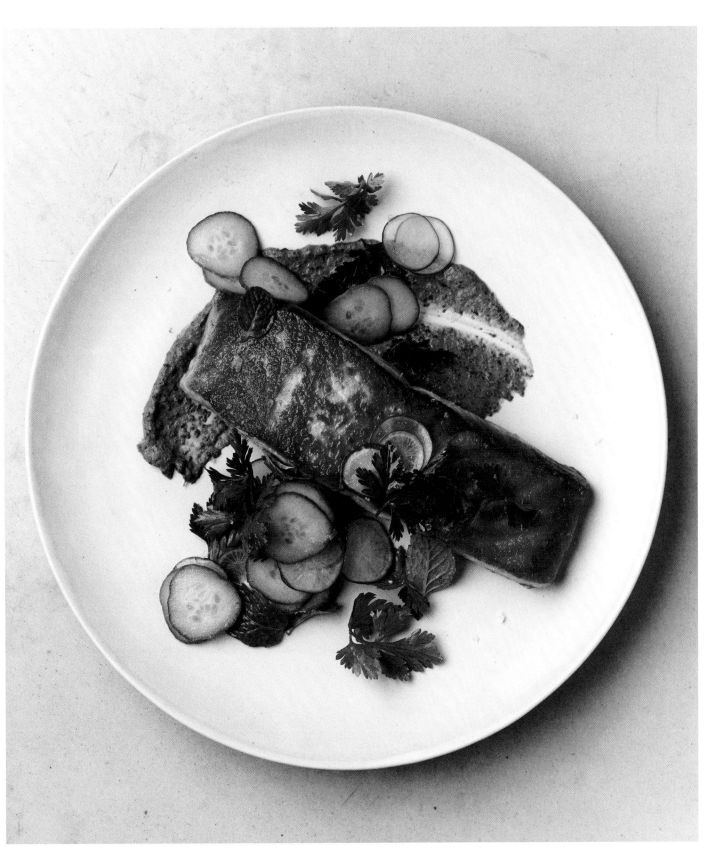

GREENEST TAHINI SAUCE

Pictured on page 63

10 MINUTES	MAKES ABOUT 1¾ CUPS

- 2 garlic cloves
- Kosher salt
- 1 bunch watercress, thick stems trimmed
- 1 cup fresh mint leaves
- ½ cup fresh flat-leaf parsley leaves
- ½ cup tahini (sesame seed paste)
- 2 tablespoons (or more) fresh lemon juice

As you might be able to tell by now, I cannot get enough green flavors in the spring. I created this sauce, rich with watercress and mint, to load vibrant color and flavor into a simple tahini sauce, one of my home staples for quick flavor. The blanching step ensures a bright green color and also makes it easier to blend together the tahini and the greens.

Cook the garlic in a medium saucepan of boiling salted water until slightly softened, about 30 seconds. Using a slotted spoon, transfer the garlic to a bowl of ice water; let cool.

Return the water in the saucepan to a boil and cook the watercress, mint, and parsley just until wilted, about 15 seconds; drain. Transfer the watercress and herbs to ice water; let cool. Drain the watercress, herbs, and garlic and squeeze between paper towels to remove as much moisture as possible; coarsely chop.

Purée the watercress, herbs, garlic, tahini, lemon juice, 1 teaspoon salt, and ¾ cup water in a blender until smooth, thinning with more water as needed to reach the desired consistency; season with salt and more lemon juice, if desired.

Do ahead: The sauce can be made 3 days ahead. Cover and chill. Shake before using.

BLACK RICE WITH COCONUT

Pictured on page 67

30 TO 35 MINUTES (7 ACTIVE)	4 SERVINGS

- ¼ cup unsweetened flaked coconut
- 1 cup black rice, such as Lotus Foods Forbidden Rice
- 1 (3-inch) lemongrass tip (optional)
- 1 (2-inch) piece of fresh ginger, peeled and cut into 2 1-inch coins
- Fine sea salt to taste

Forget little black dresses—this little black rice sharpens up nearly any meal with its striking jet color and nutty taste, set off here by the pretty ivory contrast of toasted coconut flakes. You might want to cook a double batch, too: black rice warmed through with some coconut milk and water makes for a delicious breakfast porridge. Black rice does have a sturdy composition; if you like a more tender texture, you can soak your rice overnight before cooking it with the same method.

Preheat the oven to 350°F.

Spread out the coconut on a small rimmed baking sheet and toast, stirring occasionally, until golden, about 5 minutes; let cool. When cool, keep in an airtight container at room temperature.

Combine the rice, lemongrass, if using, ginger, salt, and 1¾ cups water in a medium saucepan. Bring to a boil, reduce the heat to low, and cook, covered, until the liquid is absorbed and the rice is tender, 30 to 35 minutes. Remove from the heat and discard the ginger and lemongrass; fluff the rice with a fork. Cover and set aside for 5 minutes. (If desired, reserve ½ cup rice for lunch the next day.) Serve the hot rice topped with coconut flakes.

Do ahead: Coconut can be toasted up to 3 days ahead.

TOFU, MUSTARD GREENS, AND SHIITAKE MUSHROOM STIR-FRY

35 TO 40 MINUTES (20 ACTIVE)	4 SERVINGS AND 1 LUNCH THE NEXT DAY

- 1 (14-ounce) package firm tofu, drained and cut into 1-inch cubes
- 2 tablespoons vegetable oil
- Fine sea salt and freshly ground black pepper to taste
- 8 ounces shiitake mushrooms, stems removed and mushrooms cut in half
- 2 garlic cloves, chopped
- 1 bunch mustard greens, large stems removed, leaves cut into 2-inch pieces (about 10 cups)
- 1 bunch baby bok choy, cut into 1½-inch pieces
- 2 tablespoons reduced-sodium soy sauce
- 1 teaspoon toasted sesame oil

There are a lot of tofu nonbelievers out there, I know, but tofu is what you make it. It's great if you load it with plenty of flavor, such as garlic, sesame oil, soy sauce, and umami-radiating shiitakes. Then you need to take care to get the texture right. Whenever I'm shooting for a crispy finish, I sandwich the tofu between paper towels on a plate and then top it with another plate (or six) to weigh the tofu down. After 15 minutes, much of the surface moisture has been squished away, and it's ready to develop a deep caramel-brown crust in the pan. (You can also roast it to similar effect.)

Put a double layer of paper towels on a plate. Place the tofu on it in a single layer. Cover with another double layer of paper towels and top with two plates. Let sit at least 15 minutes.

In a large nonstick skillet, heat 1 tablespoon of the oil over high heat. Add the tofu in a single layer and season it with salt and pepper. Cook until browned, 3 to 4 minutes on the first side, and then 1 or 2 minutes on each additional side; transfer the tofu to a plate.

Heat the remaining 1 tablespoon oil in the same skillet and add the shiitakes; season with salt and pepper. Cook, stirring just once or twice, until lightly browned, about 5 minutes. Stir in the garlic and cook until fragrant, about 1 minute. Add the mustard greens, bok choy, soy sauce, and 2 tablespoons water to the skillet. Cook, tossing, until the greens are wilted and tender, about 2 minutes. Remove from the heat and stir in the sesame oil and tofu.

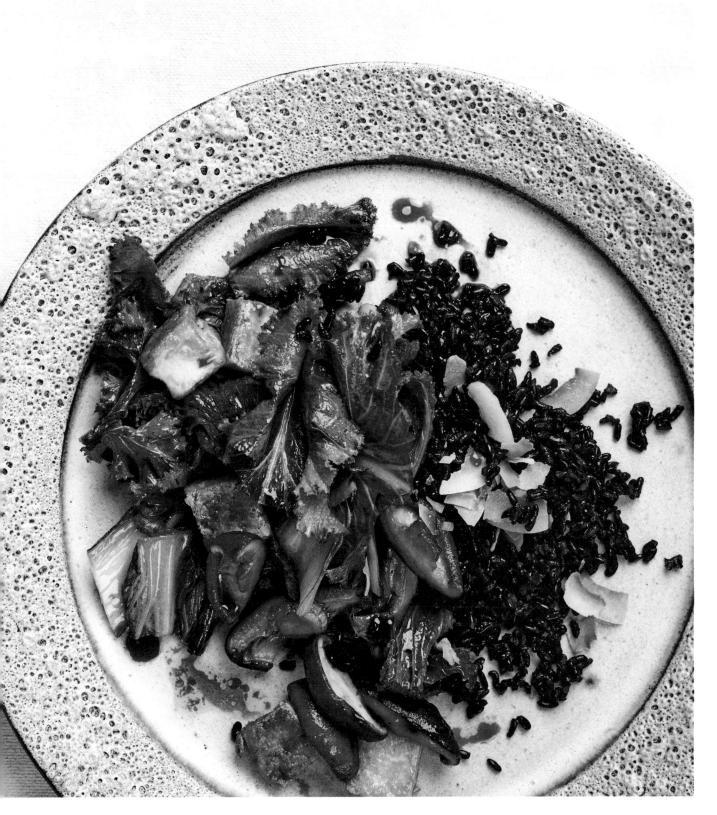

SAVOY CABBAGE WITH DILL AND PISTACHIOS

15 MINUTES (8 ACTIVE)	4 SERVINGS

- 2 tablespoons olive oil
- 1 large shallot, sliced
- 1 large Savoy cabbage head, cored, sliced into ½-inch ribbons
- 1 teaspoon fine sea salt, plus more to taste
- ¼ cup chopped fresh dill leaves
- 1 tablespoon lemon juice, plus more to taste
- 2 tablespoons chopped pistachios, toasted (see page 306)

If there's one vegetable that deserves a publicist, it's cabbage—what a lovely undersung vegetable! The heart of kimchi, sauerkraut, and summer slaws, it's also delicious showing its sweet side, as when it's quickly cooked to tenderness. Cabbage's perceived frowziness may come from its old-world tendency to be overcooked; do keep your eye on its texture and flavor as you go. A squeeze of lemon and a shower of fresh dill will keep the dish extra sunny.

In a large skillet or wide saucepan with a lid, heat the oil over medium heat. Add the shallot and cook for 1 minute, stirring frequently. Add the cabbage, 1 teaspoon of the salt, and ½ cup water and cover the pan. Cook for 3 minutes, or until the cabbage can be stirred easily, and toss well. Cover again and cook until the cabbage is tender but still toothsome, about 3 minutes. Remove from the heat and stir in the dill, lemon juice, and pistachios. Taste the cabbage and add more salt and/or lemon juice, if desired.

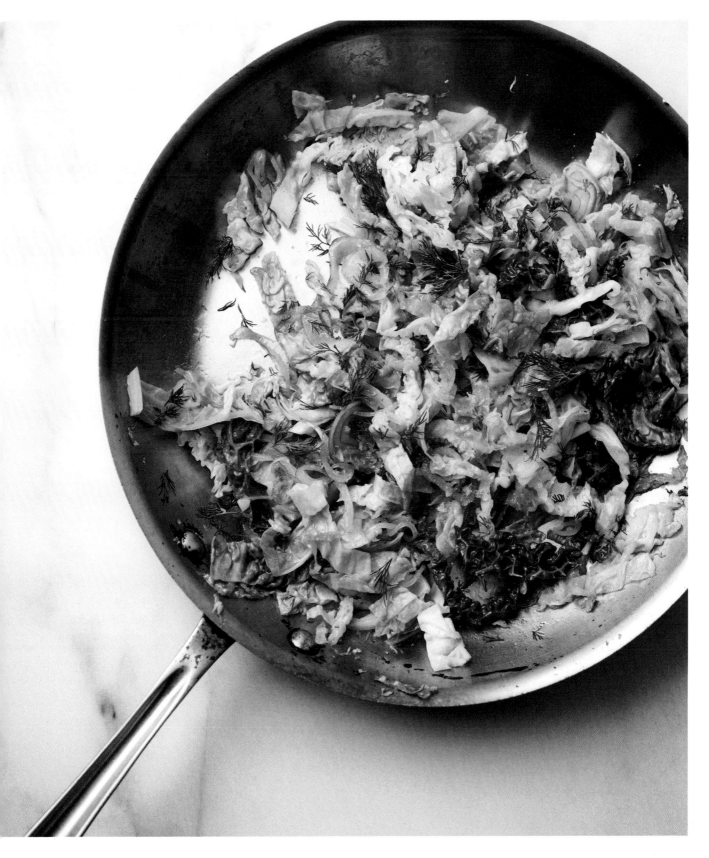

CHICKEN IN A POT WITH CARROTS, TURNIPS, AND BARLEY

60 TO 65 MINUTES (5 TO 10 ACTIVE)	4 SERVINGS AND 1 LUNCH THE NEXT DAY

- ½ cup pearled barley
- 1 (3½- to 4-pound) chicken
- Fine sea salt and freshly ground black pepper to taste
- 3 garlic cloves
- 3 fresh thyme sprigs
- 1 bay leaf
- 1 tablespoon extra-virgin olive oil
- ¼ cup brandy or dry white wine
- 3 large carrots, cut into 3-inch pieces
- 2 large leeks (white and light greens, well rinsed), trimmed and cut into 3-inch pieces
- 1 bunch peeled whole baby turnips or 1 larger turnip (about 6 ounces), peeled and cut into 1-inch wedges
- 2 cups well-washed baby spinach
- 1 tablespoon chopped fresh chives

Making steamy chicken in a broth like this is an ancient approach that's overlooked these days. But this cooking method has great benefits: you can cram the pot with vegetables to add flavor and healthy balance to the meat, plus you get a delicious soup along with the finished bird. If you have some left over, warm it up and sip it as a snack the next day: bone broth is a wildly trendy health drink these days.

Cook the barley according to the instructions in the note on page 246. Drain and set aside.

Season the chicken inside and out with salt and pepper. Place the garlic, thyme sprigs, and bay leaf inside the chicken.

In a Dutch oven or cast-iron pot, heat the oil over medium-high heat. Pat the chicken dry and place it breast side down in the pot. Cook until browned, 5 to 7 minutes per side, then transfer the chicken to a plate. Pour the brandy or wine into the pot and scrape up any browned bits from the bottom of the pan. Add the carrots, leeks, and turnips and nestle the chicken among the vegetables. Add 3 cups water and bring to a boil. Reduce the heat to low and cook, covered, until the thighs pull easily away from the bone, 45 to 55 minutes.

Remove the chicken from the pot and gently spoon out the vegetables. Skim any foam or fat from the stock and strain it through a fine-mesh sieve lined with cheesecloth or paper towels. Stir in the barley to warm it; season with salt and pepper. Carve the chicken, cutting the breast into wide slices, deboning the thighs, and cutting each thigh into two pieces.

Place a handful of spinach in each bowl, then spoon in the chicken, vegetables, and stock. Serve topped with chives.

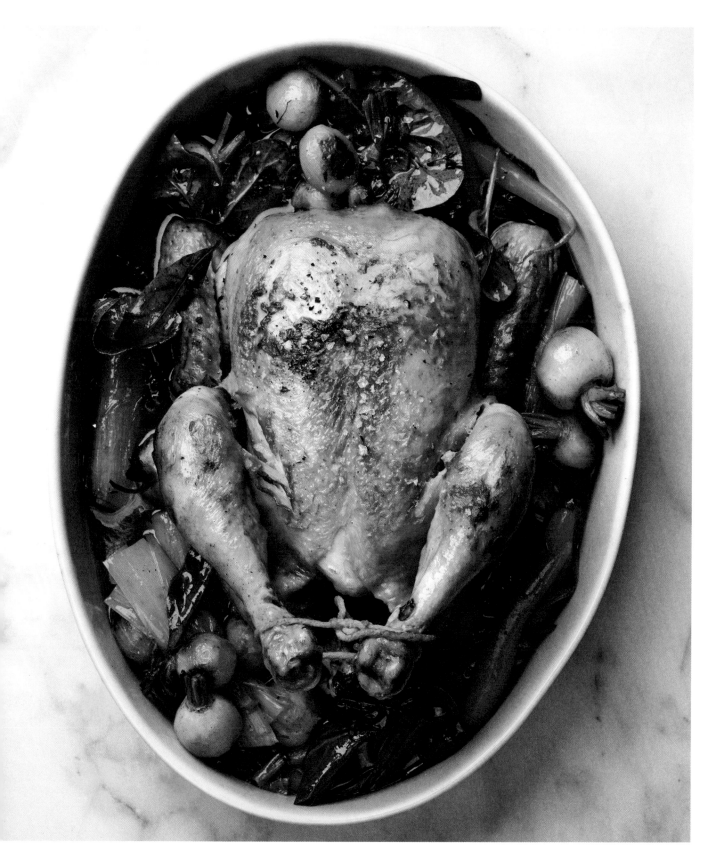

LENTILS WITH CARAMELIZED FENNEL

40 TO 45 MINUTES (10 ACTIVE)	4 SERVINGS AND 1 LUNCH THE NEXT DAY

- 1 large fennel bulb, trimmed and sliced lengthwise into ¼-inch pieces, small fronds chopped and reserved for garnish
- 2 tablespoons olive oil, plus more as needed
- Fine sea salt to taste
- 1 teaspoon fennel seeds
- 3 garlic cloves, sliced thin
- 1 pinch red pepper flakes, preferably Aleppo or Marash, or more as desired
- 1¼ cups beluga lentils or French green lentils
- ½ cup white wine (optional)
- 3 to 4 fresh thyme sprigs (optional)

Lentils are just the legume for people in a hurry. No soaking necessary, and you can still get a delicious pot cooked in about half an hour. Of course if you're not in *that* much of a rush, it's nice to add a little texture and flavor with the addition of some caramelized fennel. It's a brilliant friend to lamb and salmon, but with the help of a few walnuts or a crumble of chèvre, it could be the centerpiece of a delicious vegetarian meal. I like the plump texture and elegant color of black beluga lentils, but French green lentils work fine here, too.

Preheat the oven to 450°F.

Toss the fennel slices with 1 tablespoon of the oil and season with salt. Spread on a baking sheet and bake until the edges are browned and caramelized, about 7 minutes.

In a large saucepan, heat the remaining 1 tablespoon oil over medium-high heat. Add the fennel seeds and toast until fragrant, about 30 seconds. Add the garlic, red pepper flakes, and lentils and toss to coat well. Pour in the wine, if desired, and cook until it is evaporated, about 5 minutes. Pour in 3 cups water, add the thyme sprigs, if using, and season with salt. Turn the heat up and bring the water back to a boil, then turn the heat down to a slow simmer. Cover and cook until the lentils are tender, 30 to 35 minutes. Lentils vary in their dryness; check about 10 minutes in, and if more than a few lentils poke above the water, add a little more water to float them.

Just before serving, pluck out the thyme sprigs and toss in the caramelized fennel. Add more salt or red pepper flakes to taste and garnish with the fennel fronds.

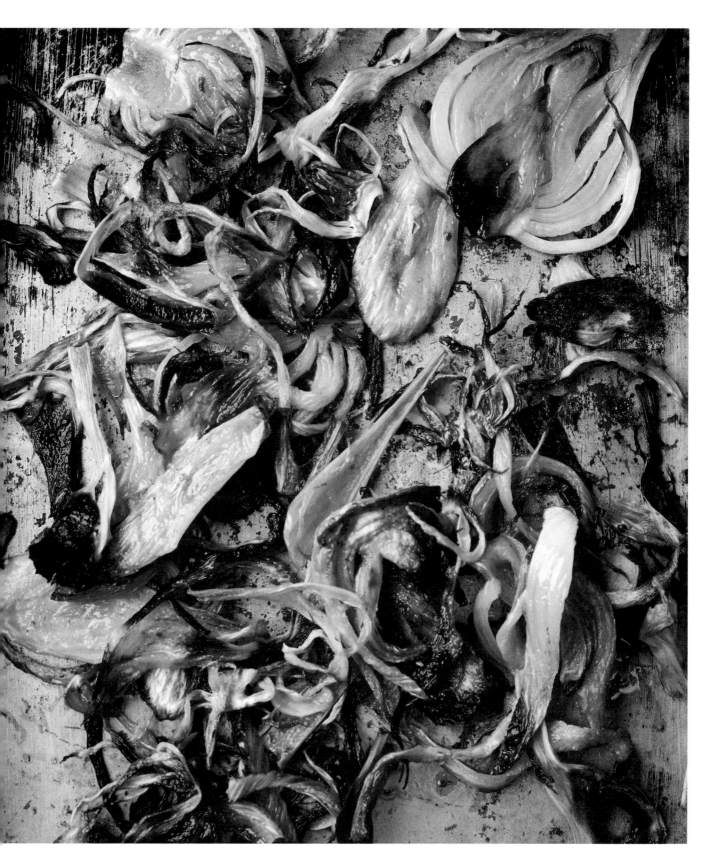

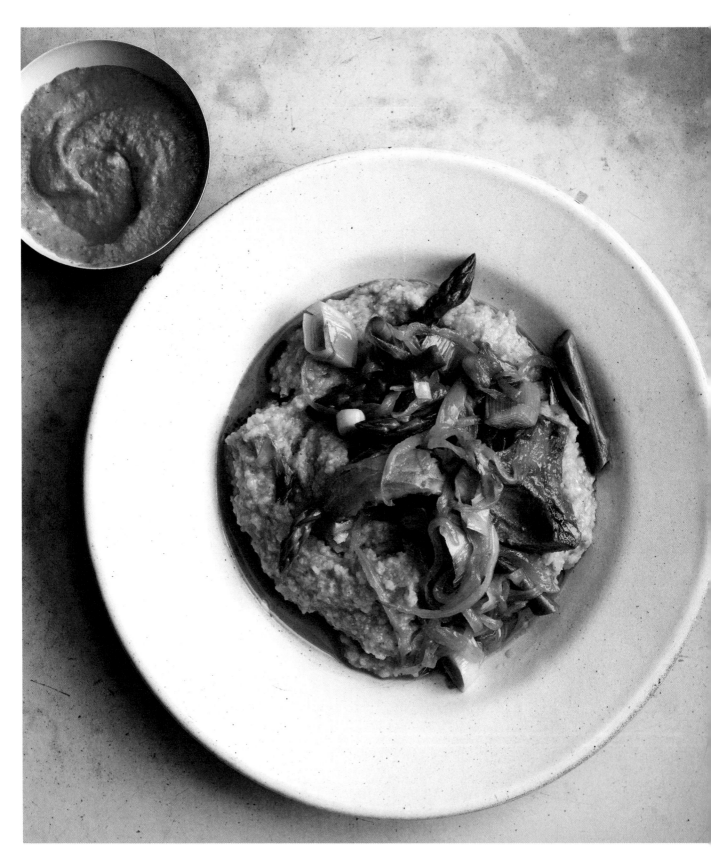

SPRING RAGOUT OF ARTICHOKES, ASPARAGUS, AND PRESERVED LEMON

18 MINUTES (10 ACTIVE) | **4 SERVINGS AND 1 LUNCH THE NEXT DAY**

- 6 teaspoons olive oil
- 1 medium onion, cut lengthwise into ¼-inch slices, or 2 spring onions, finely sliced
- 1 large leek (white and light green parts), cut into ½-inch slices
- Fine sea salt to taste
- 2 garlic cloves, chopped, or 1 teaspoon chopped green garlic
- 4 large artichokes, pared to the hearts, chokes removed, hearts cut into 2-inch wedges
- 1½ pounds asparagus, tough ends snapped off, cut on the bias into 3-inch lengths
- Freshly ground black pepper to taste
- 2 tablespoons preserved lemon peel,* julienned (from half a lemon), or 2 teaspoons grated fresh lemon peel
- 1 cup fresh flat-leaf parsley leaves
- Piquillo Romesco Sauce, for garnish (page 53)

Preserved lemons can be purchased at specialty grocers and Middle Eastern markets and online.

In my world, one measure of true love is prepping an artichoke (or several) for another person, presenting nothing but the delicious, digestible heart. You might, then, think of this recipe as an edible love note: it's a celebration of the artichoke, framed by asparagus and seasoned with salty flecks of preserved lemon. Although I encourage paring fresh artichoke hearts (search "prep baby artichokes" on bonappetit.com), there are a couple of less labor-intensive options: frozen artichoke hearts are very nice but a little hard to find. You can also prepare this dish with canned artichoke hearts or bottoms (not the marinated artichokes that are packed in vinegar, though). Rinse them well before use; two cans should work in this recipe. If you do use canned artichokes, you may want to add a bit more olive oil as a condiment before serving.

Heat 5 teaspoons of the oil in a large covered saucepan over medium heat. Stir in the onion and leek plus 1 tablespoon water and a generous pinch of salt. Cover and cook for 2 to 3 minutes, until the leek has wilted. Stir in the garlic and cook 1 more minute, then place the artichokes in the pan. Add another pinch of salt, stir to coat, and then pour in 1 cup water. Cover and cook until artichokes are tender but not mushy, about 8 minutes. (If using canned artichokes, cut the cooking time down to 5 minutes.) Add the asparagus, cover, and cook for 2 minutes, or until crisp-tender; remove from the heat. Taste the ragout and add salt and pepper, if desired.

To make the parsley salad, in a small bowl, combine the preserved lemon peel, parsley, and 1 teaspoon oil. Toss and season with salt and black pepper.

To serve, top the ragout with the parsley salad and garnish with the romesco sauce.

HANGER STEAK WITH ORANGE-OREGANO CHIMICHURRI

45 TO 55 MINUTES (20 ACTIVE)	4 SERVINGS AND 1 LUNCH THE NEXT DAY

- 1½ pounds hanger steak, center membrane removed, cut into 4 pieces
- 1 small garlic clove, grated
- 1 teaspoon dried oregano
- 1 teaspoon finely grated orange zest
- Fine sea salt
- ½ cup chopped flat-leaf parsley leaves
- 1 tablespoon freshly squeezed orange juice
- 2 teaspoons red wine vinegar, white wine vinegar, or cider vinegar
- ¼ cup extra-virgin olive oil
- Freshly ground black pepper to taste
- 2 teaspoons neutral oil, such as canola or grapeseed oil

I dream of one day trying some actual Argentine steaks, cooked over an open fire somewhere out on the Pampas. For now, I settle for some pretty delicious Pacific Northwest grass-finished beef that I can score near my house. Hanger steak, also known as the hanging tender or onglet, is a classic bistro cut that's got a chewy, loose-grained tenderness full of minerally flavor. I love it because it makes for a quick dinner that feels pretty celebratory when paired with a simple but compelling sauce like this chimichurri.

Remove the steaks from the refrigerator 30 minutes before cooking.

To make the chimichurri, combine the garlic, oregano, and orange zest in a medium bowl; using the back of a spoon, crush with ¾ teaspoon salt until fragrant. Mix in the parsley, orange juice, and vinegar. Slowly whisk in the olive oil until emulsified; season with salt and pepper.

Season the steaks with salt and pepper. Heat the neutral oil in a large skillet over medium-high heat. Add the steaks and cook, turning once, until browned and medium-rare, 4 to 6 minutes per side. Let rest at least 10 minutes, then slice against the grain. Reserve about 4 ounces for lunch the next day.

Serve with the chimichurri.

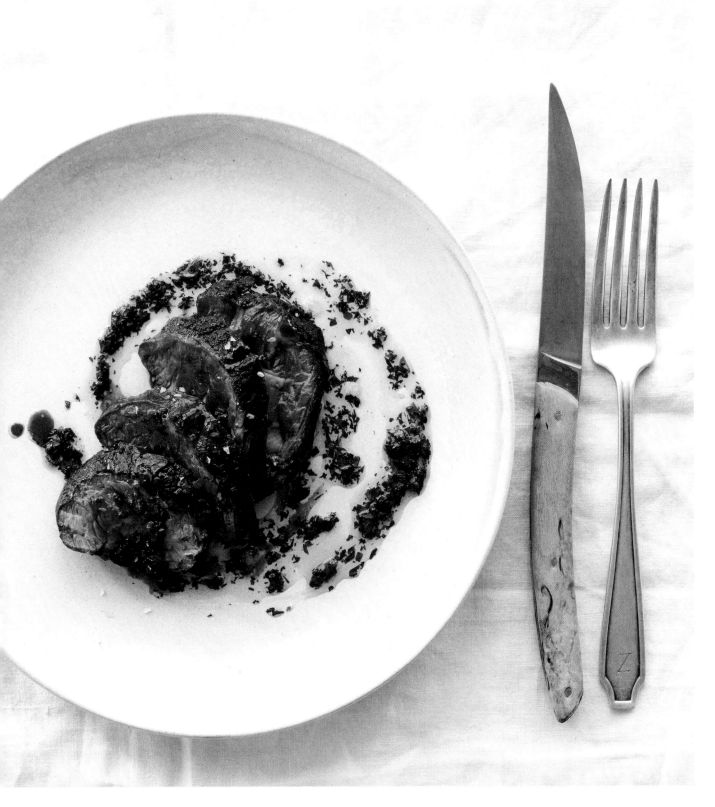

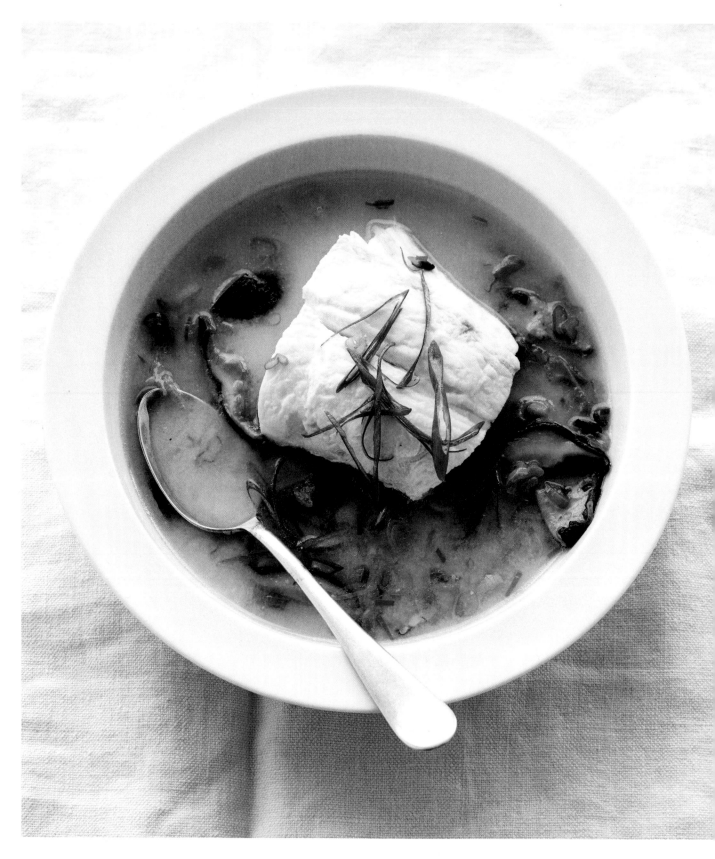

HALIBUT POACHED WITH SCALLIONS AND MISO

20 MINUTES (15 ACTIVE)	4 SERVINGS AND 1 LUNCH THE NEXT DAY

- 1½ pounds halibut fillets, skinned, cut into 5 portions
- Fine sea salt and freshly ground black pepper
- 3½ teaspoons canola oil
- 1 (2-inch) piece fresh ginger, peeled and cut into 4 disks
- 4 ounces shiitake mushrooms, stems removed and caps sliced ¼ inch thick
- 1 bunch scallions (white and light green parts), thinly sliced, dark green stalks reserved
- 2 tablespoons white miso

In spring, while the chilly weather still demands something soothing, I simultaneously crave freshness and warmth. This meal straddles both desires, with crisp-tender spears of asparagus set off against a rich-but-light miso-mushroom combination. The headliner is halibut, the first great fish of the year to reenter our Northwest markets. Snow white and flaky halibut is a lean fish, so it does well when poached in a broth like this. Feel free to substitute other fish, of course: Arctic char, turbot, striped bass, or steelhead would also work well.

Season the fish with salt and pepper.

In a large nonstick skillet, heat 2 teaspoons of the oil over medium-high heat. Add the ginger and mushrooms. Cook until the mushrooms are browned on one side, about 2 minutes, then add a pinch of salt and stir. Cook for 1 minute, then add the sliced scallions. Cook for 1 minute, stirring frequently. Add 2 cups water and the miso, whisking to dissolve the miso in the liquid. Bring to a boil, then turn off the heat. Pour the broth into a bowl or saucepan and rinse and wipe out the pan.

Heat the remaining 1½ teaspoons oil in the pan over high heat. Place the fish in the pan, top side down, and cook, undisturbed, for 1½ minutes, until lightly browned. Turn the fish over, turn the heat down to medium, and pour in the miso-mushroom broth. Top with the scallion greens, pushing gently to immerse them in the liquid. Bring the liquid to a gentle simmer and poach the fish until just opaque at the center, 1 to 2 minutes.

Serve the fish with the broth, mushrooms, and scallion tops.

SPRING FRITTATA WITH ASPARAGUS, LEEKS, AND DILL

15 MINUTES (8 ACTIVE)	6 TO 8 SERVINGS

- 5 teaspoons olive oil
- 2 large leeks (white and light green parts, well rinsed), thinly sliced
- 1 teaspoon fine sea salt, plus more to taste
- ½ pound asparagus, tough ends snapped off, cut on the bias into 2½-inch pieces
- 10 large eggs
- Freshly ground black pepper to taste
- Pinch of smoked paprika
- ¼ cup chopped fresh dill
- 2 tablespoons chopped fresh chives
- 2 ounces chèvre, crumbled

At dinner last year, my son asked what my favorite food is. At first I couldn't answer. "I like too many things," I insisted. My husband pointed to the frittata we were eating, and I reconsidered. If forced to choose, my answer would be eggs. Golden and voluptuous, they're the cheapest luxury out there, and are always around to bind together whatever delicious odds and ends I have in the fridge. Case in point, this wonderful omelet, which borrows heavily from the Persian omelet *kookoo sabzi*. Feel free to dab a little Piquillo Romesco Sauce (page 53) on the side, if you have some on hand.

Place an oven rack in the upper third of the oven and preheat the oven to 375°F.

In a 9- or 10-inch nonstick skillet, heat 1 tablespoon (3 teaspoons) of the oil over medium heat. Add the leeks, 1 tablespoon water, and 1 teaspoon of the salt and cook, stirring occasionally, until the leeks are wilted and tender, about 3 minutes. Add the asparagus and cook for 1 minute. Remove the vegetables to a plate. Wipe out the pan and let it cool until tepid.

Break the eggs into a bowl and whisk them together with salt and pepper to taste, the paprika, dill, chives, and leeks and asparagus mixture.

Heat the remaining 2 teaspoons oil in the pan over medium heat. Pour in the egg mixture and add the chèvre. Cook until the eggs begin to set on the bottom. Using a heat-resistant spatula, lift the edges of the cooked eggs and let liquid eggs run under to the pan below. Cook for another minute and repeat. When the bottom half of the eggs are cooked, place the pan in the oven and cook for 5 minutes, until the eggs are no longer wobbly at the center. Turn on the broiler and broil the frittata until lightly browned on the top, about 30 seconds.

Remove the frittata from the oven and let set at least 5 minutes in the pan, then slice and serve.

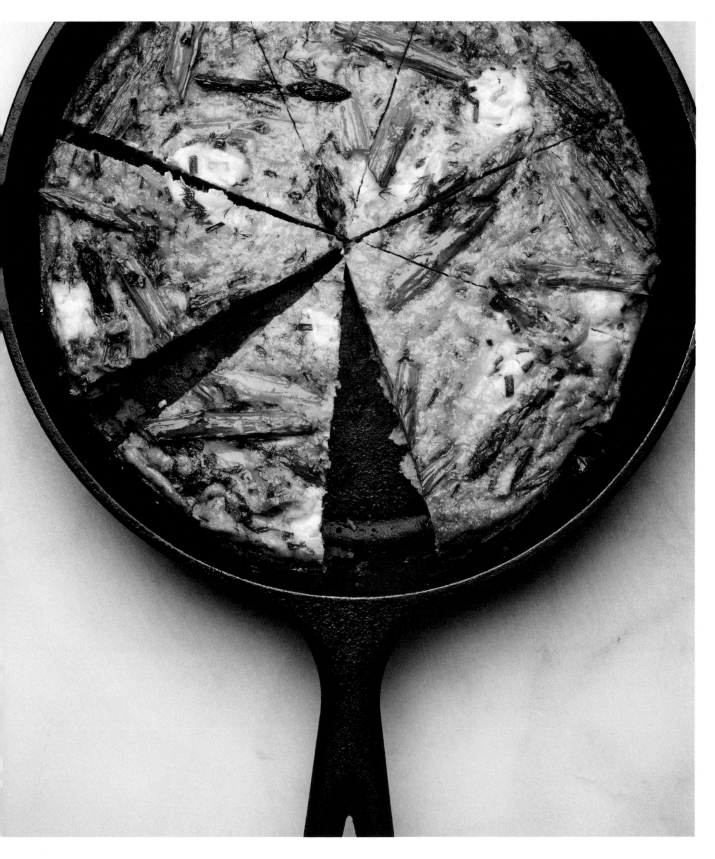

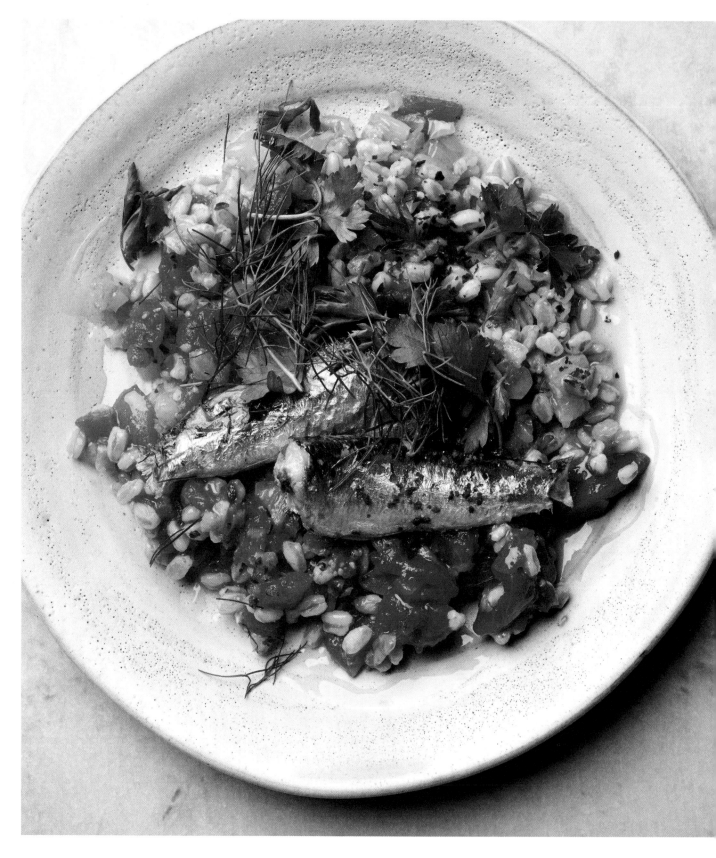

TOMATO FARROTTO WITH SARDINES

50 TO 60 MINUTES (15 ACTIVE)	4 SERVINGS AND 1 LUNCH THE NEXT DAY

- 2 tablespoons olive oil
- ½ fennel bulb, trimmed and finely chopped, plus 2 tablespoons fennel fronds
- 1 medium onion, finely diced
- 3 garlic cloves, chopped
- 1 teaspoon fennel seeds
- ¼ teaspoon red pepper flakes, preferably Aleppo pepper or Marash
- Fine sea salt and freshly ground black pepper to taste
- 2 (3.5- to 4.5-ounce) cans sardines, drained, fish bones removed, or 2 (4-ounce) cans good-quality tuna
- 1 teaspoon fresh lemon juice
- ¾ cup semi-pearled farro,* soaked overnight and drained
- 2 cups boiling water
- 1½ cups chopped canned whole tomatoes with juices
- 2 tablespoons fresh flat-leaf parsley leaves

* Semi-pearled farro is sold at Italian markets and natural foods and specialty food stores.

Farro is a deeply chewy and delicious whole grain that loves the bright acidity of tomatoes such as those in this dish. Fresh sardines are only sporadically available, so I recommend using canned sardines here. (By all means broil or grill fresh sardines if your fishmonger has them.) If you go with canned, spend a little money on them: imported Portuguese and Spanish sardines such as Cole's and Matiz taste much better than the grocery store staples. You could also use good-quality tuna—imported canned tuna or line-caught albacore from the western United States will taste best. A time-saving tip: soaking the farro overnight (or at least during the day while you're at work) will give you a running start with this dish.

Heat 1 tablespoon of the oil in a large skillet over medium heat. Add the fennel, onion, garlic, fennel seeds, and red pepper flakes and season with salt and pepper. Cook, stirring, until the vegetables are tender and translucent, 8 to 10 minutes; remove from the heat. Place the sardines in a single layer on a plate (if using tuna, break it up into small chunks and set it on the plate) and spoon 2 tablespoons of the cooked fennel mixture on top of the fish. Drizzle with lemon juice and the remaining 1 tablespoon oil.

Return the skillet to medium-high heat and stir in the soaked farro. Cook, stirring often, for 1 minute, then add the 2 cups boiling water; season with salt and black pepper. Bring to a boil, reduce the heat, and simmer until the farro is al dente, 35 to 40 minutes. Stir in the tomatoes and their juices and increase the heat to high. Cook until the liquid is absorbed, 5 to 7 minutes; season with salt and black pepper.

Serve the tomato farrotto topped with the sardines, vegetables, fennel fronds, and parsley.

LEMONGRASS SHRIMP WITH MUSHROOMS

25 TO 30 MINUTES (12 ACTIVE)	4 SERVINGS AND 1 LUNCH THE NEXT DAY

- 1 shallot, roughly chopped
- 2 garlic cloves, roughly chopped
- 2 tablespoons soy sauce
- 1 teaspoon sesame oil
- 3 tablespoons coconut oil, softened, or canola oil
- 2 teaspoons honey
- 2 teaspoons fine sea salt
- ¼ teaspoon freshly ground black pepper
- 2 lemongrass stalks, exterior leaves removed and tender bulb and lower stalk cut into 2-inch pieces
- 1½ pounds shelled, deveined jumbo or extra-jumbo shrimp, preferably wild American shrimp (about 30 per pound)
- 1 pound cultivated mushrooms, preferably king trumpet, oyster, or beech mushrooms, tough stems removed and caps cut lengthwise in ½-inch slices
- 1 tablespoon chopped fresh mint
- 1 tablespoon chopped fresh chives
- 1 tablespoon lime juice, plus more to taste
- Flaky sea salt to taste

Prepping lemongrass is therapeutic. There's the satisfying *thunk* that comes from chopping off the stubborn root end, and, most important, that invigorating lemony herbal fragrance adds gorgeous flavor to any ingredient it embellishes. I've paired juicy shrimp with plump mushrooms, but try the marinade on other ingredients, too: tofu, chicken, beef, and eggplant all benefit from the power of lemongrass.

Place an oven rack in the upper third of the oven and preheat to 450°F.

To make the marinade, in a blender or small food processor, combine the shallot, garlic, soy sauce, sesame oil, coconut oil, honey, fine sea salt, and pepper. Process into a rough puree.

Press down on the lemongrass stalks using the back of your knife until fragrant and the oils have been released.

In a medium bowl, toss half the lemongrass and half the marinade with the shrimp. Chill until ready to cook.

In a separate bowl, toss the rest of the lemongrass and marinade with the mushrooms, turning gently but thoroughly to coat the mushrooms evenly. Let sit for 10 minutes, or up to an hour. Lift the mushrooms out of the marinade and spread in a single layer on a baking sheet. Roast the mushrooms until lightly browned and tender, about 12 minutes, rotating the pan and flipping the mushrooms halfway through. Turn on the broiler to brown them a bit more, 1 or 2 minutes, watching carefully.

Pull the shrimp out of the marinade and spread them on a baking sheet. Place the sheet on the highest oven rack and broil them just until opaque at their centers, 2 to 3 minutes. It should not be necessary to flip the shrimp if they're the recommended size; larger or shell-on shrimp will do best if turned midway through the cooking.

Toss the shrimp with the mushrooms, mint, and chives. Add the lime juice, taste, and add flaky sea salt and/or more lime juice as desired.

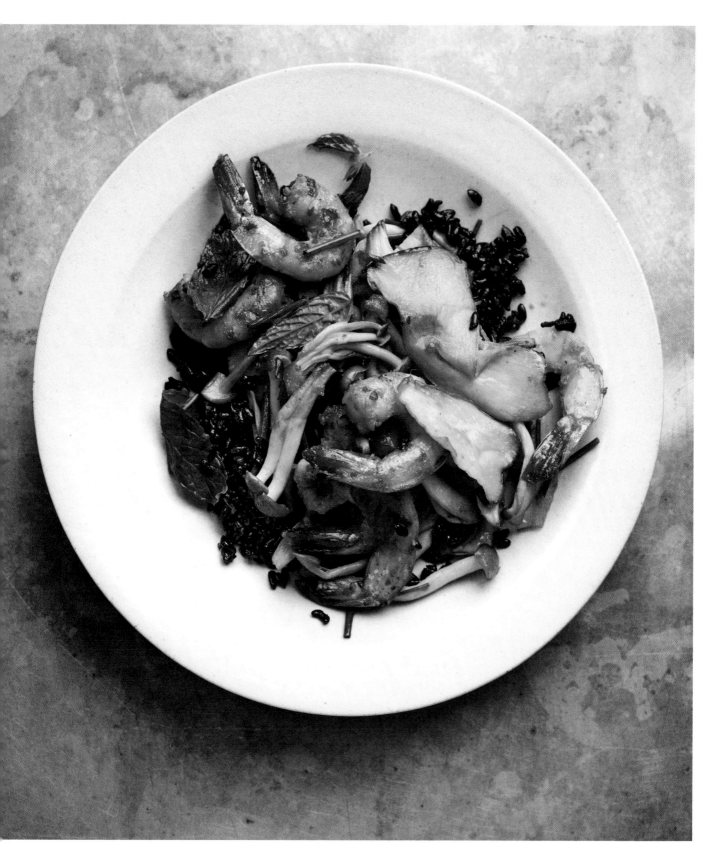

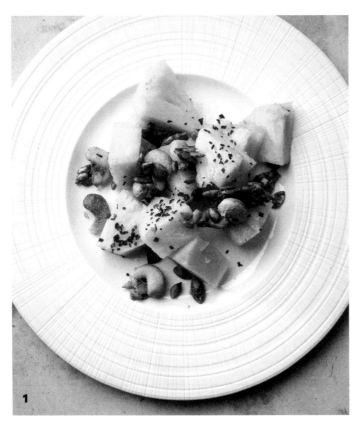

1

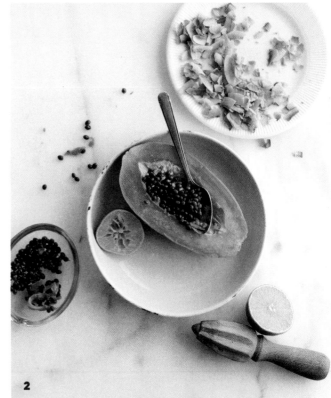

2

SPRING DESSERT SUGGESTIONS

The suggested portions below are for one person.

1. **Pineapple with Aleppo pepper and Spiced Pumpkin Seed and Cashew Crunch**
1 cup pineapple chunks with Aleppo pepper and
1 tablespoon Spiced Pumpkin Seed and Cashew Crunch
(page 316)

2. **Papaya with toasted coconut, lime, and Maldon salt**
½ papaya with 1 tablespoon toasted coconut, a squeeze of
lime, and a sprinkle of salt

3. **Strawberries with lime zest and honey**
1 cup sliced strawberries topped with lime zest and up
to 1 teaspoon honey

4. **Dried figs and apricots with almonds**
1 fig, 2 apricots, and 8 or 9 almonds (see page 306)

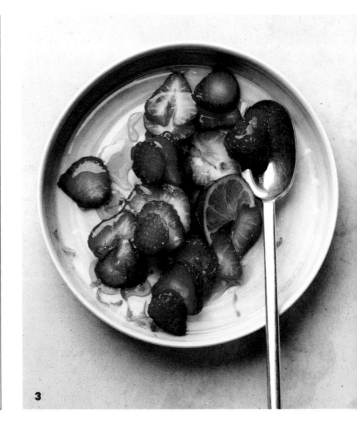

3

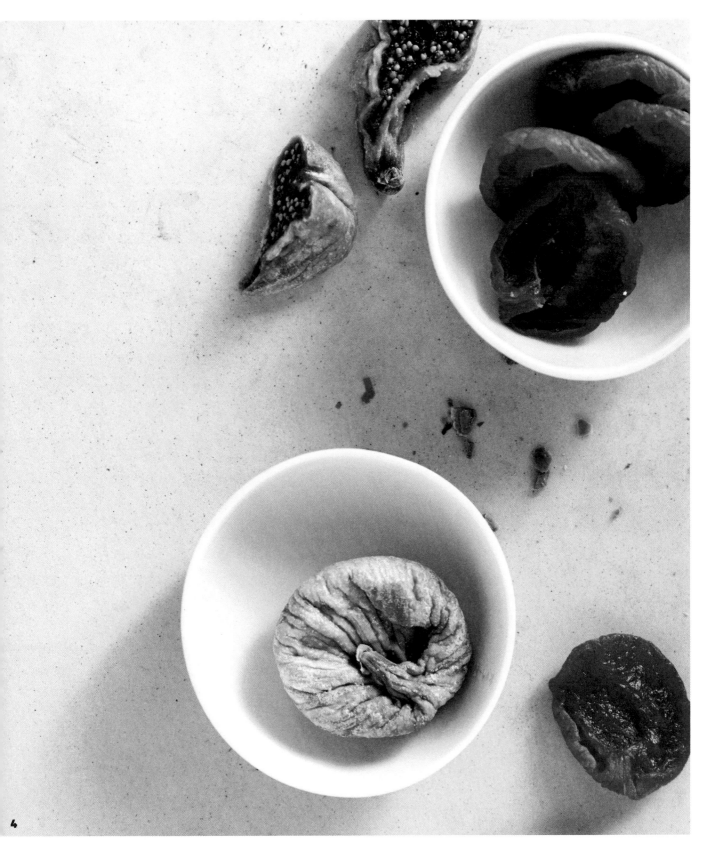

CLEANSE MENU

DAY 1

(STARTS WITH DINNER)

DINNER
Sake-Steamed Clams with Soba Noodles (page 47)

Steam-Sautéed Sesame Broccoli (page 57)

DESSERT
Papaya with toasted coconut, lime, and flaky sea salt (pictured on page 86)

DAY 2

BREAKFAST
Toasted Rye and Coconut Muesli with Apricots (page 30)

LUNCH
Chickpeas with shaved asparagus, arugula, celery, Chickpea and Hazelnut Dukkah (page 322) and Meyer Lemon–Shallot Vinaigrette (page 313)

SNACK
Herbed Yogurt Spread (page 321) with 1 cup sliced carrots

DINNER
Pork Ragout with Morels and Celery Root (page 50)

Buckwheat Polenta (page 52)

DESSERT
Raspberry-Pistachio Chocolate Bark (page 324)

DAY 3

BREAKFAST
Greek Yogurt with Strawberries, Pistachios, and Poppy and Sesame Seeds (page 33)

LUNCH
Warmed leftover Pork Ragout (page 50) with side salad of radicchio, walnuts, and Caesar-Style Vinaigrette with Figs (page 314)

SNACK
Hard-boiled egg (see page 301) with Smoked Salt Furikake (page 323)

DINNER
Salmon with the Greenest Tahini Sauce, Shaved Radishes, and Cucumbers (page 62)

Savoy Cabbage with Dill and Pistachios (page 68)

DESSERT
Pineapple with Aleppo pepper and Spiced Pumpkin Seed and Cashew Crunch (pictured on page 86)

DAY 4

BREAKFAST
Crispbread with Herbed
Yogurt Spread, Smoked
Salmon, and Radishes
(page 29)

LUNCH
Leftover pan-roasted salmon
with shaved asparagus, pink
grapefruit, butter lettuce,
pistachios, and Meyer
Lemon–Shallot Vinaigrette
(pictured on page 38)

SNACK
Rhubarb Applesauce for
Spring Breakfasts and
Snacks (page 36) with
toasted almonds

DINNER
Pan-Roasted Chicken with
Sautéed Pea Shoots and
Piquillo Pepper Romesco
(page 53)

Millet Tabbouleh (page 61)

DESSERT
Strawberries with lime
zest and honey (pictured
on page 86)

DAY 5

BREAKFAST
Fried Egg with Spinach,
Toasted Garlic, and Piquillo
Pepper Romesco (page 35)

LUNCH
Shredded leftover chicken
with leftover millet
tabbouleh, butter lettuce,
and Meyer Lemon–Shallot
Vinaigrette (page 314)

SNACK
Herbed Yogurt Spread
(page 321) with 1 cup
sliced carrots

DINNER
Tofu, Mustard Greens, and
Shiitake Mushroom Stir-Fry
(page 66)

Black Rice with Coconut
(page 65)

DESSERT
Dried figs and apricots with
cinnamon-toasted almonds
(pictured on page 86)

DAY 6

BREAKFAST
Multigrain Hot Cereal with
Cherries and Almonds
(page 32)

LUNCH
Leftover tofu and shiitakes,
shredded Napa cabbage,
cucumbers, cilantro, and
Sesame-Miso Vinaigrette
(page 310)

SNACK
Hard-boiled egg (see
page 301) with Smoked
Salt Furikake (page 323)

DINNER
Charmoula-Rubbed
Mahi-mahi (page 42)

Lentils with Caramelized
Fennel (page 72)

DESSERT
Papaya with toasted coconut,
lime, and Maldon salt
(pictured on page 86)

CLEANSE MENU

DAY 7

BREAKFAST
Steel-Cut Oats with Rhubarb Applesauce and Hazelnuts (page 36)

LUNCH
Leftover lentils and caramelized fennel with slivered kale, toasted almonds, chèvre, and Caesar-Style Vinaigrette with Figs (pictured on page 41)

SNACK
Chickpea and Hazelnut Dukkah (page 322) with radishes

DINNER
Spring Ragout of Artichokes, Asparagus, and Preserved Lemon (page 75)

Buckwheat Polenta (page 52)

DESSERT
Raspberry-Pistachio Chocolate Bark (page 324)

DAY 8

BREAKFAST
Toasted Rye and Coconut Muesli with Apricots (page 30)

LUNCH
Leftover artichokes and asparagus, white beans and spinach, and Meyer Lemon–Shallot Vinaigrette (page 313)

SNACK
Herbed Yogurt Spread (page 321) with sliced carrots

DINNER
Hanger Steak with Orange-Oregano Chimichurri (page 76)

Roasted Asparagus with Shallots, Thyme, and Almonds (page 44)

DESSERT
Pineapple with Aleppo pepper and Spiced Pumpkin Seed and Cashew Crunch (pictured on page 86)

DAY 9

BREAKFAST
Fried Egg with Spinach, Toasted Garlic, and Piquillo Pepper Romesco (page 35)

LUNCH
Leftover hanger steak, chimichurri, and asparagus with arugula, chickpeas, and Chickpea and Hazelnut Dukkah (page 322)

SNACK
Rhubarb Applesauce for Spring Breakfasts and Snacks (page 36) with toasted almonds

DINNER
Halibut Poached with Scallions and Miso (page 79)

Green Peas and Edamame (page 48)

DESSERT
Strawberries with lime zest and honey (pictured on page 86)

DAY 10

BREAKFAST
Greek Yogurt with
Strawberries, Pistachios,
and Poppy and Sesame
Seeds (page 33)

LUNCH
Leftover halibut and
shiitakes, frisée, avocado,
and Sesame-Miso Vinaigrette
(page 310)

SNACK
Hard-boiled egg (see
page 301) with Smoked Salt
Furikake (page 323)

DINNER
Spring Frittata with
Asparagus, Leeks, and Dill
(page 80)

Millet Tabbouleh (page 61)

DESSERT
Dried figs and apricots with
cinnamon-toasted almonds
(pictured on page 87)

DAY 11

BREAKFAST
Multigrain Hot Cereal with
Cherries and Almonds
(page 32)

LUNCH
Leftover frittata with
chopped salad of romaine,
parsley, sliced red onion,
piquillo peppers, and
chickpeas with Meyer
Lemon–Shallot Vinaigrette
with Figs (pictured on
page 40)

SNACK
Herbed Yogurt Spread
(page 321) with sliced carrots

DINNER
Tomato Farrotto with
Sardines (page 83)

Savoy Cabbage with Dill
and Pistachios (page 68)

DESSERT
Papaya with toasted coconut,
lime, and Maldon salt
(pictured on page 86)

DAY 12

BREAKFAST
Fried egg with leftover
farrotto (see page 83)

LUNCH
2 ounces sardines, cannellini
beans, shaved fennel,
shallots, slivered kale,
and Meyer Lemon–Shallot
Vinaigrette (page 313)

SNACK
Chickpea and Hazelnut
Dukkah (page 322)
with radishes

DINNER
Lamb Leg with Greenest
Tahini Sauce and Sautéed
Swiss Chard (page 58)

Lentils with Caramelized
Fennel (page 72)

DESSERT
Raspberry-Pistachio
Chocolate Bark (page 324)

DAY 13

BREAKFAST
Crispbread with Herbed
Yogurt Spread, Smoked
Salmon, and Radishes
(page 29)

LUNCH
Sliced leftover lamb, mâche,
avocado, mint, pistachios,
and Meyer Lemon–Shallot
Vinaigrette (page 313)

SNACK
Rhubarb Applesauce for
Spring Breakfasts and
Snacks (page 36) with
toasted almonds (see
page 306)

DINNER
Chicken in a Pot with
Carrots, Turnips, and Barley
(page 70)

DESSERT
Pineapple with Aleppo
pepper and Spiced Pumpkin
Seed and Cashew Crunch
(pictured on page 86)

DAY 14

BREAKFAST
Toasted Rye and Coconut
Muesli with Apricots
(page 30)

LUNCH
Leftover chicken from
Chicken in a Pot, pulled
and tossed with slivered
scallions, julienned carrots,
slivered Napa cabbage,
mint, and Sesame-Miso
Vinaigrette (pictured on
page 310)

SNACK
Hard-boiled egg (see
page 301) with Smoked Salt
Furikake (page 323)

DINNER
Lemongrass Shrimp with
Mushrooms (page 84)

Black Rice with Coconut
(page 65)

DESSERT
Strawberries with lime zest
and honey (pictured on
page 86)

SHOPPING LIST

We've put together a shopping list for you following the number of servings in our recipes; that means dinner recipes are for four people, but breakfasts, lunches, snacks, and desserts are portioned for one person. Please adjust according to your needs!

PANTRY

CANNED AND NONPERISHABLE GOODS

- almond milk, 1 quart
- anchovy fillets
- bonito flakes
- cannellini beans, 15-ounce can
- chicken stock, homemade or low-sodium canned, 6 cups (36 ounces)
- chickpeas, 2 (15-ounce) cans
- nori
- piquillo peppers
- preserved lemon
- sardines, 3 (3.5- to 4.5-ounce) cans (or good-quality canned tuna)
- tahini
- whole canned tomatoes, 28-ounce can

CONDIMENTS

- light soy sauce
- white miso

DRIED FRUITS

- apricots, dried, preferably California, ¾ cup
- coconut flakes, unsweetened, 1¼ cups
- figs, dried, ½ cup
- raspberries, freeze-dried

FROZEN GOODS

- edamame, frozen shelled, 2 cups

GRAINS

- all-rye crackers
- barley, pearled, ½ cup
- farro, semi-pearled, ¾ cup
- flour or cornstarch, 1 tablespoon
- kasha (roasted buckwheat groats), ½ cup
- lentils, beluga or French green, 2½ cups
- millet, 2½ cups
- multigrain hot cereal, such as Bob's Red Mill 10 Grain cereal
- polenta, 1½ cups
- rice, black, such as Lotus Foods Forbidden Rice, 2 cups
- rye flakes, 2 cups (can use rolled oats)
- soba noodles, preferably all-buckwheat, 8 ounces
- steel-cut oats, ¼ cup

NUTS AND SEEDS

- almonds, 1 cup
- cashews, ¼ cup
- hazelnuts, 1 cup
- Marcona almonds, ¼ cup
- pepitas (pumpkin seeds), ¼ cup
- pistachios, ¾ cup
- poppy seeds, 2 tablespoons
- roasted chickpeas or additional hazelnuts, ¼ cup
- sunflower seeds, shelled, ¼ cup
- sesame seeds, ½ cup
- walnuts, ¾ cup

OILS AND VINEGARS

- coconut oil
- toasted sesame oil
- canola, grapeseed, or vegetable oil
- olive oil, at least 1 quart
- olive oil, extra-virgin, small bottle
- red wine vinegar
- rice vinegar
- white wine vinegar

SPICES

- ancho chili powder, 2 teaspoons
- bay leaf, 1
- black peppercorns
- caraway seeds, 1 teaspoon
- cayenne pepper, ground, 2 teaspoons
- cinnamon, ground, a pinch
- coriander seeds, 2 tablespoons
- cumin, ground, 1 teaspoon
- cumin seeds, 2 tablespoons
- dried oregano, 1 teaspoon
- fennel seeds, 2 tablespoons
- fine sea salt, 1 container, typically 26 ounces
- flaky sea salt, small container
- garam masala (may substitute Madras curry powder), 1 teaspoon
- kosher salt
- paprika, smoked, 1 teaspoon
- red pepper flakes, preferably Aleppo or Marash, ¼ cup
- smoked sea salt, 1 tablespoon

SWEET GOODS

- agave syrup
- bittersweet chocolate, 8 ounces
- honey

WINE AND ALCOHOL

- brandy or white wine, ¼ cup
- sake, dry, small bottle
- white wine (optional)

SHOPPING LIST

DAIRY AND OTHER REFRIGERATED ITEMS

- chèvre, 4- or 5-ounce package
- plain Greek yogurt, 1 quart
- eggs, large, 1 dozen
- tofu, firm, 1 (14-ounce) package

MEAT AND SEAFOOD

- pork shoulder, 1 pound
- chicken breasts, bone in, skin on, 4 pieces
- mahi-mahi, 4 (6-ounce) fillets
- clams, small hard-shell, such as Manila or littleneck, 2½ pounds
- salmon, preferably wild-caught sockeye or king, 1¼ pounds, skin on
- smoked salmon, sliced, small package

PRODUCE

- apples, Gala or Fuji, 4 large
- artichokes, 4 large
- arugula, 2 cups
- asparagus, 2 bunches
- baby bok choy, 1 head
- broccoli, 2 small heads, about 2 pounds
- butter lettuce, 2 small heads
- cabbage, Napa, ½ medium head
- cabbage, Savoy, 1 large head
- carrots, 4 medium
- celery root, 1 large
- celery, 1 small heart
- cherries, ½ cup (fresh or frozen)
- chiles, 2 jalapeño or 1 jalapeño and 1 Fresno
- chives, 1 small bunch
- cilantro, 1 bunch
- cucumbers, 2 small
- dill, 1 small bunch
- dried morels, 1 ounce (can use porcini)
- fennel, 1 large bulb
- flat-leaf parsley, 3 bunches
- garlic, 2 heads
- ginger, 1 large piece
- grapefruit, pink, 1 small
- kale, lacinato, 2 bunches
- leek, 1 large
- lemons, 5
- lemons, Meyer, 4
- lemongrass, 1 stalk (optional)
- limes, 4
- mint, 2 bunches
- mustard greens, 1 large bunch
- onions, 4 medium
- papaya, 1
- pea shoots or vines, 6 cups (can substitute spinach)
- pineapple, 1 cup chunks
- radishes, 2 bunches
- radicchio, 1 head
- rhubarb, 3 large stalks
- scallions, 2 bunches
- shallots, 5
- shiitake mushrooms, 8 ounces
- spinach, 2 cups
- strawberries, 1 pint
- tarragon, 1 bunch
- thyme, 1 bunch (optional)
- tomatoes, 2 medium (about 10 ounces)
- watercress, 1 bunch

SHOPPING LIST

Do a quick inventory before heading out shopping for your second week—some of your dairy, produce, and sauces may be in fine shape for a second week!

DAIRY AND OTHER REFRIGERATED ITEMS

- chèvre, 4- or 5-ounce package
- eggs, large, 1½ dozen
- plain Greek yogurt, 1 pint

MEAT AND SEAFOOD

- chicken, whole, 3 to 4 pounds
- hanger steak, 1½ pounds
- lamb leg, 1½ pounds, butterflied
- halibut, skinned fillet, 1½ pounds
- shrimp, preferably wild American, 1½ pounds, shelled
- smoked salmon, sliced, 1 small package

PRODUCE

- apples, Gala or Fuji, 4 large
- arugula, 2 cups
- asparagus, 2½ pounds
- avocado, 1
- cabbage, Napa, ½ medium head
- cabbage, Savoy, 1 large head
- carrots, 5 medium, 3 large
- cherries, ½ cup (fresh or frozen)
- chives, 1 bunch
- dill, 1 bunch
- fennel, 2 large bulbs
- parsley, flat-leaf, 2 bunches
- frisée, 1 head
- garlic, 2 heads
- ginger, 1 medium piece
- kale, 1 bunch
- leeks, 4 large
- lemons, 4
- lemons, Meyer, 2
- lemongrass, 2 stalks
- limes, 2
- mâche, 3 to 4 cups
- mint leaves, 2 bunches
- mushrooms, cultivated, preferably king trumpet, oyster, or beech mushrooms, 8 ounces
- onion, 1 medium
- onion, red, 1 small
- orange, 1
- papaya, 1
- peas, freshly shelled English or frozen, 3 cups
- pineapple, 2 cups chunks (about 1 pineapple)
- radishes, 1 bunch
- rhubarb, 3 large stalks
- romaine lettuce, 1 heart
- rosemary, 1 sprig
- scallions, 2 bunches
- shallots, 8
- shiitake mushrooms, 4 ounces
- spinach, 6 cups (about 2 bunches)
- strawberries, 2 pints
- Swiss chard, 2 bunches
- tarragon, 1 bunch
- thyme, 1 bunch
- turnips, 1 bunch baby or 1 large
- watercress, 1 bunch

SUM

MER

Summertime gives you all the tools you need to eat cleaner and lighter; there's a landslide of fruits and vegetables—herbs and tomatoes, berries, peaches, and corn to name a few—and you can easily let them take over your meals. The evening light lingers, tempting you outside to cook your dinner over hot charcoal. Summer food for me is all about delivering freshness, like the cool tang of buttermilk, the juiciness of melons and cucumbers, and the chilly green bite of basil, parsley, and chives. That freshness seems all the more pronounced when it is contrasted with something earthy and charred, whether that's peppers grilled till blistered, or darkly browned eggplant, or the satisfying crust on a piece of line-caught albacore. The darkness of those well-cooked foods makes the juiciness of a tomato or garden-plucked mint just jump into relief. I also love to eat casually in these months, serving food family-style on my backyard table or having guests assemble their own tacos. If you plan your cleanse now, keep it fun, keep it social, and let the playfulness of the season lead you in the right direction.

SUMMER'S KEY INGREDIENTS

VEGETABLES

Chard

Corn

Eggplant

Green beans

Peppers of all kinds

Spinach

Summer squash

Tender herbs: tarragon, basil, parsley, chives

Tomatoes

Tomatillos

Zucchini

FRUIT

Apricots

Blackberries

Cherries

Melons

Peaches

Plums

Nectarines

Raspberries

OTHER

Buttermilk

Line-caught albacore tuna

Salmon

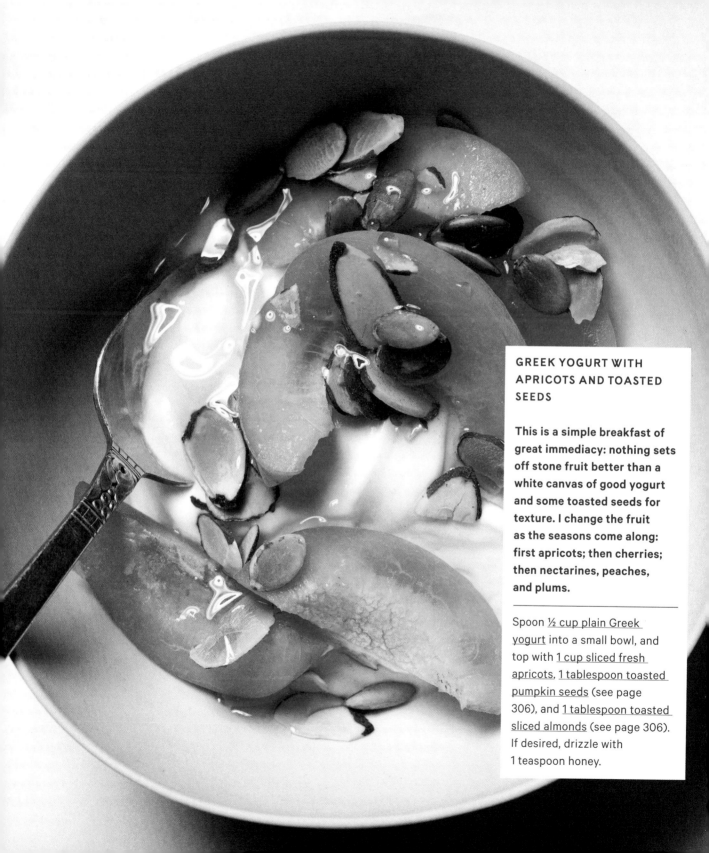

GREEK YOGURT WITH APRICOTS AND TOASTED SEEDS

This is a simple breakfast of great immediacy: nothing sets off stone fruit better than a white canvas of good yogurt and some toasted seeds for texture. I change the fruit as the seasons come along: first apricots; then cherries; then nectarines, peaches, and plums.

Spoon ½ cup plain Greek yogurt into a small bowl, and top with 1 cup sliced fresh apricots, 1 tablespoon toasted pumpkin seeds (see page 306), and 1 tablespoon toasted sliced almonds (see page 306). If desired, drizzle with 1 teaspoon honey.

SCRAMBLED EGGS WITH CHERRY TOMATOES

5 MINUTES	MAKES 1 SERVING

- ½ cup halved or quartered cherry tomatoes
- 1 teaspoon white balsamic vinegar
- 2 large eggs
- Fine sea salt and freshly ground black pepper
- 1 teaspoon canola oil
- 1 tablespoon chopped fresh basil

I can't think of a better motivation to get out of bed than a pile of simply marinated cherry tomatoes complementing a soft scramble of eggs. Last year I learned a tip to make slicing cherry tomatoes quicker. Place the tomatoes to be sliced on a plate. Set an upside-down plate of the same size on top. Using a long-bladed serrated knife, apply pressure to the top plate while guiding the knife, held parallel to the counter, through the crack in between the two plates, slicing through all the tomatoes. Once you're through the plates, remove the top one, and you've got a bunch of halved cherry tomatoes!

Combine the tomatoes and vinegar in a small, nonreactive bowl. Set aside.

Whisk the eggs and salt and pepper in a medium bowl. In a small nonstick skillet, heat the oil over medium-low heat and add the eggs. Cook the eggs, stirring with a heatproof spatula, until they are mostly set but still runny in parts, about 4 minutes, then slide them onto a plate.

Spoon the tomato mixture over the eggs, garnish with the basil, and season with more salt, if desired.

Note: If you end up with extra tomatillo sauce from your albacore dinner (page 136), it goes brilliantly with this simple breakfast.

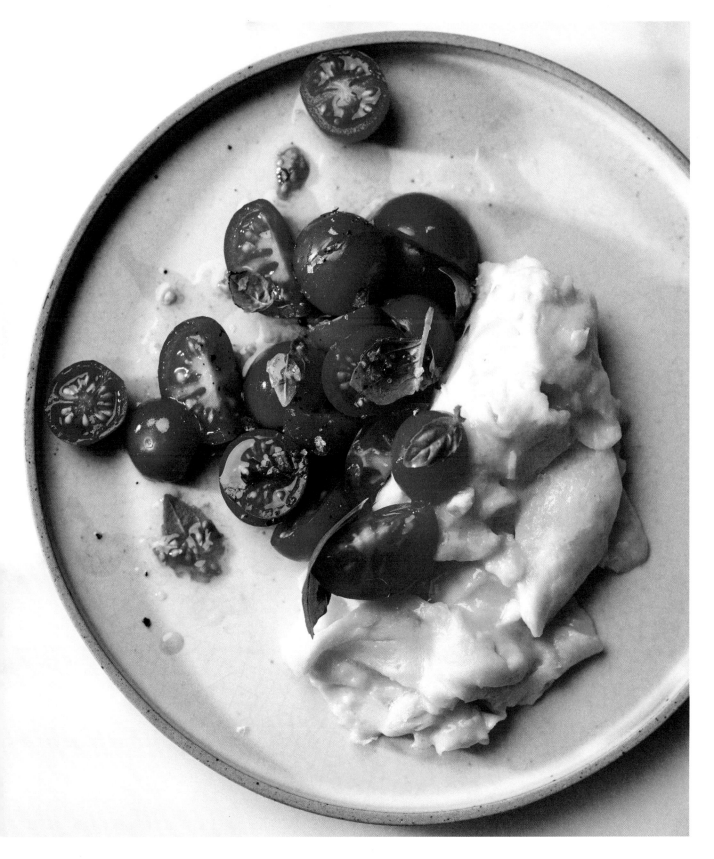

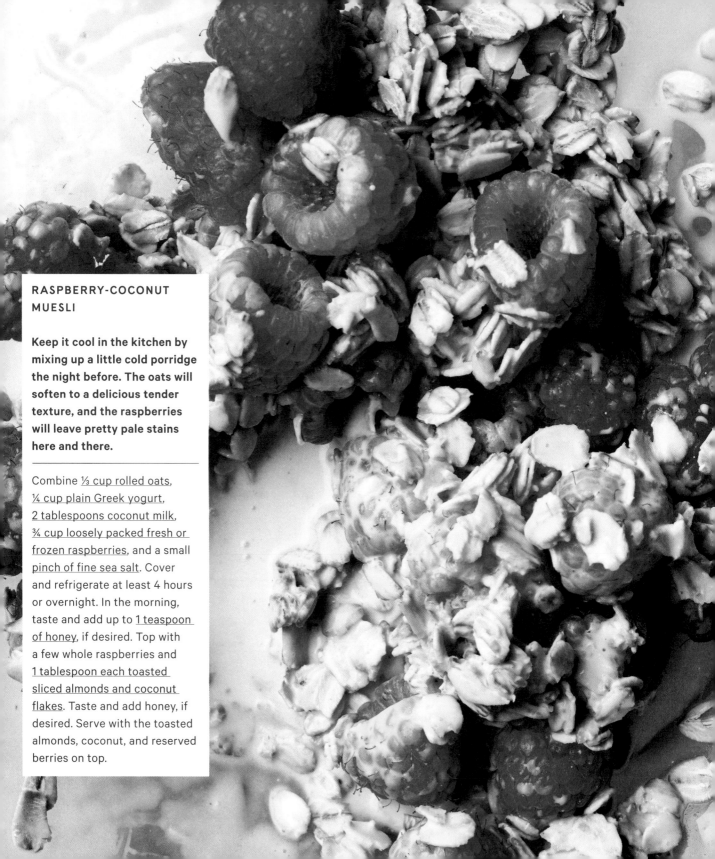

RASPBERRY-COCONUT MUESLI

Keep it cool in the kitchen by mixing up a little cold porridge the night before. The oats will soften to a delicious tender texture, and the raspberries will leave pretty pale stains here and there.

Combine ⅓ cup rolled oats, ¼ cup plain Greek yogurt, 2 tablespoons coconut milk, ¾ cup loosely packed fresh or frozen raspberries, and a small pinch of fine sea salt. Cover and refrigerate at least 4 hours or overnight. In the morning, taste and add up to 1 teaspoon of honey, if desired. Top with a few whole raspberries and 1 tablespoon each toasted sliced almonds and coconut flakes. Taste and add honey, if desired. Serve with the toasted almonds, coconut, and reserved berries on top.

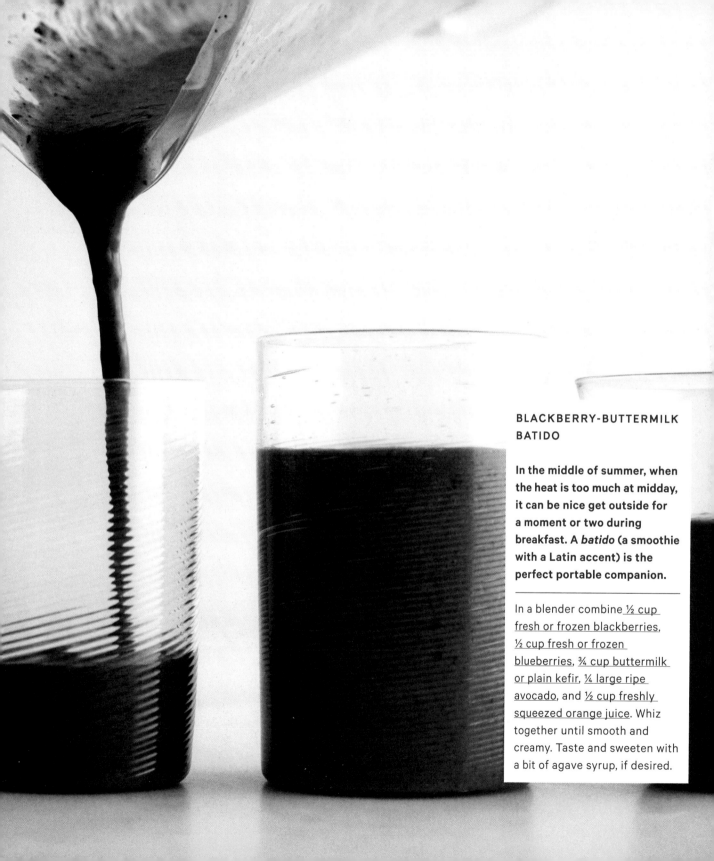

BLACKBERRY-BUTTERMILK BATIDO

In the middle of summer, when the heat is too much at midday, it can be nice get outside for a moment or two during breakfast. A *batido* (a smoothie with a Latin accent) is the perfect portable companion.

In a blender combine ½ cup fresh or frozen blackberries, ½ cup fresh or frozen blueberries, ¾ cup buttermilk or plain kefir, ¼ large ripe avocado, and ½ cup freshly squeezed orange juice. Whiz together until smooth and creamy. Taste and sweeten with a bit of agave syrup, if desired.

FRIED EGG WITH SPICY BEANS, SHAVED ZUCCHINI, AND TORTILLA

6 TO 7 MINUTES	MAKES 1 SERVING

- 1 tablespoon olive oil
- 3 scallions (white, pale green, and dark green parts), sliced thinly, tough middle reserved for stock or discarded
- 1 teaspoon minced serrano chile
- 1 (15-ounce) can pinto beans, drained
- Fine sea salt to taste
- 1 corn tortilla
- 1 large egg
- Julienned zucchini, for garnish
- Hot sauce (optional)

This is a California breakfast to me, a stripped-down version of the huevos rancheros that I feel I've eaten along Highway 1 sometime in my road-tripping past. Feel free to add an extra egg if you've just gotten back from a dawn surf session or simply need a little more sustenance.

Please note that this recipe makes more beans than you need for a single breakfast, but you might as well season all the beans in the can while you've got it open. Save the rest for another breakfast, or use them as a little crudité dip in a snack sometime.

In a small skillet, heat ½ tablespoon of the oil over medium heat. Add the scallions and serrano chile and cook, stirring frequently, for 1 minute. Stir in the beans and cook until warmed through, about 2 minutes. Season with salt to taste.

Heat the tortilla in a dry skillet over high heat until flexible and browned in spots. Wrap in a clean kitchen towel until ready to use.

Place a nonstick pan over medium-high heat. Heat the remaining ½ tablespoon oil, break the egg into the pan, and let it bubble and crisp a bit on the edges, about 1½ minutes. Add 2 teaspoons water and cover with a lid. Cook until the yolk is the desired firmness: a runny yolk with well-set whites takes about 1 minute.

Place a scoop of the beans on a plate and sprinkle with shreds of zucchini. Top with the egg and hot sauce, if desired. Serve with the tortilla on the side.

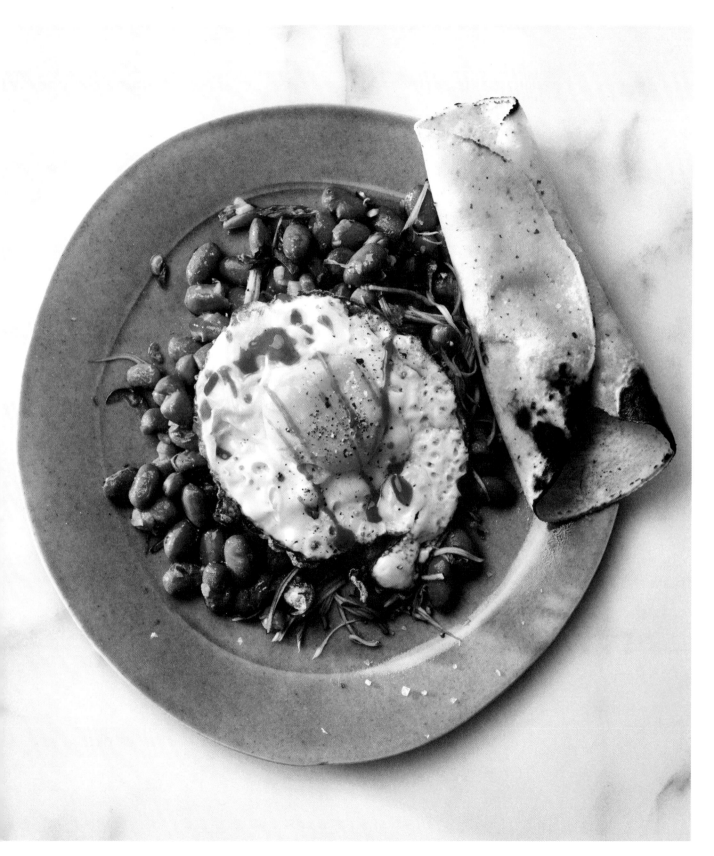

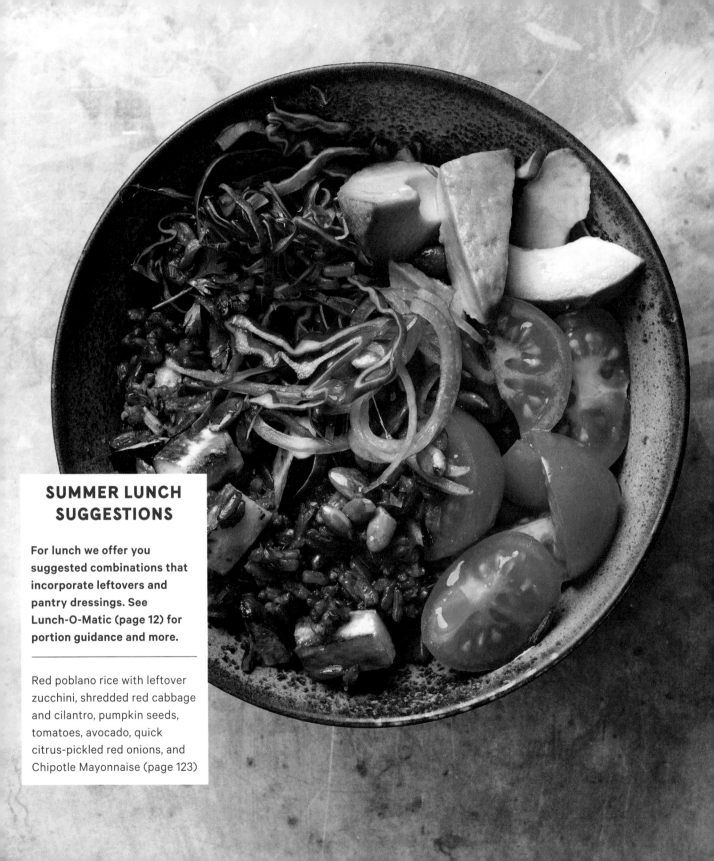

SUMMER LUNCH SUGGESTIONS

For lunch we offer you suggested combinations that incorporate leftovers and pantry dressings. See Lunch-O-Matic (page 12) for portion guidance and more.

Red poblano rice with leftover zucchini, shredded red cabbage and cilantro, pumpkin seeds, tomatoes, avocado, quick citrus-pickled red onions, and Chipotle Mayonnaise (page 123)

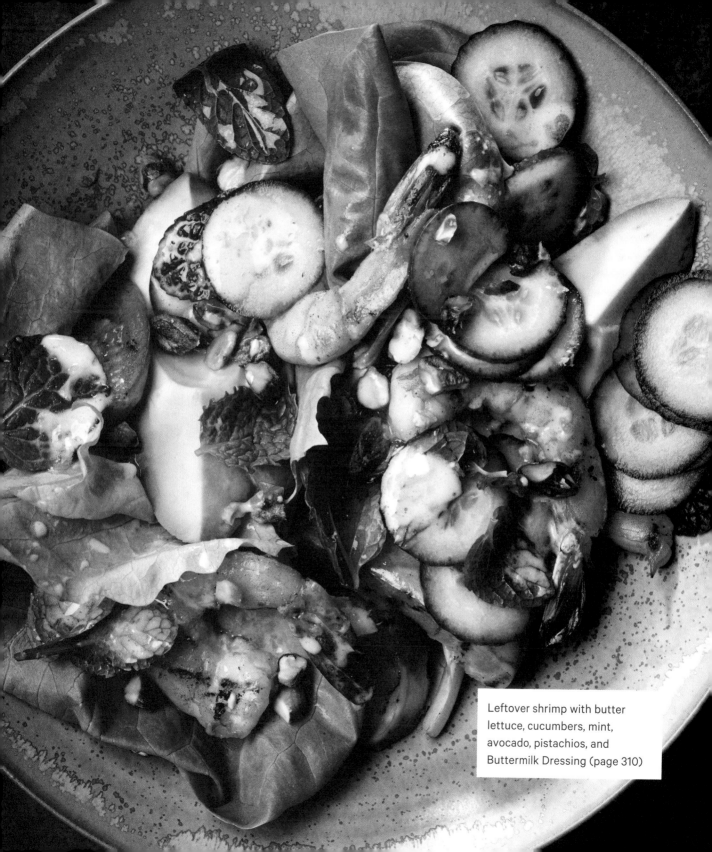

Leftover shrimp with butter lettuce, cucumbers, mint, avocado, pistachios, and Buttermilk Dressing (page 310)

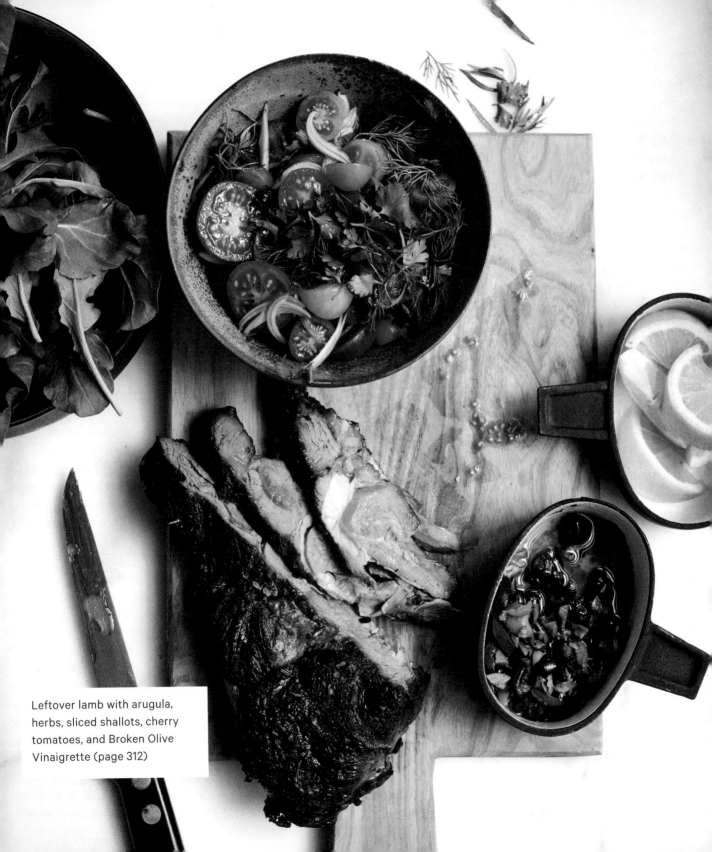

Leftover lamb with arugula, herbs, sliced shallots, cherry tomatoes, and Broken Olive Vinaigrette (page 312)

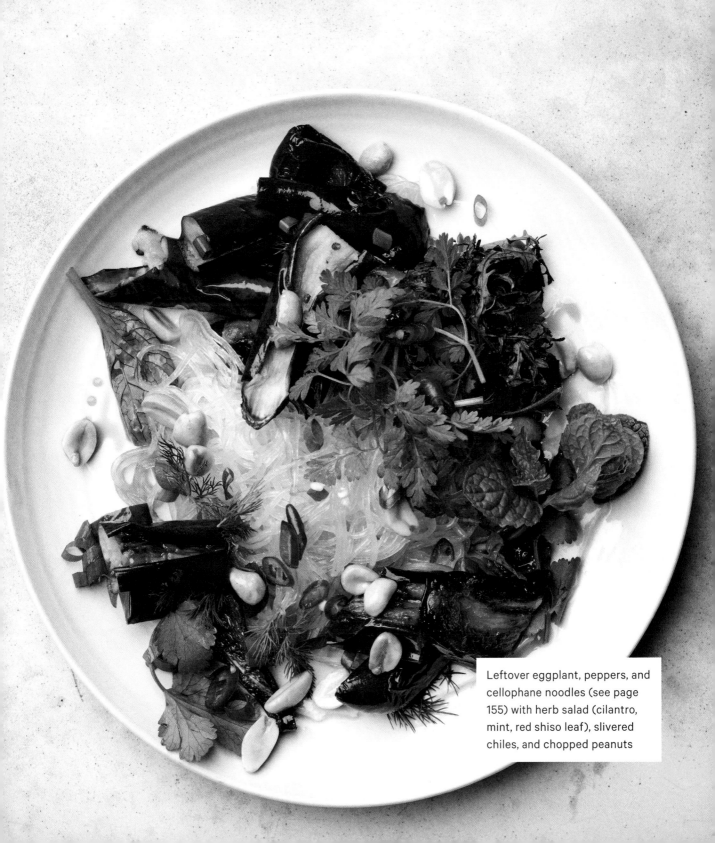

Leftover eggplant, peppers, and cellophane noodles (see page 155) with herb salad (cilantro, mint, red shiso leaf), slivered chiles, and chopped peanuts

BLACK RICE SALAD WITH CORN, TOMATOES, AND SPINACH

40 MINUTES (8 ACTIVE)	4 SERVINGS AND 1 LUNCH THE NEXT DAY

- 1 cup black rice
- Fine sea salt to taste
- 2 garlic cloves, finely minced
- 1 tablespoon minced jalapeño chile (no seeds or pith)
- Finely grated zest of 1 lime
- 2 tablespoons olive oil
- Kernels from 2 ears corn (about 1 cup)
- 1 bunch spinach, well washed, roots and thick stems removed, leaves cut into 3- to 4-inch strips
- 1 pint cherry tomatoes, halved
- 1 teaspoon lime juice, plus more to taste
- 2 tablespoons chopped fresh cilantro leaves
- Red pepper flakes, preferably Aleppo or Marash, to taste

Black rice is a brilliant canvas for color on the plate; its purple-black darkness beautifully punctuates the greens, yellows, and tomatoes of summer. We tested recipes with the Chinese-style rice sold as Forbidden Rice. It's so striking that it makes you forget that it's also a whole-grain rice, full of the fiber and nutrients that get polished off of white rice. In this dish, it plays the role of a pasta, tossed together with a garlic-kissed sauté of corn, spinach, and tomatoes.

In a 2- or 3-quart saucepan with a lid, bring the rice, 1¾ cups water, and about ½ teaspoon salt to a boil. Turn the heat down to a low simmer and cover the pan. Cook for 30 minutes, turn off the heat, and stir the rice. Cover and let steam for 5 minutes.

In a small bowl, combine the garlic, jalapeño, and lime zest.

In a large skillet with a lid, heat 1 tablespoon of the oil over medium heat. Add half the garlic mixture and stir frequently until fragrant, about 1 minute. Add the corn, season with salt, and cook for 1 minute, stirring frequently. Add the spinach, another pinch of salt, and 2 tablespoons water. Cover the pan and let the spinach steam for 2 minutes, until the spinach is easy to stir. Mix the corn and spinach well and cook for 1 or 2 minutes, until all the spinach leaves have softened. Stir in the remaining garlic mixture, the cherry tomatoes, cooked rice, lime juice, cilantro, and the remaining 1 tablespoon oil. Turn off the heat, taste, and add pepper flakes or more salt or lime juice, if desired.

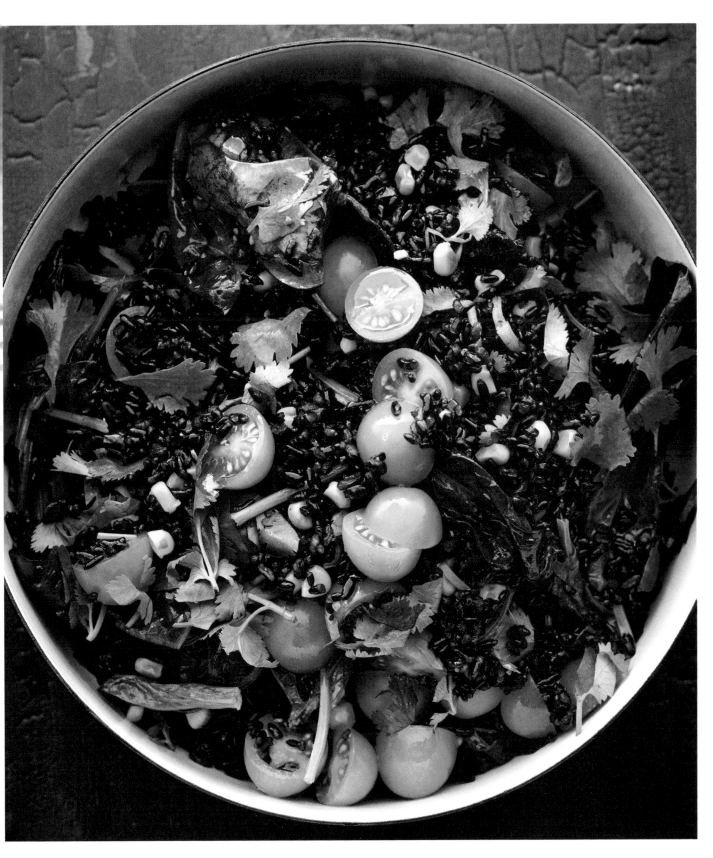

MIXED BEAN SALAD WITH CILANTRO AND PEPITAS

10 TO 15 MINUTES	MAKES 4 TO 6 SERVINGS

- Fine sea salt
- ½ pound green beans, trimmed
- ½ pound yellow wax beans, trimmed
- ¼ cup pepitas (pumpkin seeds)
- 1 tablespoon freshly squeezed lime juice, plus more to taste
- ½ tablespoon white wine vinegar
- 1 tablespoon olive oil
- Pinch of dried oregano
- ¼ cup roughly chopped fresh cilantro leaves
- Flaky sea salt and freshly ground black pepper to taste

The bean salads I grew up with were made with canned green, yellow, and kidney beans tossed with a bottled vinaigrette, and the dish scared me off picnic beans for a long time. But I came back around to bean salads at precisely the same time that I started blanching market-fresh beans until crisp but tender and dressing them just before serving with sharp vinaigrettes of all sorts. In this recipe, I keep it simple and dress the beans with lime juice, cilantro, and crispy pepitas, which go well with Mexican and Latin American flavors. One more bean salad trick: dress the beans right before serving, since the acid in the lime will cause the beans to discolor over time.

Bring a large pot of fine-sea-salted water to a boil. Have ready a slotted spoon or spider and a large plate or baking sheet lined with a clean kitchen towel or a double layer of paper towels. When the water reaches a rolling boil, add the green beans and cook until crisp-tender (about 1 minute). Use the slotted spoon or spider to remove them to the towel-lined plate to cool to room temperature. Repeat with the yellow wax beans, which tend to take a bit longer to cook, about 1½ minutes.

In a small dry skillet, toast the pepitas over medium heat until they start to crackle, about 1 minute. Remove from the pan and let cool.

In a large salad bowl, whisk together the lime juice, vinegar, oil, and 1 teaspoon fine sea salt. Toss with the cooled beans, pepitas, oregano, and cilantro. Taste and adjust the seasoning with flaky sea salt and pepper, and more lime juice, if desired.

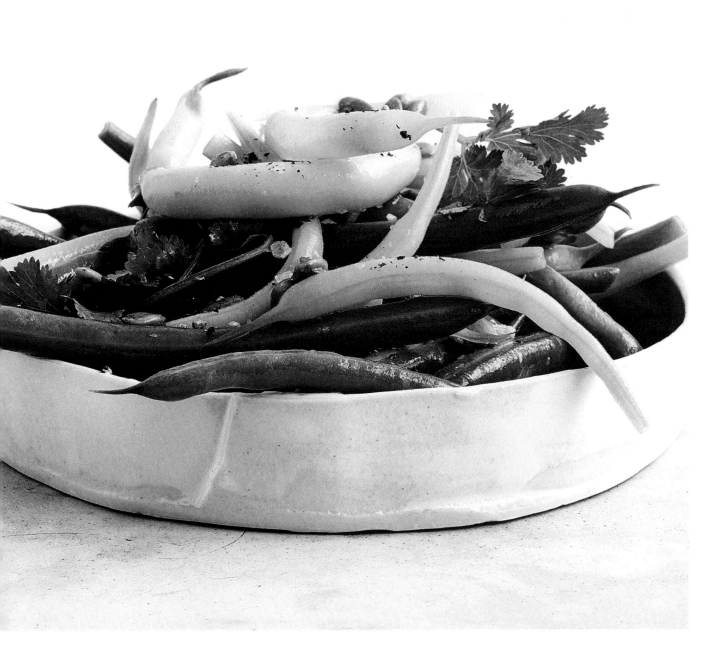

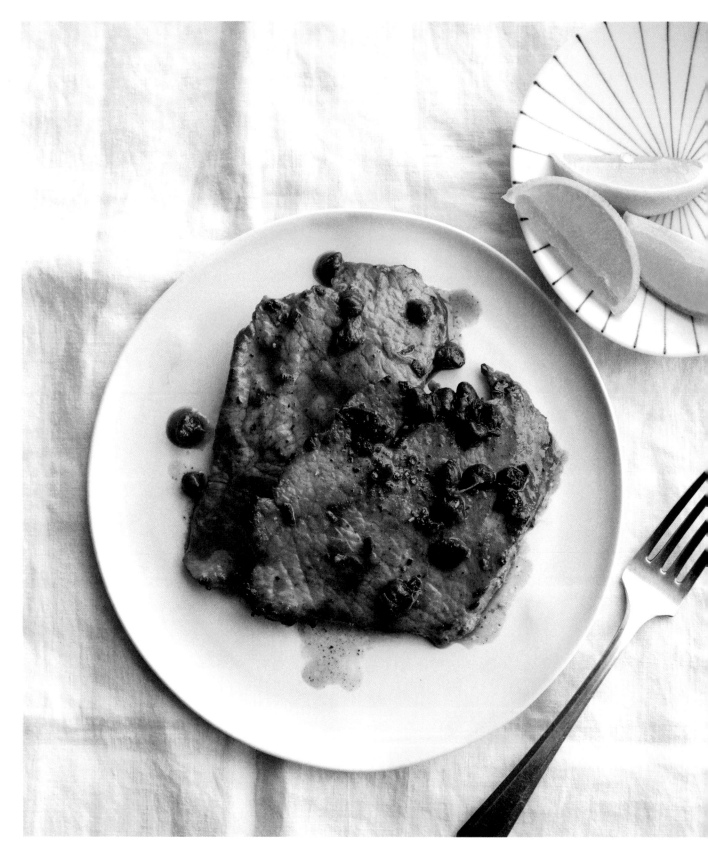

VEAL CUTLETS WITH SAGE-CAPER RELISH

20 MINUTES	4 SERVINGS

- 8 thin veal cutlets (about 1 pound)
- Fine sea salt and freshly ground black pepper
- 5 tablespoons olive oil
- ¼ cup capers, soaked and drained if packed in salt, rinsed if packed in vinegar
- ½ cup dry vermouth
- 1 tablespoon lemon zest
- 1 tablespoon lemon juice, plus more to taste
- 8 fresh sage leaves
- Mixed well-washed delicate salad greens, for garnish

A quick pan-fried meal is a great option on a hot night. You're done cooking before you can break a sweat. I'd spent years away from veal, but I've recently found sources of veal raised outside of crates, and so I feel fine about eating it from time to time. I often keep a few cutlets in the freezer for last-minute dinners (it takes just 20 minutes or so to defrost in their packaging under cold running water). Pork or chicken cutlets would work well, too; just pound them thin and adjust your cooking time as needed. What does a flash-sautéed cutlet need? Not much more than the pickle-y bite of capers and a splash of vermouth.

Pat the veal cutlets dry with paper towels, and then season with salt and pepper.

Heat a large nonstick skillet over medium-high heat. Add 1 tablespoon of the oil and place 2 cutlets in the pan. Cook until golden brown on one side, about 1 minute, then flip the cutlets and cook them 2 minutes on the second side, until they're just a shade pinker in the interior than the exterior. Set them aside on a plate and repeat to cook the remaining cutlets.

Pour the remaining 1 tablespoon oil into the pan and turn the heat to medium. Add the capers and cook until slightly browned, about 5 minutes, then add the vermouth. Reduce the heat to low and cook until the vermouth is reduced to a glaze, about 2 minutes. Stir in the lemon zest, lemon juice, and sage and turn off the heat. Taste and season with more salt or lemon juice, if desired.

Serve the cutlets (2 per person) with some delicate salad greens and top with the capers and sage.

QUINOA SALAD WITH BROCCOLI AND PISTACHIOS

30 MINUTES (8 ACTIVE)	4 SERVINGS AND 1 LUNCH THE NEXT DAY

- Fine sea salt
- 1 shallot, finely minced
- 6 tablespoons Buttermilk Dressing (page 310)
- 2 small broccoli heads, trimmed, cut into bite-size florets
- 1 cup white, red, or black quinoa (if using cooked quinoa, about 2½ cups)
- ½ cup roughly chopped fresh parsley leaves
- ¼ cup roughly chopped fresh tarragon leaves
- ¼ cup roughly chopped pistachios

Quinoa is the ingredient everyone—even I—turn to when someone asks for a *healthy* side: it's nutty, delicious, and full of protein, but it isn't usually very fresh and summery. I often find quinoa recipes stuffed with dried fruit, nuts, and other autumnal ingredients. This past summer, I thought about pairing tarragon with quinoa, a wholly untraditional combination. Still, the quinoa took well to the herbaceous treatment, and some lively broccoli branches added crispness and more greenery to the salad, which ages well overnight in the refrigerator. Keep the nuts out until the last minute, to preserve their crunch.

Bring a large pot of salted water to a boil. Have ready a bowl of ice water and a slotted spoon or spider near the pot of water.

In a small bowl, toss the shallot with 2 tablespoons of the buttermilk dressing.

Drop the broccoli in the boiling water and cook until tender but still crispy, about 1 minute. Remove the broccoli from the pot to the ice water. When cool, remove the broccoli from the cold water and drain it on a clean kitchen towel laid on a baking sheet.

Bring the water back to a boil and pour in the quinoa. Cook for 12 minutes, or until slightly al dente. Drain.

In a large bowl, toss the warm quinoa with 2 tablespoons of the buttermilk dressing and sea salt to taste. Let the quinoa cool to room temperature, about 10 minutes.

Toss the quinoa with the broccoli, macerated shallots, parsley, tarragon, pistachios, and the remaining 2 tablespoons of dressing. Taste for seasoning and add more salt to taste.

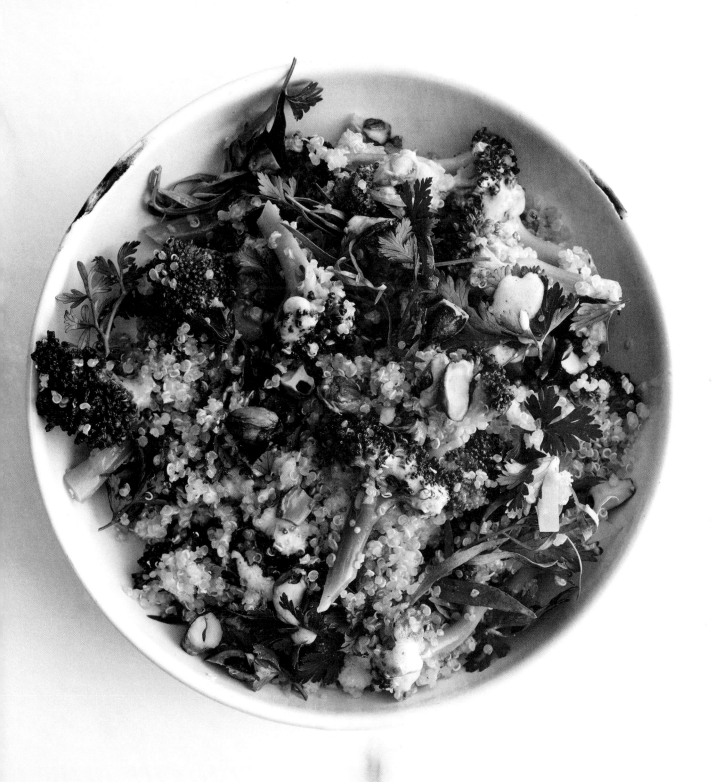

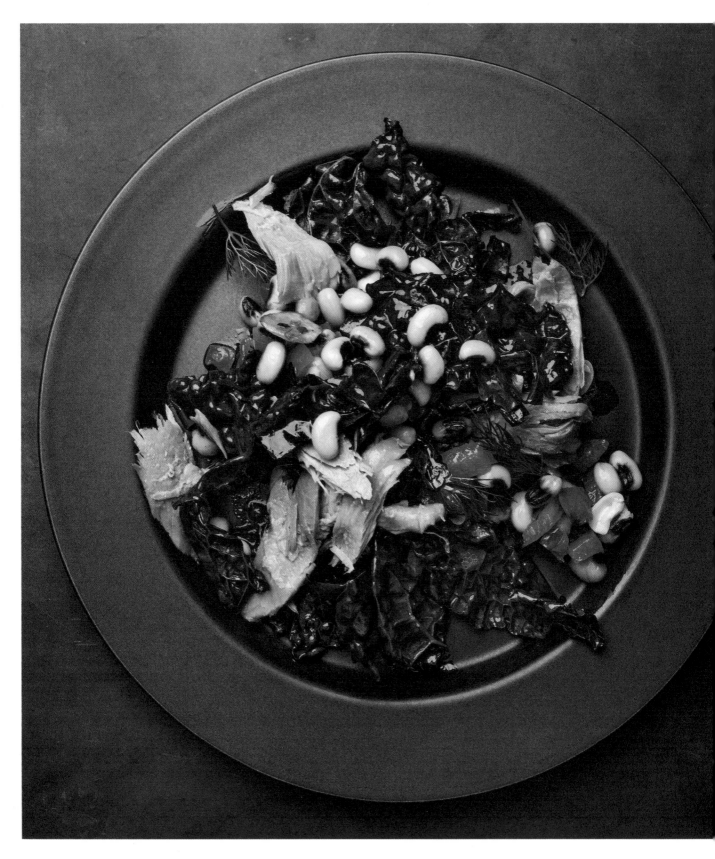

KALE WITH BLACK-EYED PEAS AND TUNA

12 MINUTES (10 ACTIVE)	4 SERVINGS AND 1 LUNCH THE NEXT DAY

- 2 tablespoons olive oil
- 2 garlic cloves, thinly sliced
- Pinch of red pepper flakes, preferably Aleppo or Marash
- 1 red bell pepper, cored and chopped
- Fine sea salt to taste
- 5 ounces tuna, preferably oil-packed, line-caught albacore, drained
- 2 cups frozen black-eyed peas
- 12 ounces lacinato kale, well washed, large stems removed, leaves cut crosswise into ½-inch strips
- Grated zest of 1 lemon
- 1 tablespoon lemon juice, plus more to taste
- ¼ cup roughly chopped dill fronds

I often use tuna as I would bacon, stirring it into the pan at the start of cooking and letting it suffuse the oil. It gives a hard-to-pinpoint richness to a really simple last-minute meal. Case in point: this wholesome dish, which emerged from a household crisis. It was August and there was a heat wave. I had, perhaps ill-advisedly, gotten a new puppy right as work on this book commenced in earnest, and he was getting into trouble a dozen times a day. The fish I had bought for dinner had gone bad. I looked in the cupboard, where I always have a can of line-caught albacore tuna. I used it to season this satisfying one-pot meal, and no one complained about the change in menu. In fact, my husband now requests it.

In a large skillet with a lid, heat 1 tablespoon of the oil over medium heat. Add the garlic and red pepper flakes. Stir in the bell pepper, season with salt, and cook until tender, 2 to 3 minutes. Stir in the tuna, breaking it up into small chunks, and cook for 1 minute. Add the black-eyed peas and another pinch of salt and cook 2 minutes, stirring frequently. Place the kale in the pan and add 3 tablespoons of water. Cover and cook for 2 minutes. Season with salt and stir the greens well. Cook, uncovered, for 1 or 2 minutes, until the kale is tender.

Stir in the lemon zest, lemon juice, dill, and the remaining 1 tablespoon oil. Taste the mixture and add more salt or lemon juice, if desired. Serve warm or at room temperature.

MUSSELS WITH HARISSA, CHARD, AND CHICKPEAS

15 MINUTES	4 SERVINGS

- 2½ pounds black mussels
- 2 tablespoons olive oil
- 2 garlic cloves, sliced
- 1 cup homemade chicken stock (see page 301), low-sodium canned, or water
- 1 tablespoon Preserved Lemon Harissa (page 320) or prepared harissa or 2 teaspoons sriracha, plus more for serving
- 12 ounces chard, well washed, stems removed and cut crosswise into ¼-inch slices, and leaves cut into 1-inch ribbons
- 1 (15-ounce) can chickpeas, drained, or 1½ cups cooked chickpeas
- Fine sea salt to taste

A bowl of mussels is such an easy summer meal: they cook in a flash, and they're perfect for a long, chatty meal in the late-dying sun. They're just the right amount of work to eat to slow things down for conversation (and help you fill up on a balanced amount of food). The only problem from a cleanse perspective is that a dinner of mussels usually calls out for lots of crusty bread. So I've loaded up this stew with tasty chickpeas and chard, along with garbanzo-flour crepes for sopping up those delicious juices.

Clean the mussels under running water. Discard any broken shells or mussels that will not close quickly when gently squeezed. Using a clean kitchen towel, pinch and pull away any stringy beards from the mussels.

Have a large bowl ready near the stovetop. In a large skillet or saucepan with a lid, heat 1 tablespoon of the oil over medium-high heat. Stir in the garlic, cook for 20 to 30 seconds, and add the mussels. Stir to coat the mussels with oil, add the stock, and cover the pan. Cook the mussels until they begin to open, 3 to 4 minutes. Use tongs or a slotted spoon to remove the mussels from the pan to the bowl as they open. Continue cooking with the cover on to coax open the slower mussels; if they don't open in 2 more minutes, discard them.

Stir 1 tablespoon of the harissa into the cooking liquid in the pan. Add in the chard stems and leaves and the chickpeas and cover the pan. Cook until the chard begins to wilt, about 1 minute. Taste the chard, stir in the remaining 1 tablespoon oil, and season with salt to taste (be sure to taste before adding salt; the mussels will exude some salt into the cooking broth). Cook until the chard is tender, about 1 more minute, then add the mussels back to the pan. Cover the pan and steam the mussels for 1 minute to warm them through.

Distribute the mussels and stock among 4 bowls and serve with harissa on the side.

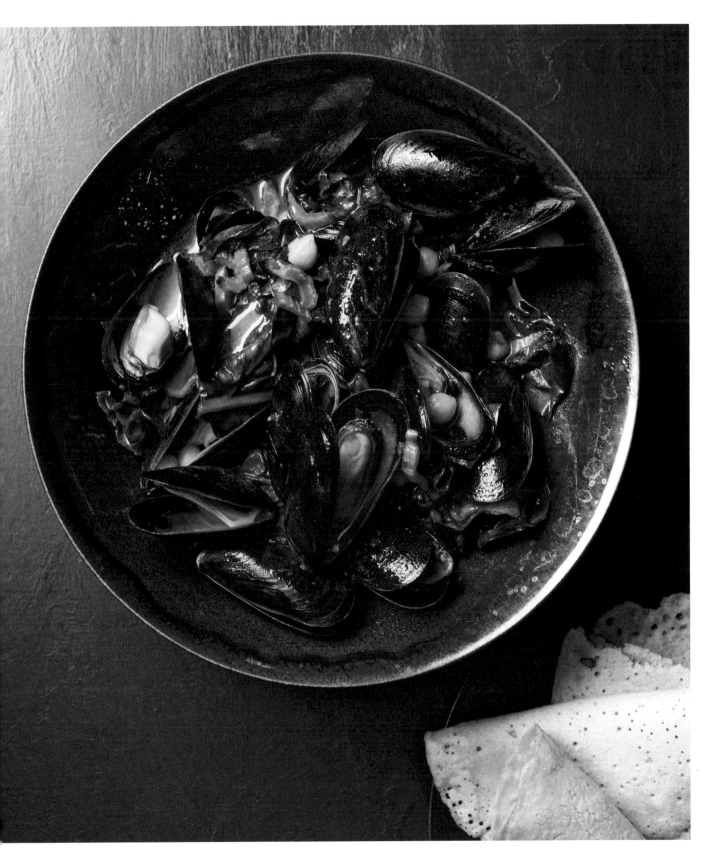

ROSEMARY SOCCA

Pictured on page 121

40 MINUTES (25 ACTIVE)	MAKES 4 SERVINGS

- 1 cup chickpea flour*
- 2 tablespoons olive oil, plus more for cooking
- ¾ teaspoon salt
- Pinch of freshly ground black pepper
- ½ teaspoon finely minced fresh rosemary

* You can find garbanzo flour in the gluten-free section of many stores, online at bobsredmill.com, or in Indian groceries, where it may be labeled gram flour.

Socca are Provençal garbanzo flour flatbreads; they have a wonderful caramel color and nutty deliciousness. What's more, they are a lifesaver if you or any of your friends have a gluten-free diet and you need a little starchy something to dip into a stock. They're good for entertaining because they can be made ahead in two ways. First off, the batter is best if it sits a long time before cooking (even in the fridge overnight), and second, you can cook them early in the day before serving, too. Just put a little parchment paper between each layer to keep them from sticking. I don't have the traditional wood oven to make them in, so I use my nonstick skillet on the stovetop as I would with any other crêpe.

In a large measuring cup or bowl, whisk together the flour, 2 tablespoons of the oil, the salt, pepper, rosemary, and 1 cup plus 2 tablespoons water. Let the batter sit for at least 15 minutes before cooking.

Have a warm plate ready. Heat a small (6- to 8-inch) nonstick skillet over medium-high heat. Drizzle ½ teaspoon of oil into the pan when warm. Pour about ¼ cup batter into the pan; tilt the pan to spread the batter evenly, and cook the crêpe until lightly browned on one side, about 1 minute; use a spatula to flip the crêpe and cook until dappled brown on the second side (about 1½ to 2 minutes total time). Remove the crêpe to the plate and repeat with the remaining batter, placing a sheet of parchment between crêpes if possible. The crêpes can be made several hours in advance and warmed in a skillet before serving.

CHIPOTLE MAYONNAISE

Pictured on page 147

7 MINUTES (1 MINUTE ACTIVE)	MAKES 1½ CUPS

- 3 black garlic cloves or 3 fresh garlic cloves
- 2 to 3 tablespoons chipotle peppers in adobo (1 to 2 roughly chopped peppers with sauce)
- 2 teaspoons rice vinegar
- 8 ounces silken tofu
- 1 teaspoon fine sea salt
- 3 teaspoons canola oil

I've long been a fan of mixing chipotle peppers with mayonnaise to hype up sandwiches and salads, and I thought I'd see if I could make a lighter version that I could use a little more liberally. This year I started playing around with silken tofu, and I realized that the creamy vegan version could do the same job as the traditional mayo, smoothing and softening the heat of the chipotles while keeping their flavor front and center. The sauce is very good with fresh garlic, but if, like me, you've picked up some caramelized "black" garlic out of curiosity, feel free to throw that in instead—it will lend a sweet and funky note to the versatile sauce.

If using fresh garlic, bring a small pot of water to a boil, add the garlic cloves, and blanch them for 1 minute. Drain.

In a blender, whizz together the chipotles (more chiles = more spice), garlic, and vinegar until the chiles are roughly chopped. Add the tofu, salt, and oil and blend for 2 minutes, until the mixture is very smooth and homogenized. Store in an airtight container in the refrigerator for up to a week; the mayonnaise can be eaten right away, but it will thicken and set better if it chills first for several hours.

ZUCCHINI TACOS WITH CABBAGE AND QUESO FRESCO

10 MINUTES	4 SERVINGS AND 1 LUNCH THE NEXT DAY

- 2 cups slivered red cabbage
- 3 teaspoons freshly squeezed lime juice, plus more to taste
- Fine sea salt to taste
- 1 tablespoon Chipotle Mayonnaise (page 123), plus more for serving
- 2 to 3 tablespoons olive oil
- 2 pounds zucchini (about 4 medium), cut into 1-inch sticks
- 2 small garlic cloves, minced
- 2 teaspoons minced jalapeño chile (no seeds or pith)
- 8 small corn tortillas
- ¼ cup crumbled queso fresco
- Fresh cilantro sprigs, for garnish (optional)
- Hot sauce, for serving (optional)

I have always loved Baja-style fish tacos with their crunchy fringe of slivered cabbage and a bit of creamy sauce to smooth it all out. In this case, they've inspired a delicious vegetarian taco combination. Of course, you can always have bowls of pulled chicken, sautéed ground beef, and/or grated cheese off to the side to meet the desires of everyone at the table. A make-your-own-taco meal is a great way to satisfy cleansers and noncleansers, vegetarians and carnivores, suspicious kids and omnivorous adults alike.

In a large bowl, toss the cabbage with 1 teaspoon of the lime juice, salt, and the chipotle mayonnaise. Set aside.

Heat 1 tablespoon of the oil in a large skillet over high heat, place half the zucchini in the pan, and add half the garlic and half the jalapeño. Cook undisturbed for 1 minute, then season the zucchini with salt and stir. Cook for another 30 seconds, until the zucchini is crisp-tender and browned. Repeat with the remaining zucchini, garlic, and jalapeño. Toss the zucchini with 2 teaspoons lime juice.

Have a plate covered with a cloth napkin ready. To warm the tortillas, place a dry skillet over a high flame and heat each tortilla individually for about 20 seconds on each side. Place each tortilla underneath the napkin as it's finished.

To assemble the tacos, place some zucchini on the warm tortillas and top with a big pinch of cabbage and a few crumbles of queso fresco. Top with cilantro and hot sauce, if desired. Serve with additional chipotle mayonnaise on the side.

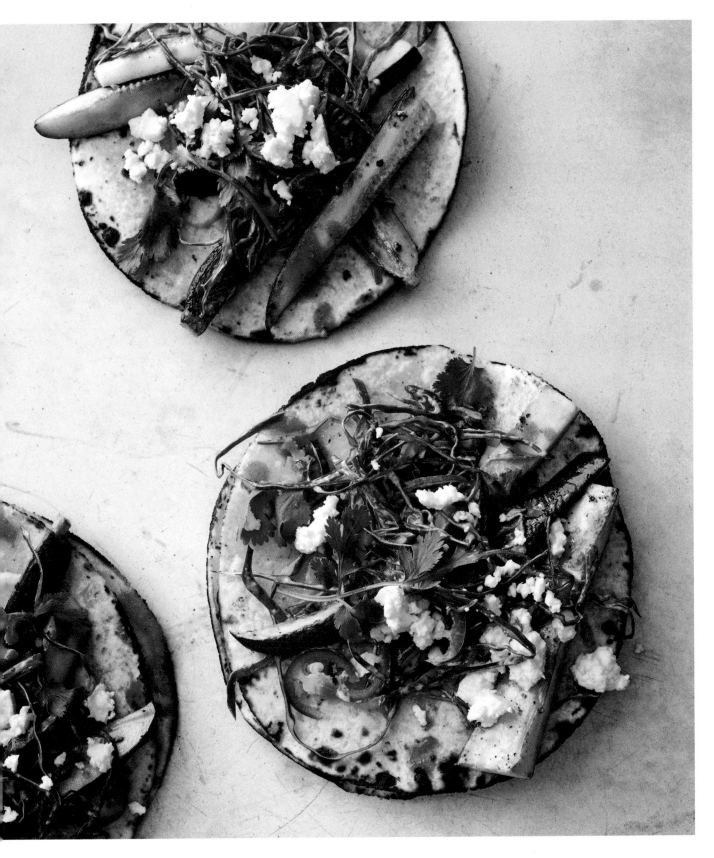

SLOW-BAKED SALMON WITH FENNEL

30 TO 45 MINUTES (5 ACTIVE)	4 SERVINGS AND 1 LUNCH THE NEXT DAY

- 1½ pounds salmon fillet,* preferably wild-caught king or sockeye, skin on, pin bones removed
- Fine sea salt and freshly ground black pepper
- 1 teaspoon fennel seeds (optional)
- 1 fennel bulb, trimmed, sliced thinly, fronds chopped and reserved
- 1 medium sweet onion, cut into ¼-inch slices
- 1 garlic clove, thinly sliced
- 2 tablespoons olive oil
- 2 cups well-washed arugula, for garnish

*If you work with individual fillets, the cooking time will be less, about 25 minutes total.

Every salmon-eating household should have this method in its repertoire. Think of it as a salmon sauna: longish cooking at a very low temperature. It's very hard to overcook when the temperature is this gentle, and the resulting salmon flesh is gloriously lush. I placed it on a bed of aromatic fennel before cooking, but you can change the setting as easily as an outfit. Try it with a heap of basil and onions on top of the fish. It is hard to eyeball doneness on this salmon, since it won't get as pale as fish cooked at a higher temperature. It's done when it flakes when gently pressed.

Preheat the oven to 275°F. On a low rack, place a small ovenproof dish or pan filled with ½ cup water.

Season the salmon with salt and pepper and, if using, fennel seeds. Lay the fennel slices, onion, and garlic on a baking sheet. Place the salmon on top of the fennel mixture and pour the oil over the fish. Sprinkle the salmon with half the chopped fennel fronds.

Bake the salmon until it flakes when gently pressed, 30 to 40 minutes: it will be much darker at the interior than when cooked at a higher heat. Peel the skin off the salmon and break the flesh into casual chunks.

Arrange the salmon on plates with the fennel, onion, and arugula. Drizzle the cooking juices on the salad and sprinkle with the reserved fennel fronds.

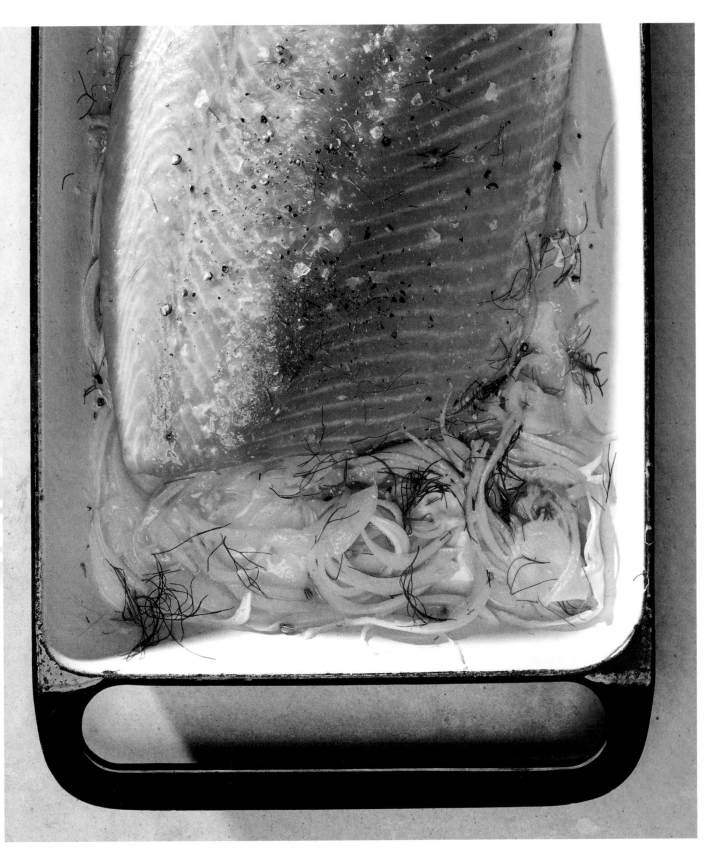

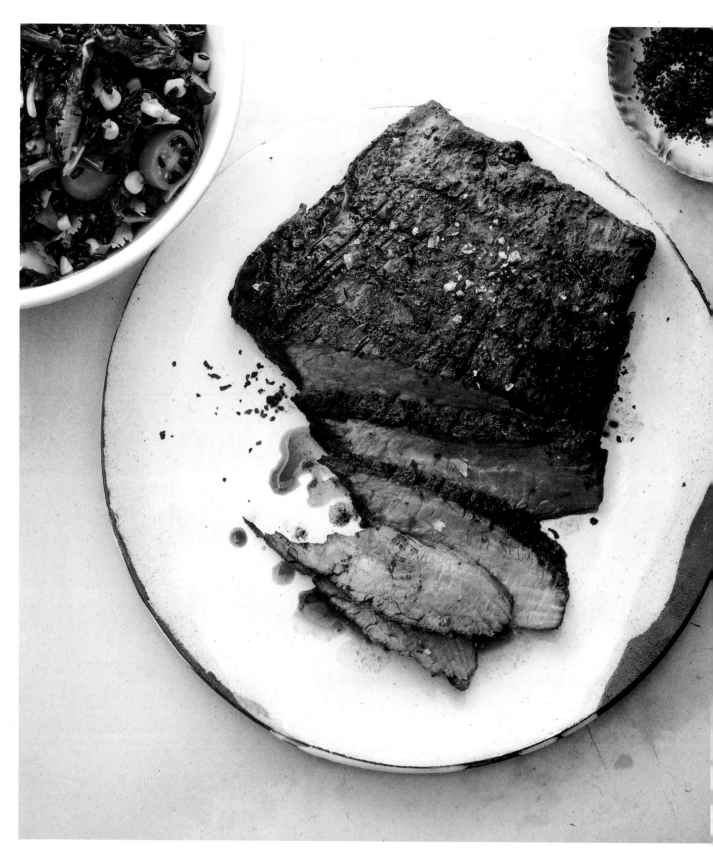

SMOKY GRILLED FLANK STEAK

25 MINUTES (10 ACTIVE)	MAKES 4 SERVINGS AND 1 LUNCH THE NEXT DAY

- 1 teaspoon fine sea salt
- ⅛ teaspoon freshly ground black pepper, plus more to taste
- ⅛ teaspoon smoked paprika
- 1¼ pounds grass-fed flank steak, large fat pieces trimmed
- 2 tablespoons plus 1 teaspoon olive oil
- Black Rice Salad with Corn, Tomatoes, and Spinach (page 110), for serving
- Flaky sea salt to taste

Flank steak may be my favorite picnic steak: the lean cut tastes good hot and cold, and it can always be sliced thinner to feed a crowd. I love paper-thin slices of steak: I use a long, thin flexible knife that's made for slicing sashimi, and I tilt it on the bias to get gorgeous rosy ruffles of the steak. You can use any thin, sharp knife for the same effect. I often choose flank steak when I'm in a dinner crunch because it cooks so quickly and it's easy to find in ordinary groceries. That said, I favor grass-finished flank steaks when I can find them, since they have a more minerally, brisk flavor than conventionally raised beef.

In a small bowl, combine the fine sea salt, pepper, and paprika. Season the beef with the spice mixture.

Preheat a grill to high (and scrape the grill well) or place an oven rack in the upper third of the oven and heat the broiler. Rub the steak with 1 teaspoon of the oil. If grilling, cook the flank steak to the desired temperature (about 4 minutes on each side for medium-rare). If using the broiler, place the meat on a baking sheet and broil, turning the meat over once, until it reaches the desired temperature (about 5 minutes on each side for medium-rare). Let the steak rest for at least 10 minutes, then cut it thinly on the bias.

Serve the steak on top of the black rice salad and season with flaky sea salt and more pepper, if desired.

ORANGE-BRAISED CARROTS AND BEETS

45 TO 50 MINUTES (10 ACTIVE)	4 SERVINGS AND 1 LUNCH THE NEXT DAY

- 2 tablespoons extra-virgin olive oil
- 1 large garlic clove, chopped
- ¼ teaspoon red pepper flakes, preferably Aleppo or Marash
- 1½ pounds beets (about 3 medium), peeled and cut into 1-inch wedges
- 1 (4-inch) slice of orange peel (no pith)
- Fine sea salt to taste
- 1 pound carrots (about 4 large), cut on the bias into 1½-inch pieces
- ¼ cup freshly squeezed orange juice
- Flaky sea salt to finish

Strolling through the summer markets, I'm always a little torn by the beets: they look so gorgeous with their burnished skin and glossy leaves. On the other hand, I rarely want to do a big long roast to heat up the kitchen. Sometimes, with my daughter at the helm of the juicer, I liquidize them with fennel, oranges, and ginger. But here's another option: cut them relatively small and cook them on the stovetop with some carrots, which they will stain the most fetching shade of magenta. Orange peel and juice keep the dish sunny and bright.

In a large skillet, heat the oil over medium heat. Add the garlic and red pepper flakes and cook until fragrant. Add the beets, orange peel, and a pinch of fine sea salt. Stir to coat and cook for 1 minute. Cover the beets with 3 cups water, turn the heat to high, and bring to a boil. Turn the heat down to a simmer, and cook until slightly tender but still crisp, 15 minutes. Add the carrots, season with another pinch of fine sea salt, and cook until the vegetables are tender, 20 to 25 minutes.

Drain out the water and remove the orange peel. Add the orange juice, toss it with the vegetables, remove from the heat, and season to taste with flaky sea salt.

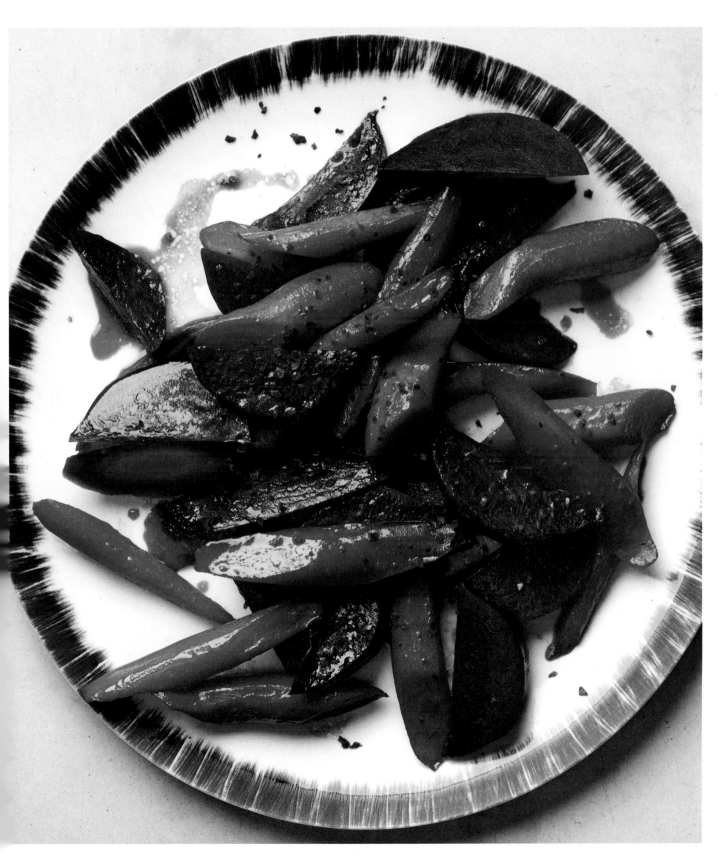

GRILLED SWORDFISH WITH CHARRED TOMATILLO SALSA

30 MINUTES	4 SERVINGS AND 1 LUNCH THE NEXT DAY

- 1 teaspoon ancho chili powder
- 1 garlic clove, grated
- ½ teaspoon dried oregano
- 2½ tablespoons canola oil, plus more for the grill
- 1½ pounds swordfish fillets, about 1 inch thick
- Fine sea salt and freshly ground black pepper
- 1 medium onion, sliced into ½-inch rings
- ¾ pound tomatillos (about 5 medium), husks on
- 1 unpeeled garlic clove
- 2 tablespoons chopped fresh cilantro leaves
- 2 teaspoons lime juice, plus more to taste
- 1 medium ripe avocado, pitted, peeled, and cut into 1-inch chunks
- Flaky sea salt to finish (optional)

I've always loved the tangy-fruity taste of tomatillo salsas, but when I invited Seattle chef Matt Dillon over once, he showed me just how casually I could throw one together. He dumped a whole bagful of tomatillos onto the grill and toasted them until they were blistered and burned. Then, of course, because he likes things earthy and rusticated and travels with a large sharp knife, he chopped them together with a small mountain of grilled onions and mixed them with no small amount of lime juice. He served it with grilled pork from his Vashon Island farm.

Here's my blenderized version, served with delicious rich swordfish (the pork chop of the sea). Sustainable swordfish is tricky to figure out, but there are several swordfish fisheries on the best choice list at seafoodwatch.org. If you can't find them at your fish counter, go with another steak-like fish: wild salmon, ono, or mahi-mahi would all work.

Heat a gas grill to medium-high heat or build a medium-hot fire in a charcoal grill. (Alternatively, you can use a broiler to make both the salsa and the fish.)

In a small bowl, combine the chili powder, grated garlic, oregano, and 1½ tablespoons of the oil. Rub onto all surfaces of the fish. Season the fish with fine sea salt and pepper.

If you have skewers, insert one or two into each onion slice to keep the rings together. Rub 1 tablespoon of the oil onto the onion slices. Season with fine sea salt. Chill the fish until about 15 minutes before cooking it.

Scrape the grill well and use tongs to rub a paper towel coated with oil onto the grate to create a stick-resistant surface. Have a large heatproof bowl ready by the side of the grill.

Lay the onion rings, tomatillos, and whole garlic clove on the grate. Grill the garlic until it is browned and softened at the interior, about 2 minutes.

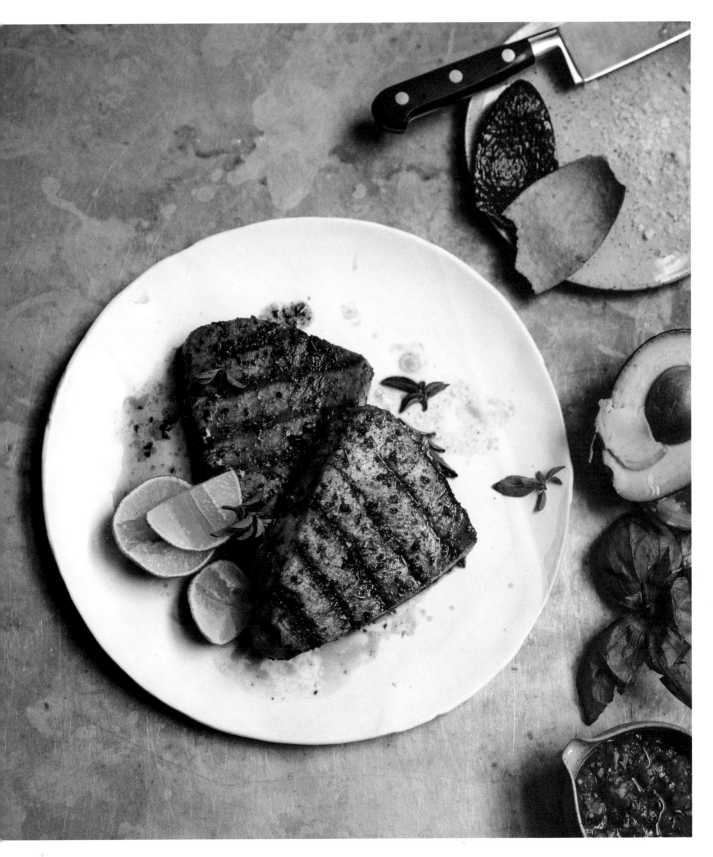

Grill the onion rings until tender and charred in spots, rotating as they cook, about 15 minutes total; remove them to the bowl. Grill the tomatillos until the husks are browned and blistered, turning them as needed. Remove them to the bowl when softened and juicy, 18 to 20 minutes. Set the bowl aside while you cook the fish.

If necessary, add more charcoal to the grill to maintain a medium-high heat. Scrape the grill well and, using tongs, rub once again with an oil-coated paper towel. Lay the fish on the grill and cook until the fish is just opaque at the center, about 6 minutes per side.

When the grilled vegetables are cool enough to handle, remove any skewers from the onion rings, remove the husks from the tomatillos, and peel the garlic. Add the vegetables, 1 teaspoon fine sea salt, the cilantro, and the lime juice to a food processor and pulse for 1 minute to make a chunky puree. Taste the salsa and add more fine sea salt or lime juice to taste.

Serve the fish with a dollop of sauce and the avocado chunks. Season the fish and avocado with flaky sea salt, if desired.

TOMATO SALAD WITH BUTTERMILK DRESSING

Pictured on page 137

12 MINUTES	4 SERVINGS AND 1 LUNCH THE NEXT DAY

- ¼ cup Buttermilk Dressing (page 310)
- ¼ medium red onion, finely sliced
- 2½ pounds various tomatoes (about 6 medium), cored, cut into bite-size wedges, slices, or halves
- Flaky sea salt and freshly ground black pepper to taste
- 1 loose cup torn well-washed mixed tender herbs, such as any combination of mint, basil, tarragon, dill, cilantro, and parsley leaves, with a few small whole leaves for garnish

Sometimes you just need to submit to the avalanche of tomatoes at the August market. They're so good, and they won't be this way for long, so it's okay to have them at more than one meal. And it's more than okay not to do too much with them—as in this salad—to show off their extraordinary flavor in a minimalist fashion. Choose beautiful tomatoes and serve them with nothing but a mass of tender herbs and a lick of gently tart buttermilk dressing to show off their sun-ripened flavor. Don't let the raw onions scare you off; their snappy flavor and texture make for a delightful contrast to the yielding tomatoes. Whenever I toss raw onions into a dish, I soak them first in something acidic (here it's buttermilk) to blunt their pungency.

In a large bowl, mix the dressing with the onion and let sit for 10 minutes while prepping the rest of the salad. Gently toss the tomatoes with the onion-vinaigrette mixture and torn herbs. Season with salt and pepper and garnish the salad with a few whole leaves.

GRILLED ALBACORE WITH TOMATO-HERB SALAD

15 TO 20 MINUTES (12 ACTIVE)	4 SERVINGS AND 1 LUNCH THE NEXT DAY

- 1½ pounds albacore or yellowtail tuna fillets
- 1 teaspoon coriander seeds, crushed
- Fine sea salt and freshly ground black pepper to taste
- 1 tablespoon olive oil
- Olive or canola oil, for the grill
- Flaky sea salt to taste
- 1 batch Tomato Salad with Buttermilk Dressing (see page 135)

My husband rolls his eyes at me (lovingly, I'm sure) when I get on the subject of tuna. I went albacore fishing once, and I now act like Ernestine Hemingway. It *was* a truly exciting fight with those silvery fish (and my balance) as they dove down, down, down into the open ocean. It was also a thrill to eat my bounty in dozens of different dishes. Albacore tuna is the West Coast's secret summer fish. It shows up late in the season and gets incredibly inexpensive at the market. It's a brilliant grilling fish, and it tastes great cold the next day, too. The best thing about line-caught Pacific albacore is that, for the moment at least, it's not heavily overfished like bluefin, and because it's a smaller fish, it doesn't accumulate as much mercury as its bigger cousins. Line-caught yellowtail is also a good choice.

A bright and vibrant assortment of the summer's best tomatoes is the perfect accompaniment to fish stories of all sorts.

Build a charcoal fire or preheat a grill to medium-high heat.

If the tuna loin is very wide, cut it lengthwise into 2 sections, so that no piece is wider than 3 inches across. Combine the coriander and fine sea salt and pepper. Rub the tuna with the oil and season it with the coriander mixture.

Scrape the grill well with a brush and, using tongs, rub the grate with an oil-coated paper towel. Lay the tuna on the grate and cook each side until opaque and lightly browned, 2 to 3 minutes per side. Continue cooking until medium-rare, about 3 more minutes: the meat should be a bit translucent at the center but not chilly and raw.

Cut the tuna loin into 1-inch-wide slices, garnish with flaky sea salt, and serve with the tomato salad.

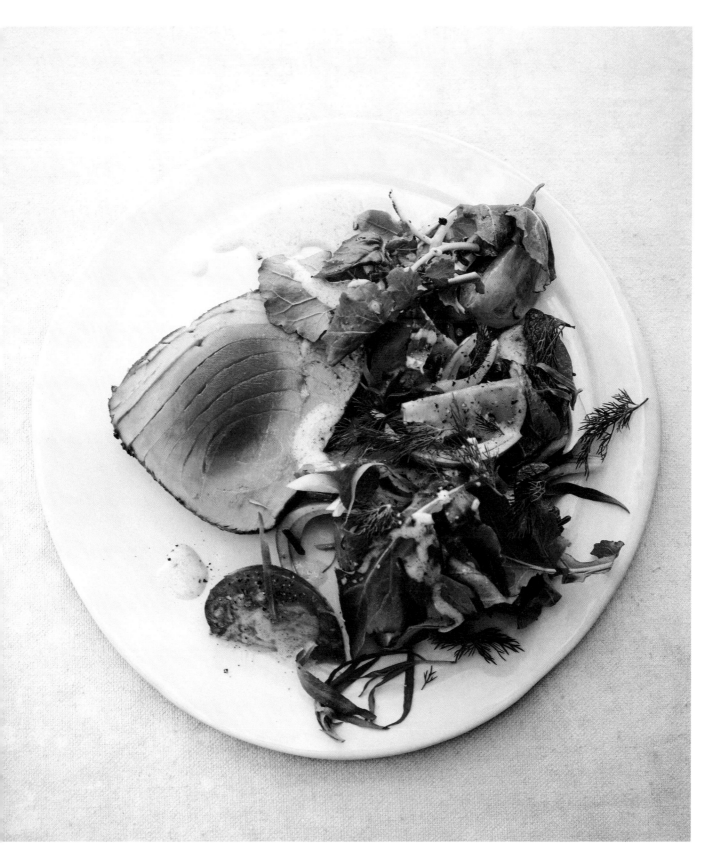

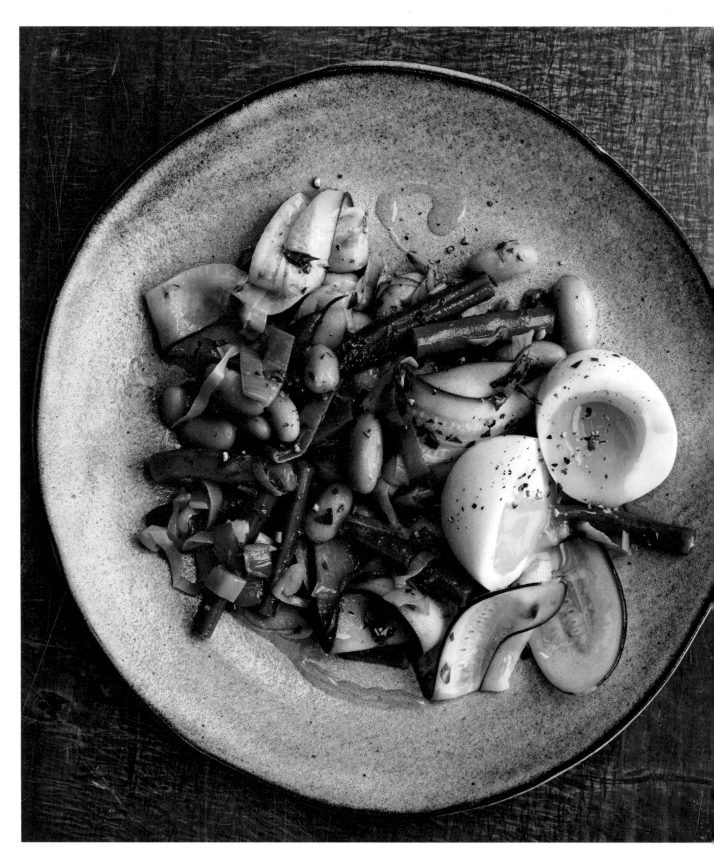

PISTOU SALAD WITH EGGS

25 TO 30 MINUTES (15 ACTIVE)	4 SERVINGS AND 1 LUNCH THE NEXT DAY

- Fine sea salt
- 2 cups finely chopped fresh basil leaves
- 1 teaspoon dried oregano
- 1 garlic clove, grated
- ¼ cup extra-virgin olive oil
- 1 tablespoon freshly squeezed lemon juice, plus more to taste
- 8 ounces green beans, trimmed and halved crosswise
- 5 large eggs
- 1 large leek (white and light green parts), cut into ⅛-inch slices, rinsed
- 3 garlic cloves, sliced
- 1 (15-ounce) can cannellini beans, drained and rinsed, or 1¼ cup beans cooked from dry (see page 303)
- 1½ pounds green zucchini (about 4 medium), shaved into thin ribbons
- Freshly ground black pepper and flaky sea salt to taste

Pistou is the wonderful Provençal sauce made of pounded basil and garlic. Pistou is best known as the killer garnish in a gorgeous summer vegetable soup. But since you don't always want to eat a hot soup, I've turned those same elements—beans, summer squash, and pistou—into a hearty dinner salad that you can prep well before serving. For the freshest flavor and color, wait to dress the salad until just before serving.

Bring a large pot of fine-sea-salted water to a boil. Lay 2 kitchen towels out on 2 large plates or baking sheets. Have ready a slotted spoon or spider to remove ingredients from the water and a bowl of ice water for the eggs.

In a small bowl, combine herbs, grated garlic, fine sea salt to taste, and 3 tablespoons of oil. Stir in the lemon juice. Set aside the pistou.

When the water comes to a boil, add the green beans and cook until crisp-tender, about 1 minute. Using the slotted spoon or spider, remove the green beans to one of the kitchen towels.

Gently lower the eggs into the water and bring it back to a boil. Turn off the heat and let the eggs sit for 7 minutes for a soft-set egg. Remove the eggs to the bowl of ice water to cool.

Heat the remaining 1 tablespoon oil in a large heavy skillet over medium heat. Add the leek, sliced garlic, and ½ teaspoon fine sea salt and cook, stirring occasionally, until the leek has softened but is still a bit chewy, about 2 minutes. Stir the cannellini beans into the warm leek slices, turn off the heat, add the shaved zucchini, and toss to combine.

In a large bowl, combine the green beans, leek, bean and zucchini mixture, and the pistou. Toss well and taste the vegetables, adding more lemon juice or salt, if desired. Peel the eggs and cut them in quarters, season them with pepper and flaky sea salt, and use them to garnish the salad.

LAMB WITH ROASTED FIGS AND LIMA BEAN PESTO

30 MINUTES (20 ACTIVE)	4 SERVINGS AND 1 LUNCH THE NEXT DAY

- Canola oil, for the grill
- 3 tablespoons extra-virgin olive oil
- 3 garlic cloves, minced
- 1 teaspoon finely minced rosemary leaves
- 2 pounds leg of lamb, trimmed and cut into 1½-inch pieces
- 10 ripe Black Mission figs
- Fine sea salt and freshly ground black pepper
- 1½ cups frozen baby lima beans
- ½ cup roughly chopped walnuts, toasted (see page 306)
- 1 tablespoon lemon juice, plus more to taste
- ¼ cup chopped fresh mint leaves (from 4 to 5 sprigs)
- Flaky sea salt to finish
- Special equipment: bamboo skewers, soaked in water for at least 15 minutes

Even though kids are supposed to hate them, I grew up loving lima beans—frozen ones no less—and I still love their flavor and their starchiness set off by their snappy green vigor. I underscore that flavor with mint in this simple lima pesto, which complements kebabs of summery lamb. If you can get fresh lima beans, feel free to substitute them. I might not puree them in that case, but serve them quickly steamed with the walnuts and mint on top.

Prepare a medium-hot fire in a charcoal grill or heat a gas grill to high. Clean the grate well and, using tongs, lightly coat the grate with canola oil.

Mix 1 tablespoon olive oil with about one-third of the garlic and all the rosemary. Toss the meat and figs with the olive oil mixture, then season it generously with 2 teaspoons of fine sea salt and ½ teaspoon black pepper. Place the lamb chunks and a fig or two on each skewer, leaving a little gap between each piece of meat. Leave the skewers at room temperature for at least 20 minutes before grilling.

In a 2-quart saucepan, heat 1 tablespoon of the olive oil over medium heat. Add the remaining garlic and cook, stirring frequently, for 30 seconds. Add the lima beans, season with fine sea salt, stir to coat, and add ¾ cup water. Bring the water to a boil, then turn the heat down to a simmer. Cook until the beans are warmed through, about 1 minute. Turn off the heat.

Add the lima beans, half the toasted walnuts, the cooking liquid, and the remaining 1 tablespoon olive oil to a food processor. Pulse to a medium-coarse paste. Pour the puree to a bowl and add the lemon juice, mint, and remaining chopped walnuts. Fold to combine, and add more salt, if desired.

Grill the skewers over the fire until the lamb is browned on all sides, turning every 1 or 2 minutes, until the lamb reaches your desired doneness, 7 to 8 minutes for rare to medium-rare.

Serve lamb with 2 or 3 fig halves and a dollop of the pesto.

Garnish the meat and figs with flaky sea salt and a grinding of pepper.

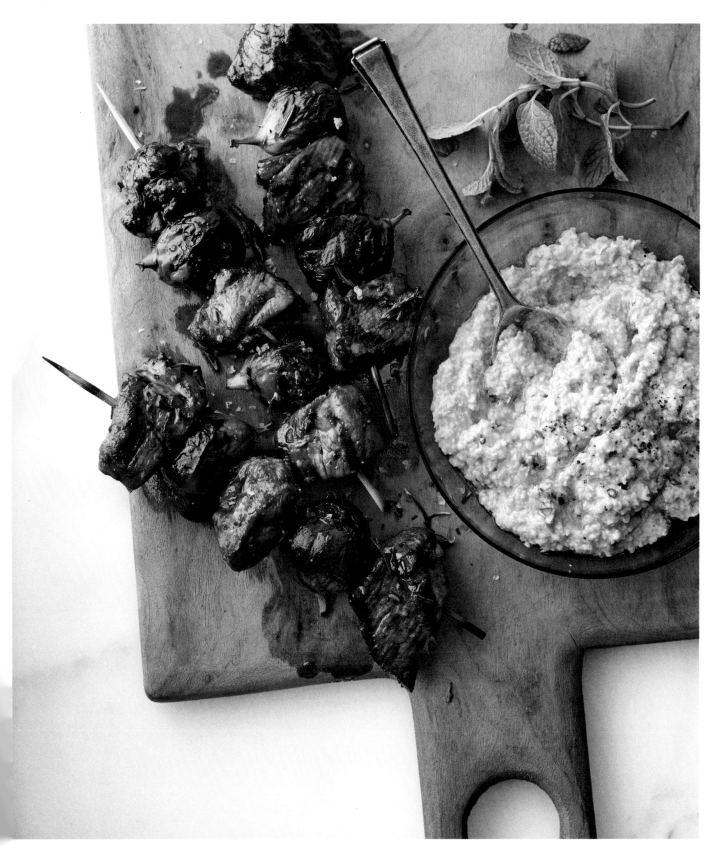

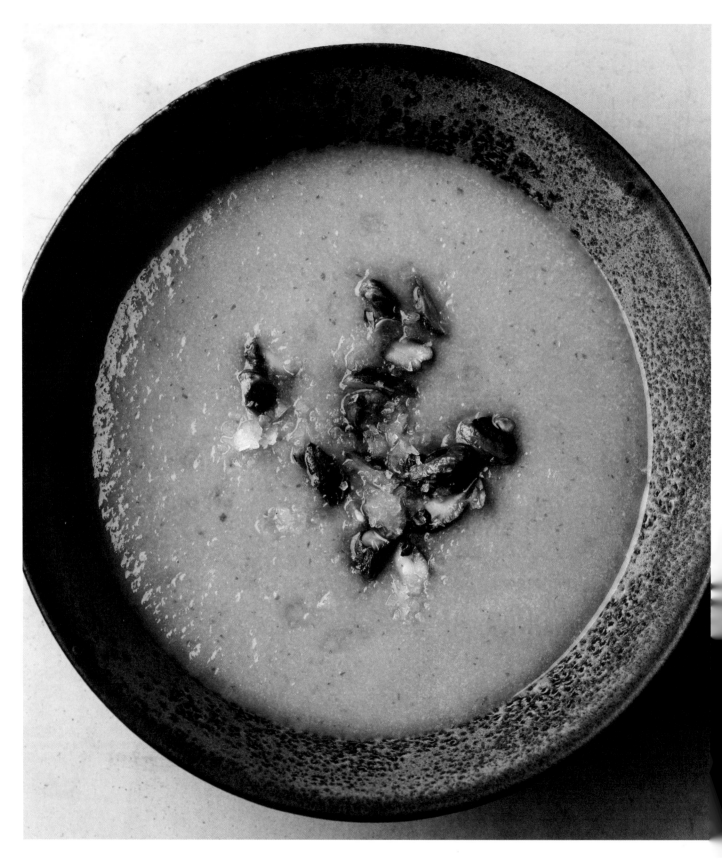

HONEYDEW, CUCUMBER, AND AVOCADO SOUP

1 HOUR 8 MINUTES (8 ACTIVE)	4 SERVINGS

- 4 cups cubed honeydew or other white/green sweet melon
- 1 ripe avocado, pitted, peeled, and cut into medium chunks
- 1 cucumber, peeled, seeded, and cut into medium chunks
- 1 tablespoon minced jalapeño chile (without seeds and pith), plus a pinch more for garnish
- 1 teaspoon fine sea salt, plus more to taste
- 2 tablespoons rice vinegar, plus more to taste
- 1 tablespoon chopped pistachios
- Flaky sea salt to taste (optional)

Blame it on the *The Silver Palate Cookbook,* maybe, but fruit soups— melon, strawberry, blueberry—were all the rage when I worked for a caterer during my Reagan-era high school years. They were easy to make ahead, and gorgeous to serve in little demitasse cups. They got overdone, as most trends do, but enough time has passed that it's okay to go a little retro, especially since it's such a refreshing way to start or finish a hot summer's meal. Almost as easy to make as a smoothie, this cool green soup gets a bit of an edge from jalapeño and rice wine vinegar.

In a blender, puree the melon, avocado, cucumber, jalapeño, salt, and vinegar. If necessary, add ¼ cup water to get the blender going. Puree until very smooth. Taste and adjust the seasoning with a bit more salt and/or rice vinegar to balance the sweetness of the melon.

Chill and serve with a few chopped pistachios, a bit of minced jalapeño, and flaky sea salt, if desired.

RED POBLANO RICE

40 MINUTES (12 ACTIVE)	4 CUPS

- 1¼ cups Bhutanese red rice
- ¾ cup homemade chicken stock (see page 301), low-sodium canned, or water
- 2 garlic cloves, roughly chopped
- 1 poblano (pasilla) chile, cored and roughly chopped
- 1 small onion, roughly chopped
- Fine sea salt to taste
- 6 to 8 fresh cilantro sprigs, plus fresh cilantro leaves for garnish
- 1 tablespoon canola oil
- 1 tablespoon lime juice, plus more to taste

This is a variation on the celebratory Mexican rice dish *arroz verde*, but it's not all that green, since it's made with nutty whole-grain red rice, mixed with a green poblano-cilantro salsa. In the States, we tend to use cilantro as a fresh garnish, but it takes on a rather different taste when it's cooked; it's more floral, less aggressive, and adds just the right note of complexity to a hearty but summery side dish. You can make the rice 2 or 3 days ahead and keep it in the fridge, warming it in a saucepan with the salsa over medium heat when you're ready to serve it.

Note: You can use any remnants of the poblano sauce to season your eggs in the morning.

Cook the rice according to the directions on the package. Set aside to cool.

In a 2-quart saucepan, combine the stock, garlic, poblano, and onion. Season with salt, bring to a boil over medium-high heat, and turn the heat down to a simmer and cook until the chile and onion are soft, about 6 minutes.

Place the stock mixture and cilantro in a blender and puree until very smooth. Take care when pureeing hot liquids; do not fill the blender more than halfway full, leave the blender lid ajar, and place a kitchen towel and then your hand over it. Start the blender slowly and only gradually increase the speed.

Combine the cooled rice with 1 cup of the sauce and 1 tablespoon each of oil and lime juice. Taste and add more salt or lime juice, if desired. Garnish with fresh cilantro leaves to serve.

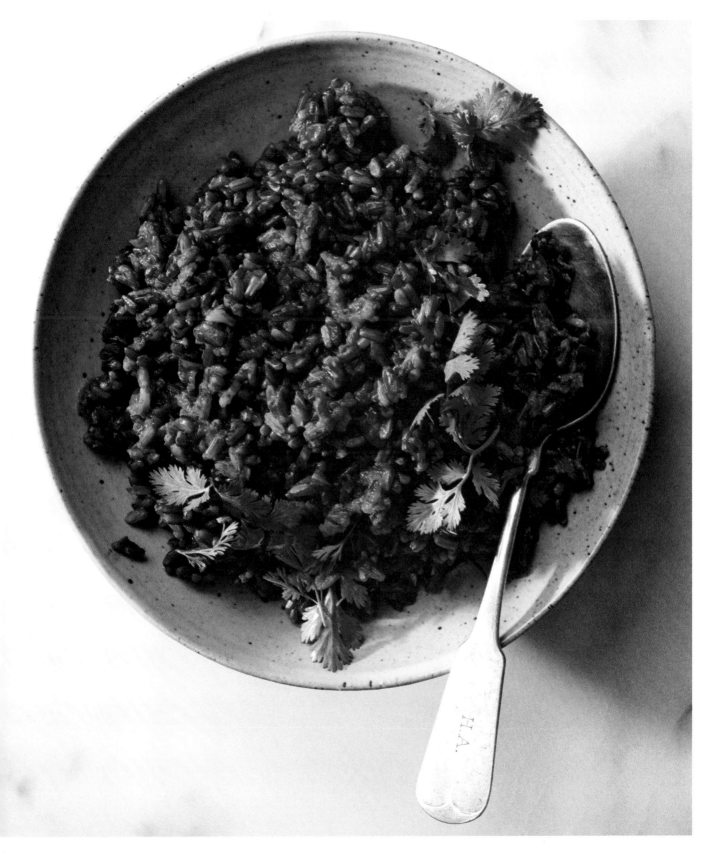

CHICKEN THIGHS WITH CHIPOTLE MAYO

25 TO 30 MINUTES (13 ACTIVE)	4 SERVINGS AND 1 LUNCH THE NEXT DAY

- 2 tablespoons olive oil
- 1 teaspoon ground cumin
- 1 garlic clove, minced
- 5 chicken thighs on the bone (about 2½ pounds)
- Fine sea salt and freshly ground black pepper to taste
- 1 large sweet onion, sliced into 8 wedges, each with some core attached
- ½ pound small shishitos or other small mild or medium-spicy peppers
- Canola oil, for the grill
- Flaky sea salt to finish
- ¼ cup Chipotle Mayonnaise (page 123), for serving

Shishito, Gypsy, Lipstick, banana, Padrón—I can't get enough of the wide-ranging peppers of summer (and their names!). And there is no better treatment for them than throwing them on the grill until they faint into a tender state. This recipe calls for shishitos, the herbaceous Japanese peppers. If your market doesn't sell them, first ask your favorite farmer to plant them for next season, and then feel free to substitute your own favorites. Serve them with sweet, char-kissed onions and chicken thighs, which are a dream to grill. Thigh meat, with a little more internal fat than breast meat, is hard to overcook, so it can spend a lazy time over moderate smoke and the flames, gathering flavor as it goes. To finish it all, serve with a bit of smoky-hot Chipotle Mayonnaise.

Heat a gas grill to medium-high or build a medium-hot fire in a charcoal grill.

In a large mixing bowl, combine 1 tablespoon of the olive oil, the cumin, and the garlic. Add the chicken thighs and massage the oil mixture onto the chicken. Season to taste with fine sea salt and black pepper.

Lay the onion and peppers out on a plate and drizzle with the remaining 1 tablespoon olive oil. Turn them gently to coat. Season with fine sea salt.

Brush the grill and use tongs to rub it with paper towels oiled with canola oil. Place the chicken on the grill skin side down and cover the grill. Cook for 4 minutes, then turn the meat, keeping it skin side down. Cook for about 5 more minutes, until the skin is lightly charred. Turn the thighs and cook until the flesh along the bone is no longer pink, 10 to 12 minutes total.

While the chicken is grilling, lay the onion wedges on the grill and cook until brown on one side, about 4 minutes. Turn over gently and cook until tender, another 4 minutes. Place the peppers on the grill and cook until the skin is browned and lightly charred on one side. Turn each pepper and cook until browned and blistered on all sides, 5 to 6 minutes total, depending on the size of peppers.

Sprinkle the chicken with flaky sea salt to taste and serve with onion wedges, peppers, and a heaping tablespoon of chipotle mayonnaise on the side.

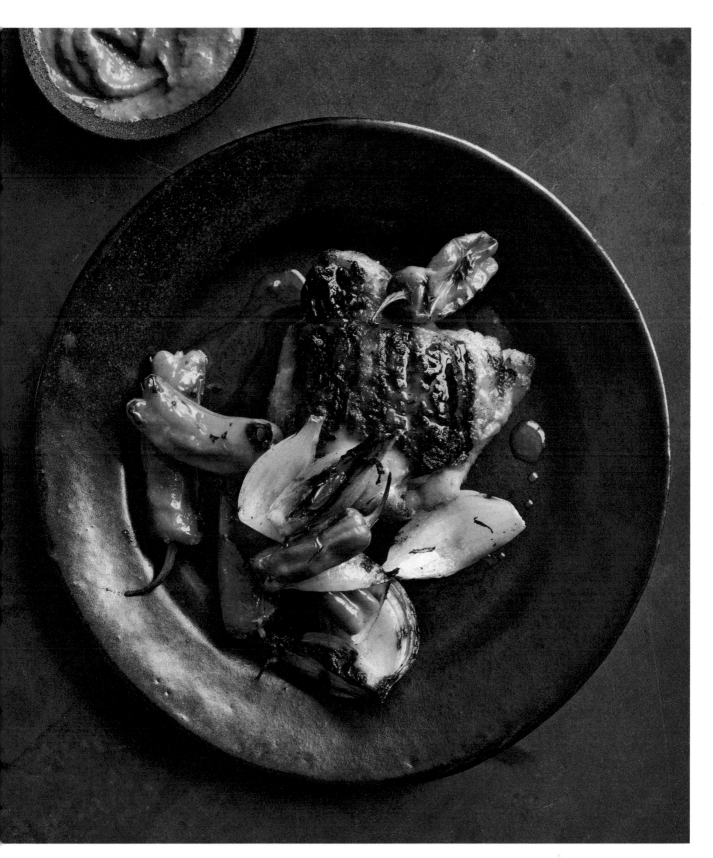

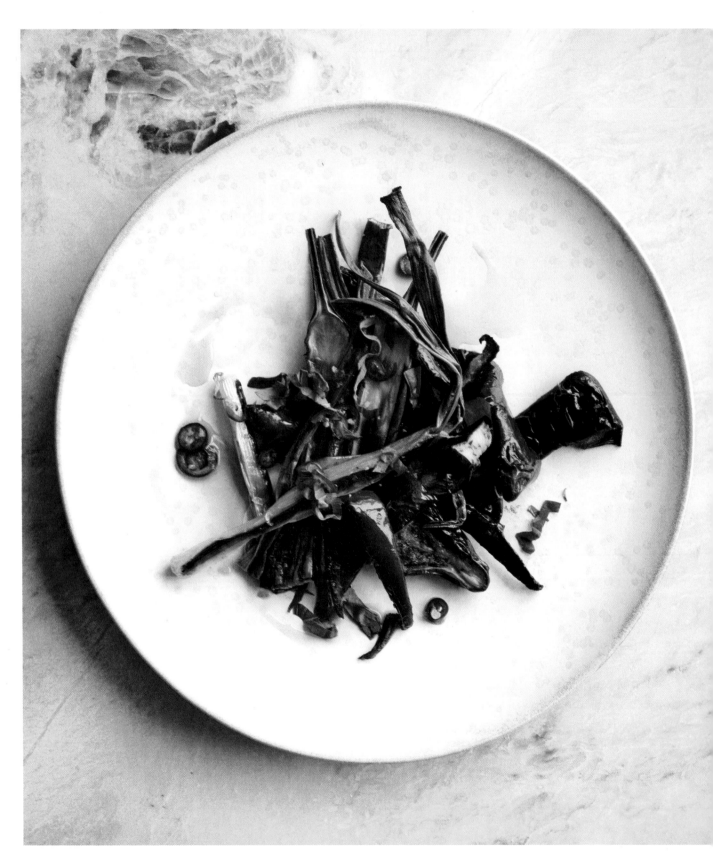

ROASTED EGGPLANT AND GREEN PEPPERS WITH NUOC CHAM

35 TO 45 MINUTES (8 ACTIVE)	4 SERVINGS AND 1 LUNCH THE NEXT DAY

- 1 pound Japanese eggplant, halved
- 1 teaspoon fine sea salt, plus more to taste
- 2 tablespoons canola oil or shallot oil, if cooking in tandem with the noodle salad on page 155
- 1 bunch scallions, roots trimmed
- 1 poblano (pasilla) chile, cored, seeded, and cut into strips
- 1 large green bell pepper, cored, seeded, and cut into strips
- ¼ cup lime juice, plus more to taste
- 2½ teaspoons fish sauce, such as Red Boat brand
- 1 tablespoon finely minced jalapeño chile
- 1 small garlic clove, grated
- 1 teaspoon honey
- 1 cup loosely packed Thai or conventional basil leaves (about 1 small bunch)

As you might know by now, I'm an inveterate sheet-pan vegetable roaster. There's nothing like the method to free up your stovetop for another part of dinner. The key is dressing the vegetables when they're still hot with something a bit assertive, like nuoc cham, a tart, savory Vietnamese-style dressing. Here it snaps eggplant and peppers to attention, but it works equally well on root vegetables, squash, and asparagus. Currently I'm partial to Red Boat brand fish sauce, which manages to deliver a strong hit of umami funk with a clean finish.

Preheat the oven to 450°F.

Season the eggplant with 1 teaspoon salt and let it stand 15 minutes. Blot the eggplant with paper towels or a clean kitchen towel and lay it on a baking sheet. Using a brush or your fingertips, paint the eggplant with 1 tablespoon of the oil.

Toss the scallions, poblano, and bell pepper with the remaining oil and lay them on another baking sheet. Roast both sheets of vegetables, rotating the position once or twice, for 15 to 20 minutes, or until tender and browned in spots.

Meanwhile, in a small bowl, whisk together the lime juice, fish sauce, jalapeño, garlic, and honey. When the vegetables are done, spoon 2 tablespoons of the lime juice mixture on top. Let cool for 5 to 10 minutes.

Taste the vegetables, and plate them, adding more salt or lime mixture, if desired. Top with the basil leaves and serve warm or at room temperature.

BUCKWHEAT NOODLES WITH ZUCCHINI AND GOLDEN FLOWERS

10 TO 12 MINUTES (10 ACTIVE)	4 SERVINGS AND 1 LUNCH THE NEXT DAY

- Fine sea salt
- 8 ounces buckwheat soba noodles or buckwheat-corn noodles from Italy
- 2 medium zucchini
- 2 tablespoons extra-virgin olive oil
- 1 garlic clove, minced
- Pinch of red pepper flakes
- 2 tablespoons rice vinegar
- 1 tablespoon black sesame seeds
- 8 squash or nasturtium blossoms, for garnish (optional)

Sometimes I get totally fixated on a color combination. The nasturtium blossoms here add peppery flavor and a wonderful jolt of color to the sober buckwheat noodles. You could substitute squash blossoms for a more delicate flourish, but flowers come and go quickly in the market. If you're not cooking at just the right time in the summer, you might not catch these beautiful blooms, but the noodles, draped with slivers of zucchini, still taste great. If you're dead set on having a bit of orange color in the mix—and I wouldn't blame you—grate some carrots and toss them in with the squash slivers.

Bring a large pot of salted water to a boil and cook the noodles al dente according to the package instructions. Drain the noodles, rinse them in cool water, drain them well again, and place them in a large bowl.

Meanwhile, julienne the zucchini by slicing off the stem and flower end of each squash. Slice the squash crosswise in half. Slice each half lengthwise into ⅛-inch slices and then slice each of those slices lengthwise into ⅛-inch ribbons. Don't worry if the strips aren't perfect, but aim for long, thin sticks of roughly the same size.

In a heavy 10- or 12-inch skillet, warm 1 tablespoon of the oil over medium heat. Add the garlic and red pepper flakes and cook until just fragrant, about 15 seconds. Take the pan off the heat and add the julienned zucchini, tossing well to coat in the garlicky oil. Season the zucchini with salt to taste.

Add the zucchini mixture to the drained buckwheat noodles. Add the remaining 1 tablespoon olive oil, the rice vinegar, and the sesame seeds. Toss with tongs to combine and coat the noodles well; add more salt to taste. Garnish with blossoms, if using.

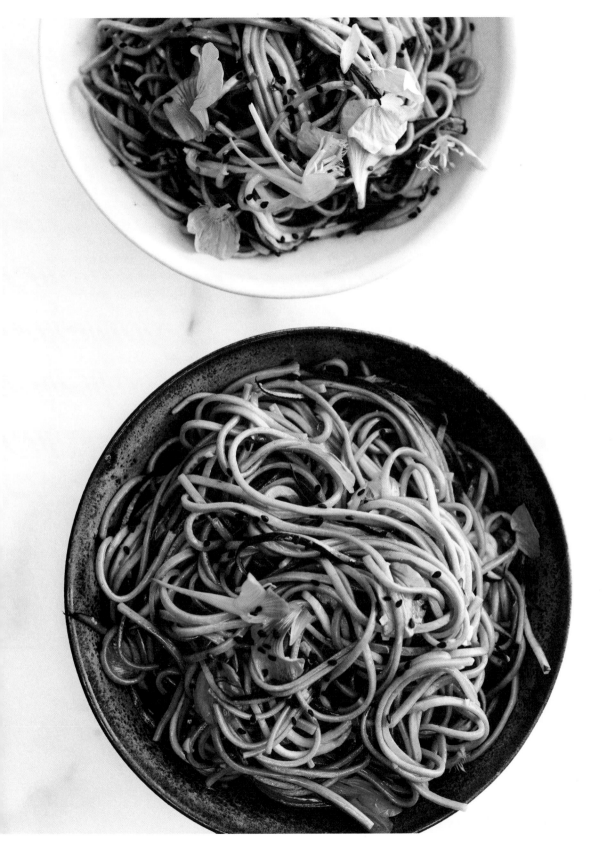

GARLICKY GRILLED SHRIMP WITH GRILLED NECTARINES AND GREEN TOMATOES

12 TO 15 MINUTES	4 SERVINGS AND 1 LUNCH THE NEXT DAY

- 2 large nectarines, pitted and quartered
- 2 large (or 6 small) tomatillos, quartered
- 2 tablespoons olive oil, plus more for garnish
- Fine sea salt and freshly ground black pepper to taste
- 1½ pounds shelled, deveined jumbo or extra-jumbo shrimp, preferably wild American (about 30 per pound)
- 2 garlic cloves, grated
- 1 small red onion, cut into ⅛-inch-thick slices
- 1 tablespoon rice vinegar
- 24 fresh mint leaves
- Flaky sea salt to taste

When stone fruit comes on in the summer, I can't get enough of it, and nectarines, which have a distinctive tart-crisp heartiness, just may be my favorite. I throw them in yogurt in the morning, crunch them for my afternoon snack, and when I'm not on a cleanse, I make rough, rustic galettes with them. They also slip into savory dishes like this one, where a little tomatillo (or an unripe tomato from the garden) helps the relish from going too sweet. It's gorgeous with grilled shrimp (though it would work just fine with pork, fish, or grilled calamari, too).

If you do use shrimp, look for wild-harvested domestic shrimp, which is a better environmental choice than crustaceans that have been shipped around the globe.

Heat a gas grill to medium high or build a medium-hot fire in a charcoal grill.

In a large bowl, toss the nectarines and tomatillo quarters with 1 tablespoon of the oil and season with fine sea salt and pepper. Grill until browned, softened, and slightly charred, rotating frequently to cook evenly, about 6 minutes total. Remove from the heat.

In the same bowl, combine the shrimp with 1 tablespoon oil and the garlic. Grill the shrimp until they're browned and slightly charred, rotating frequently to cook evenly, about 3 minutes total.

In a large, clean bowl, combine the nectarines, tomatillos, shrimp, and onion. Toss in the vinegar and mint and season with flaky sea salt and more pepper. Serve with a drizzle of oil, if desired.

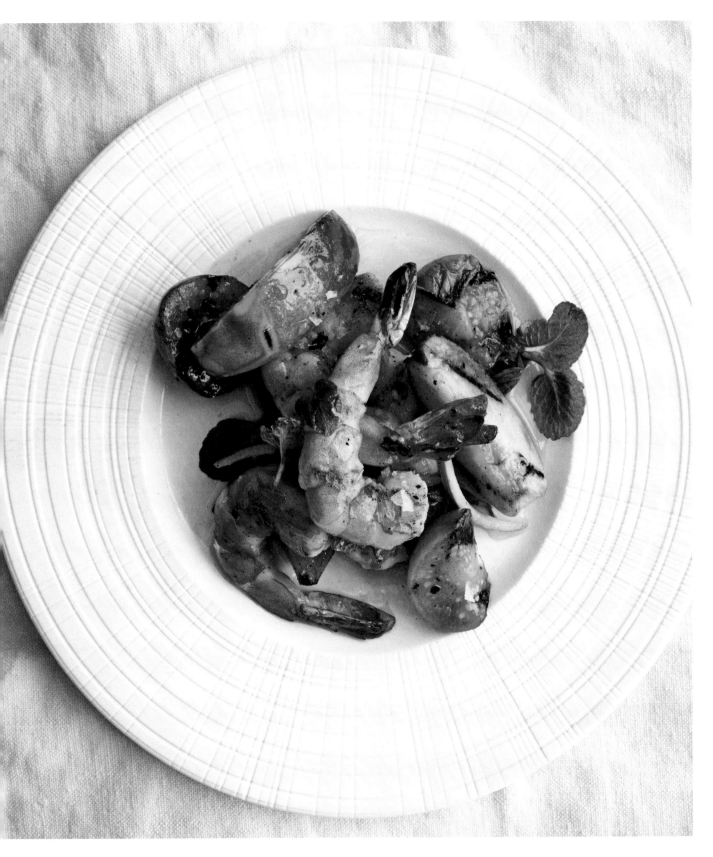

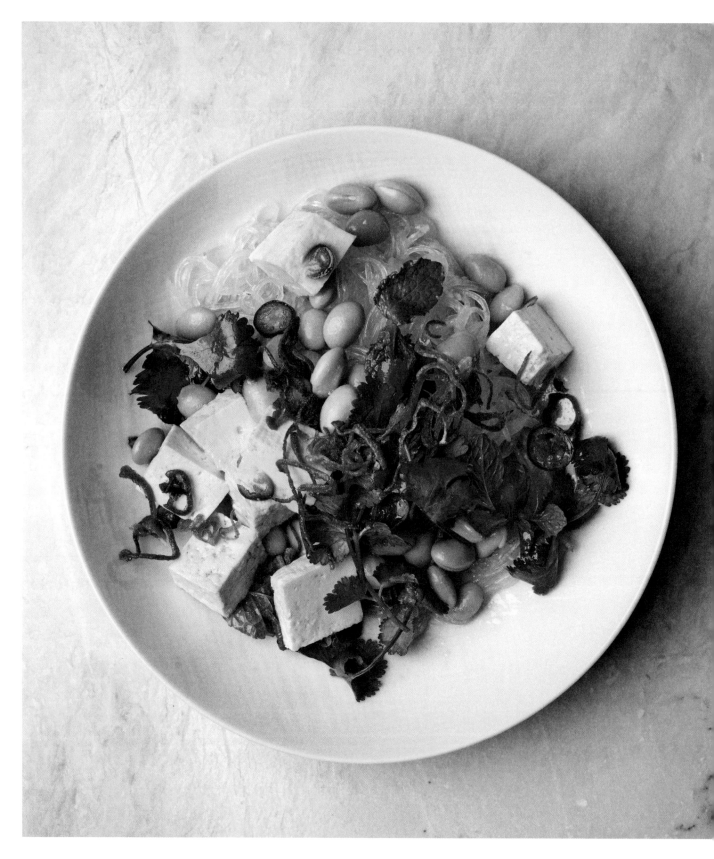

CELLOPHANE NOODLE SALAD WITH TOFU, EDAMAME, AND CRISPY SHALLOTS

20 MINUTES	4 SERVINGS AND 1 LUNCH THE NEXT DAY

- Fine sea salt to taste
- 1 cup frozen shelled edamame
- 6 ounces dry cellophane noodles (also marketed as saifun)
- ¼ cup lime juice (from about 2 large limes)
- 2½ teaspoons fish sauce, such as Red Boat brand
- 1 tablespoon finely minced jalapeño chile
- 1 teaspoon honey
- ¼ cup canola oil
- 2 shallots, cut crosswise into ¼-inch slices
- 8 ounces firm tofu, cut into ½-inch cubes
- ½ cup torn fresh cilantro leaves
- ¼ cup torn fresh mint leaves
- Flaky sea salt to taste (optional)

Cellophane noodles always remind me of Wonder Woman's invisible jet: totally transparent yet substantial, a stealthy ally to have around. They cook in a flash and are ready to take on bold flavors, like this tangy lime and fish sauce dressing. (They are, by the way, gluten-free, and surprisingly filling.) The key is to play the springy texture of the noodles against the crunch of fried shallots, the tenderness of tofu, and the fresh crispness of mint and cilantro.

Bring a pot of salted water to a boil and have ready a bowl of ice water. Pour in the edamame and cook for 1 minute. Using a slotted spoon or a strainer, remove the beans to a large bowl.

Place the cellophane noodles in the water, remove the pan from the heat, and let soak until tender but not mushy, 12 to 15 minutes. Strain and place the noodles in the bowl of ice water. Drain when cooled.

In a small bowl, whisk together the lime juice, fish sauce, jalapeño, and honey. Set aside.

Have ready a strainer set over a small heatproof bowl. In a small saucepan, heat the oil over medium heat. Add the shallots and cook for 5 to 6 minutes, stirring frequently, until they turn a golden brown. Strain the shallots into the bowl, letting them drip oil for several minutes. Drain the shallots further on a piece of paper towel.

Add 3 tablespoons of the shallot oil to the lime juice mixture and whisk to combine.

Place the tofu in a large bowl and gently stir in 1 tablespoon of the lime-oil mixture. Add the edamame, noodles, cilantro, and mint and pour in the rest of the dressing, tossing well with tongs to coat the noodles and other ingredients. Taste the noodles and season with flaky sea salt, if desired.

Top the salad with the fried shallots.

PORK SKEWERS WITH THYME AND SMOKED PAPRIKA

24 MINUTES (10 ACTIVE)	4 SERVINGS AND 1 LUNCH THE NEXT DAY

- Canola oil, for the grill
- 2 tablespoons olive oil
- 1 garlic clove, grated
- ½ teaspoon smoked paprika
- 1 tablespoon fresh thyme leaves (from 4 to 5 sprigs)
- Fine sea salt to taste
- 1 pork tenderloin (about 1¼ pounds), trimmed and cut into 1½-inch pieces
- 6 tablespoons Broken Olive Vinaigrette (page 312)
- Special equipment: bamboo skewers, soaked in water for at least 20 minutes.

Pork tenderloin is the leanest pork around, and without a little boost, it can taste a bit washed out compared with other fattier cuts like chops and shoulders. It's a gem, though, if you treat it right. You have to love its quick-cooking nature, and the sweet, bright flavor it gets when grilled till just a bit pinkish inside. Pair it with something feisty, such as this chunky olive vinaigrette, and you'll have an easy and vibrant grilling dish in your back pocket.

Prepare a medium-hot charcoal fire or heat a gas grill to medium heat. Clean the grill grate well with a brush and use tongs to grease it with a paper towel coated in canola oil.

In a large bowl, whisk together the olive oil, garlic, paprika, thyme, and salt. Toss the pork chunks with the oil mixture, coating them evenly.

Thread the pork chunks on the soaked bamboo skewers, leaving a little space between each one. Grill the pork skewers for 12 to 14 minutes, turning as needed, until all sides are browned and slightly charred and the pork is just a bit rosy at the center of each chunk. Remove and serve with the vinaigrette.

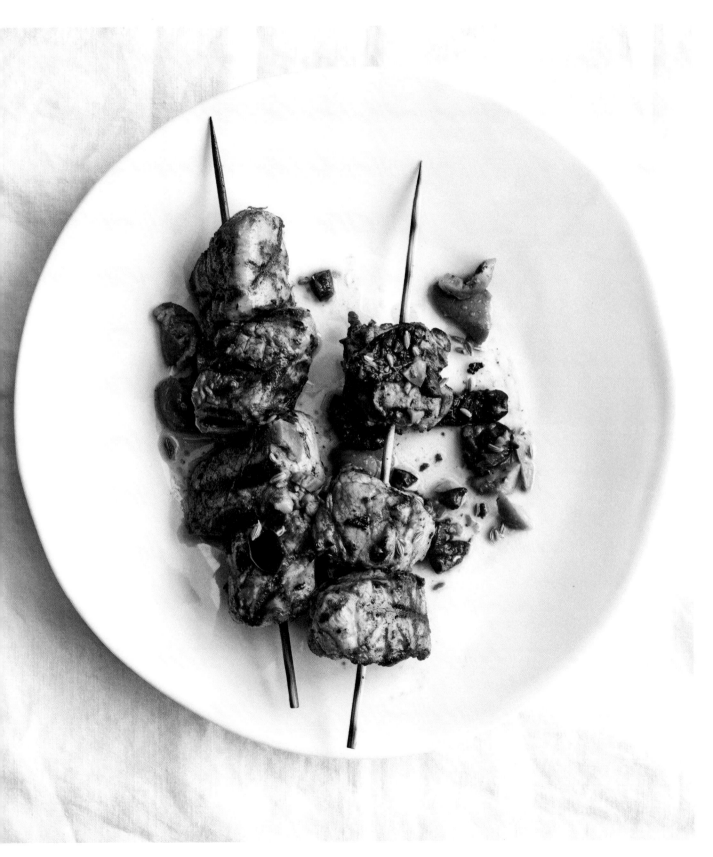

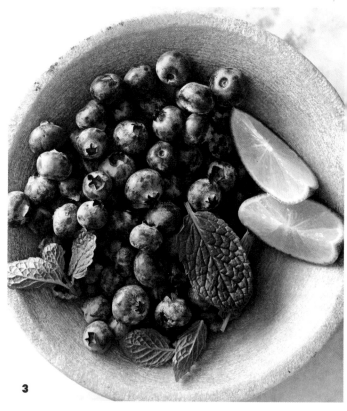

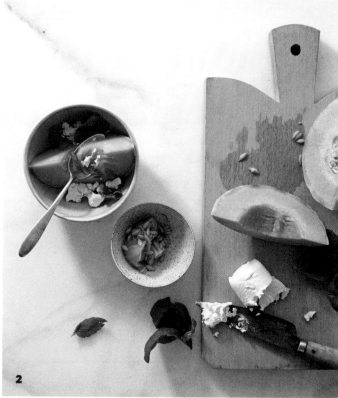

SUMMER DESSERTS

The suggested portions below are for one person.

1. **Raspberries with Honey-Chamomile Dressing (page 312)**
1 cup raspberries with 1 tablespoon dressing

2. **Melon with chèvre and basil**
1 cup melon with 1 or 2 teaspoons crumbled chèvre and torn basil

3. **Fresh blueberries with mint and lime**
1 cup blueberries with 7 or 8 torn mint leaves and 2 lime wedges

4. **Fruit salad with plums, black cherries, and Marcona almonds**
1 plum, 4 cherries, and 1 tablespoon almonds

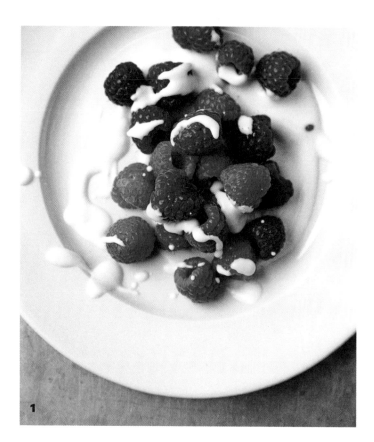

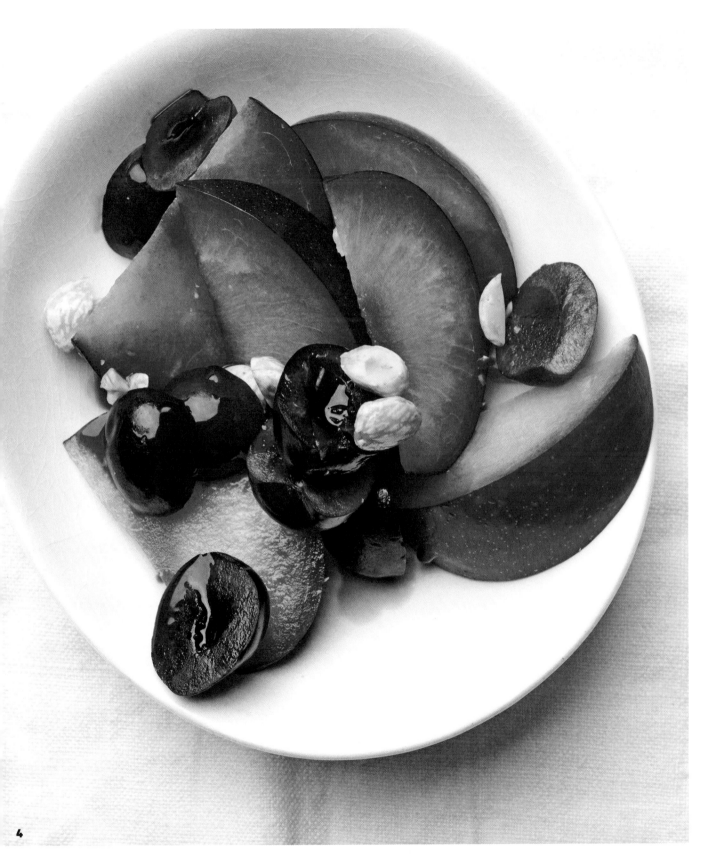

CLEANSE MENU

DAY 1

(STARTS WITH DINNER)

DINNER
Grilled Albacore with Tomato-Herb Salad (page 136) and Buttermilk Dressing (page 310)

DESSERT
Fruit salad with plums, black cherries, and Marcona almonds (pictured on page 159)

DAY 2

BREAKFAST
Scrambled Eggs with Cherry Tomatoes (page 100)

LUNCH
Leftover albacore with arugula, shaved zucchini, black olives, and Sherry Vinaigrette (page 315)

SNACK
Blanched green beans (see page 304) with White Bean Dip (page 316)

DINNER
Veal Cutlets with Sage-Caper Relish (page 115)

Quinoa Salad with Broccoli and Pistachios (page 116)

DESSERT
Fresh blueberries with mint and lime (pictured on page 158)

DAY 3

BREAKFAST
Blackberry-Buttermilk Batido (page 103)

LUNCH
Leftover quinoa broccoli salad, butter lettuce, avocado, and Buttermilk Dressing (page 310)

SNACK
Grilled Caponata Relish (page 319) with chèvre

DINNER
Slow-Baked Salmon with Fennel (page 126)

Orange-Braised Carrots and Beets (page 130)

DESSERT
Melon with chèvre and basil (pictured on page 158)

DAY 4

BREAKFAST
Fried Egg with Spicy Beans, Shaved Zucchini, and Tortilla (page 104)

LUNCH
Leftover salmon with beets, sunflower seeds, frisée, and Sherry Vinaigrette (page 315)

SNACK
Nectarine with toasted almonds

DINNER
Pistou Salad with Eggs (page 139)

Honeydew, Cucumber, and Avocado Soup (page 143)

DESSERT
Honey-Toasted Quinoa and Amaranth Bark (page 326)

DAY 5

BREAKFAST
Greek Yogurt with Apricots and Toasted Seeds (page 99)

LUNCH
Leftover pistou salad, slivered kale, pine nuts, golden raisins, olive oil, and lemon juice

SNACK
Cucumber slices with 1 ounce smoked salmon and black olives

DINNER
Zucchini Tacos with Cabbage and Queso Fresco (page 124)

Red Poblano Rice (page 144)

DESSERT
Raspberries with Honey-Chamomile Dressing (pictured on page 158)

DAY 6

BREAKFAST
Raspberry-Coconut Muesli (page 102)

LUNCH
Leftover red poblano rice with leftover zucchini, shredded red cabbage and cilantro, pumpkin seeds, tomatoes, avocado, quick citrus-pickled red onions, and Chipotle Mayonnaise (pictured on page 106)

SNACK
Blanched green beans (see page 304) with White Bean Dip (page 316)

DINNER
Smoky Grilled Flank Steak (page 129)

Black Rice Salad with Corn, Tomatoes, and Spinach (page 110)

DESSERT
Fruit salad with plums, black cherries, and Marcona almonds (pictured on page 159)

DAY 7

BREAKFAST
Blackberry-Buttermilk Batido
(page 103)

LUNCH
Leftover steak, romaine
lettuce, cilantro, Sesame-
Miso Vinaigrette (page 310),
and sesame seeds

SNACK
Grilled Caponata Relish
(page 319) with chèvre

DINNER
Mussels with Harissa, Chard,
and Chickpeas (page 120)

Rosemary Socca (page 122)

DESSERT
Honey-Toasted Quinoa and
Amaranth Bark (page 326)

DAY 8

BREAKFAST
Fried Egg with Spicy Beans,
Shaved Zucchini, and Tortilla
(page 104)

LUNCH
Leftover mussels, shelled
and marinated in Sherry
Vinaigrette (page 315); frisée,
shaved fennel, tarragon, and
other herbs

SNACK
Cucumber slices with
1 ounce smoked salmon and
black olives

DINNER
Lamb with Roasted Figs and
Lima Bean Pesto (page 140)

Orange-Braised Carrots and
Beets (page 130)

DESSERT
Melon with chèvre and basil
(pictured on page 158)

DAY 9

BREAKFAST
Scrambled Eggs with Cherry
Tomatoes (page 100)

LUNCH
Leftover lamb with arugula,
tender herbs, sliced shallots,
cherry tomatoes, and Broken
Olive Vinaigrette (pictured
on page 108)

SNACK
Nectarine with toasted
almonds

DINNER
Chicken Thighs with Chipotle
Mayo (page 146)

Mixed Bean Salad with
Cilantro and Pepitas
(page 112)

DESSERT
Fruit salad with plums,
black cherries, and Marcona
almonds (pictured on
page 159)

DAY 10

BREAKFAST
Greek yogurt with Apricots and Toasted Seeds (page 99)

LUNCH
Shredded leftover chicken tossed with Chipotle Mayonnaise (page 123) and extra cilantro with blanched green beans (see page 304)

SNACK
Spicy Carrot Dip (page 318) with zucchini spears

DINNER
Kale with Black-Eyed Peas and Tuna (page 119)

DESSERT
Honey-Toasted Quinoa and Amaranth Bark (page 326)

DAY 11

BREAKFAST
Blackberry-Buttermilk Batido (page 103)

LUNCH
Leftover kale and black-eyed peas, tomatoes, and Broken Olive Vinaigrette (page 312)

SNACK
Blanched green beans (see page 304) with White Bean Dip (page 316)

DINNER
Garlicky Grilled Shrimp with Grilled Nectarines and Green Tomatoes (page 152)

Black Rice Salad with Corn, Tomatoes, and Spinach (page 110)

DESSERT
Fresh blueberries with mint and lime (pictured on page 158)

DAY 12

BREAKFAST
Raspberry-Coconut Muesli (page 102)

LUNCH
Leftover shrimp with butter lettuce, cucumbers, mint, avocado, pistachios, and Buttermilk Dressing (pictured on page 107)

SNACK
Spicy Carrot Dip (page 318) with zucchini spears

DINNER
Roasted Eggplant and Green Peppers with Nuoc Cham (page 149)

Cellophane Noodle Salad with Tofu, Edamame, and Crispy Shallots (page 155)

DESSERT
Honey-Toasted Amaranth and Quinoa Bark (page 326)

DAY 13

BREAKFAST
Fried Egg with Spicy Beans, Shaved Zucchini, and Tortilla (page 104)

LUNCH
Leftover eggplant, peppers, cellophane noodles, and nuoc cham with herb salad (cilantro, mint, red shiso leaf), slivered chiles, and chopped peanuts (pictured on page 109)

SNACK
Nectarine with toasted almonds

DINNER
Pork Skewers with Thyme and Smoked Paprika (page 156)

Buckwheat Noodles with Zucchini and Golden Flowers (page 150)

DESSERT
Melon with chèvre and basil (page 158)

DAY 14

BREAKFAST
Greek Yogurt with Apricots and Toasted Seeds (page 99)

LUNCH
Leftover pork, romaine lettuce, cantaloupe cubes, cucumber, pistachios, and Buttermilk Dressing (page 310)

SNACK
Blanched green beans (see page 304) with White Bean Dip (page 316)

DINNER
Grilled Swordfish with Charred Tomatillo Salsa (page 132)

Red Poblano Rice (page 144)

DESSERT
Raspberries with Honey-Chamomile Dressing (pictured on page 158)

SHOPPING LIST

We've put together a shopping list for you following the number of servings in our recipes; that means dinner recipes are for four people, but breakfasts, lunches, snacks, and desserts are portioned for one person. Please adjust according to your needs!

PANTRY

CANNED AND DRIED GOODS
- cannellini beans, 15-ounce can or 1¼ cups cooked (as for dip)
- capers, preferably salt-packed
- cellophane noodles (saifun), 6-ounce package
- chicken stock, 2½ cups homemade or 20-ounce low-sodium can
- chickpeas, 15-ounce can
- chipotle peppers in adobo, small can
- coconut milk
- dried white beans, 4 cups
- olives, mixed, ½ cup
- olives, black, ¼ cup
- pinto beans, 3 (15-ounce) cans
- tuna, 5-ounce tin, preferably oil-packed, line-caught albacore, drained

CONDIMENTS
- Dijon mustard
- harissa, prepared (or Preserved Lemon Harissa, page 320)
- hot sauce, optional
- white miso
- fish sauce such as Red Boat Brand

DRIED FRUIT
- coconut flakes, unsweetened, 2 tablespoons
- golden raisins, 1 tablespoon

FROZEN GOODS
- black-eyed peas, frozen, 2 cups
- edamame, frozen, 1 cup, peeled
- lima beans, frozen, 1½ cups

GRAINS
- amaranth, 2 tablespoons
- garbanzo flour, 1 cup
- quinoa, white or other color, 1¼ cups
- rice, Bhutanese red, 2½ cups
- rice, black (often sold as Forbidden Rice), 2 cups
- rolled oats, ⅔ cup
- soba noodles, preferably all-buckwheat, 8 ounces

NUTS AND SEEDS
- almonds, sliced, ½ cup
- marcona almonds, ¼ cup
- peanuts, 1 tablespoon
- pine nuts, 1 tablespoon
- pistachios, ⅔ cup
- pumpkin seeds (pepitas), ½ cup
- sesame seeds, 1 tablespoon
- sesame seeds, black, 1 tablespoon
- sunflower seeds, shelled, 1 tablespoon
- walnuts, ½ cup

OILS AND VINEGARS
- canola, grapeseed, or vegetable oil, 16 ounces
- olive oil, 1 quart
- olive oil, extra-virgin, 1 quart
- sesame oil
- red or white wine vinegar
- rice vinegar, unseasoned
- sherry vinegar
- white balsamic vinegar, (can substitute rice vinegar)

SPICES
- ancho chile powder, 1 teaspoon
- black peppercorns
- chamomile flowers, ¼ cup or 12 teabags
- cinnamon, ground, ½ teaspoon
- coriander seed, 1 teaspoon
- cumin, ground, 2 teaspoons
- dried oregano, 2 teaspoons
- fennel seed, 2 teaspoons
- fine sea salt
- flaky sea salt
- medium-hot red pepper flakes, such as Aleppo or Marash, ¼ cup
- small dried chiles such as chile de arbol or japones, 4
- smoked paprika, 1 teaspoon

SWEET ITEMS
- agave syrup
- bittersweet chocolate, 8 ounces
- honey

WINE
- dry vermouth, white, small bottle
- white wine

SHOPPING LIST

DAIRY AND OTHER REFRIGERATED ITEMS

- buttermilk or plain kefir, 1 quart
- chèvre, 4- or 5-ounce package
- corn tortillas, 10
- eggs, 1 dozen
- orange juice, 1 cup
- plain Greek yogurt, 1 pint
- queso fresco, ¼ cup (can substitute chèvre)
- sheep's milk yogurt, ½ cup (can substitute plain Greek yogurt)
- tofu, silken, 8 ounces

MEAT AND SEAFOOD

- flank steak, preferably grass-finished, 1¼ pounds
- veal, 8 thin cutlets
- albacore tuna or yellowtail tuna loins, fresh, 1½ pounds
- mussels, black, 2½ pounds
- salmon, preferably wild-caught king or sockeye, 1½ pounds
- smoked salmon, sliced, small package

PRODUCE

- apricots, 2
- arugula, 6 cups (about 2 bunches)
- avocado, 2
- basil, 2 bunches
- beets, 1½ pounds
- blackberries, 1 cup (frozen okay)
- blueberries, 1 pint
- broccoli, 2 small heads (1¼ pounds)
- butter lettuce, 1 small head
- cabbage, red, 1 small head
- carrots, 5 large
- celery, 1 heart
- chard, 1½ bunches
- cherries, ¼ pound
- cherry tomatoes, 3 pints
- chiles, 4 jalapeños or 3 jalapeños and 1 Fresno
- chile, poblano (pasilla), 1
- chile, serrano, 1
- cilantro, 1 bunch
- corn, 2 ears
- cucumbers, 2
- eggplant, Japanese or Chinese, 1 pound
- fennel, 1 bulb
- frisée, 1 small head
- garlic, 2 heads
- ginger, 1 teaspoon
- green beans, 1 pound
- kale, 1 bunch
- leeks, 3 large
- lemon, 5
- limes, 4
- melon, cantaloupe, 1 small
- melon, honeydew, 1
- mint, 1 bunch
- mixed delicate salad greens, 2 cups
- nectarine, 1
- onions, 2 medium
- onion, red, 1 large
- onions, sweet, 2 medium, 1 large
- orange, 1 large
- parsley, flat-leaf, 1 bunch
- plums, 2
- raspberries, 1 pint
- romaine lettuce, 1 heart
- rosemary, 1 sprig
- sage, small bunch
- scallions, ½ bunch
- shallots, 2
- spinach, 1 bunch
- tarragon, small bunch
- thyme, small bunch
- tomatoes, various, 2½ pounds (about 6 medium)
- zucchini, 4 pounds, about 8 medium

SHOPPING LIST

Do a quick inventory before heading out shopping for your second week—some of your dairy, produce, and sauces may be in fine shape for a second week!

DAIRY AND OTHER REFRIGERATED ITEMS

- buttermilk or plain kefir, 1 pint
- eggs, large, ½ dozen
- orange juice, ½ cup
- plain Greek yogurt, 1 pint
- sheep's milk yogurt, ½ cup (can substitute plain Greek yogurt)
- tofu, firm, 1 (14-ounce) package
- corn tortillas, 2 (may have enough left over from week 1)

MEAT AND SEAFOOD

- chicken thighs, skin on, bone in, 5 pieces (2½ pounds)
- lamb, leg, 2 pounds boneless
- pork tenderloin (about 1¼ pounds)
- shrimp (preferably wild and American-harvested), shelled, 1½ pounds (about 30 jumbo or extra-jumbo)
- smoked salmon, 1 ounce
- swordfish fillets, 1½ pounds, about 1 inch thick

PRODUCE

- apricots, 4
- arugula, 3 cups
- avocados, 2
- basil, 1 small bunch
- basil, Thai or conventional, 1 bunch
- beets, 1½ pounds
- blackberries, ½ cup (frozen okay)
- blueberries, 1 pint
- butter lettuce, 1 small head
- carrots, 2½ pounds (10 to 12 large)
- cherries, ¼ pound
- cherry tomatoes, 2 pints
- chiles, jalapeño, 3
- chiles, poblano (pasilla), 2
- chiles, serrano, 2
- cilantro, 1 bunch
- corn, 2 ears
- cucumbers, 2 small
- dill, 1 small bunch
- fennel, 1 small bulb
- figs, Black Mission, 10 (about 1 pint)
- frisée, 1 small head
- garlic cloves, 2 heads
- green beans, 1¼ pounds
- Japanese eggplant, 1 pound
- kale, lacinato, 1 bunch
- leek, 1 large
- lemons, 4
- limes, 8
- melon, cantaloupe, 1 large or 2 small
- mint, 1 bunch
- nectarines, 4
- onions, 3 medium
- onion, red, 1
- onion, sweet, 1 large
- orange, 1 large
- pepper, green bell, 1
- pepper, red bell, 1
- peppers, shishitos or other small, mild or medium chiles, 8 ounces
- plum, 1
- raspberries, 1½ pints
- romaine lettuce, 1 heart
- rosemary, 1 sprig
- sage, 1 small bunch (likely to have some left over from week 1)
- scallions, 2 bunches
- shallots, 3
- spinach, 1 bunch
- squash or nasturtium blossoms, 8 (optional)
- thyme, 1 small bunch (likely to have some left over from week 1)
- tomatillos, 1 pound, husks on (about 7 large)
- tomatoes, 3
- yellow wax beans, ½ pound
- zucchini, 3 small, 2 medium

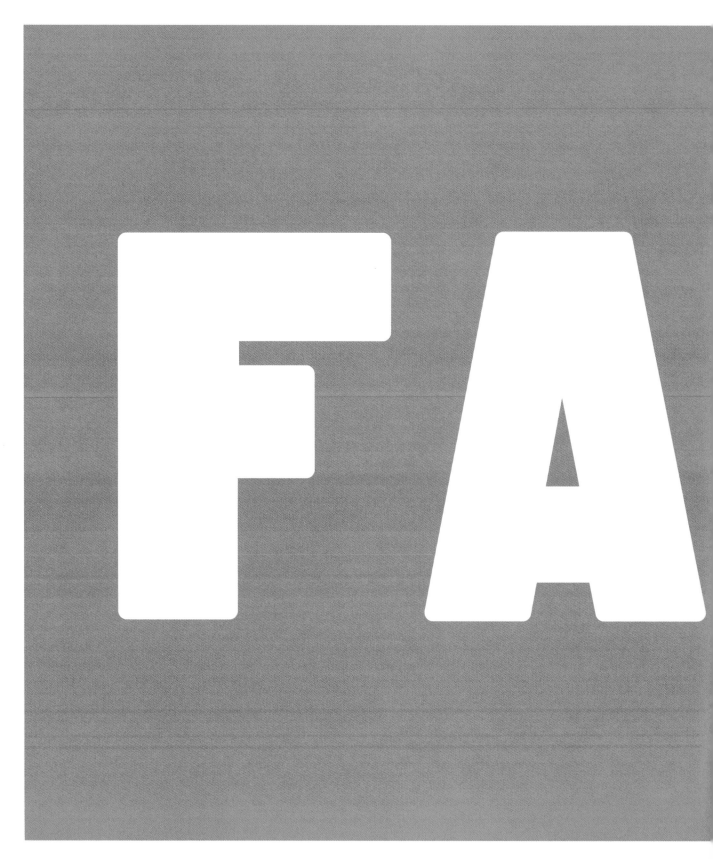

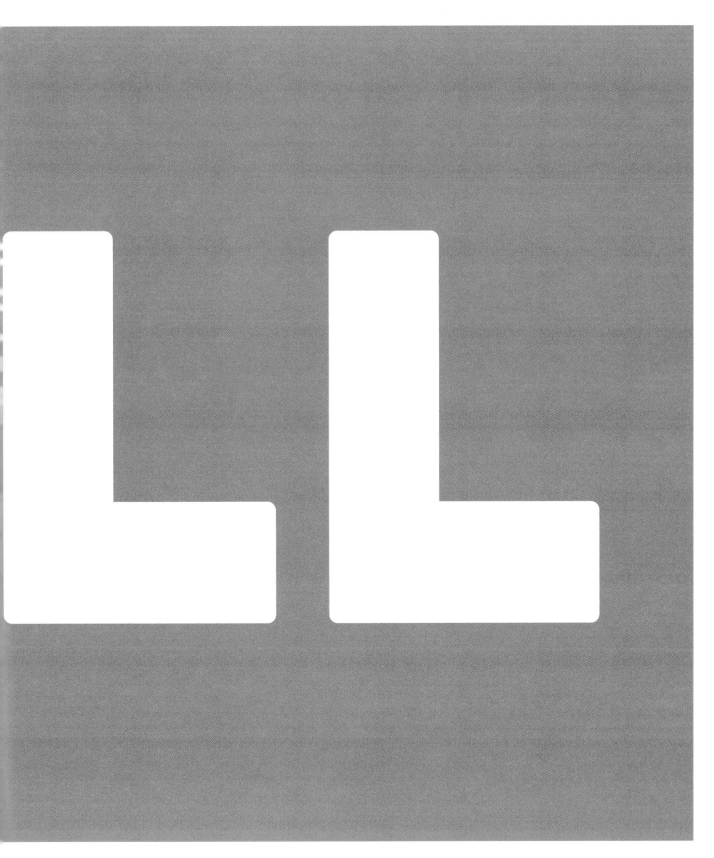

When summer ends, it can be hard to return from all those picnics on the beach (or the sidewalk stoop), but there may be no better time to commit to produce-packed home cooking. So much of what feels like summer harvest is actually hitting maximum ripeness in the fall: tomatoes, figs, grapes, peppers. At the same time, all those golden vegetables—the squashes and the carrots and such—are bringing a new depth to the mix. Because of that golden feeling, I always crave food with lots of warming qualities in the autumn: rich curries and dishes shot through with Mexican chiles. It's easy to work whole grains into your fall meals because nutty brown grains, such as bulgur, brown basmati, and buckwheat, feel just right alongside these big flavors. And nothing tastes better for breakfast, dessert, or snacks than apples at their freshest.

FALL'S KEY INGREDIENTS

VEGETABLES

Bell peppers

Black-eyed peas

Cabbage

Carrots

Cauliflower and Romanesco

Chicories

Cranberry and cannellini beans

Eggplant

Kale

Leeks

Mushrooms

Parsnips

Poblano (pasilla) chiles

Tomatoes

FRUIT

Apples

Figs

Fuyu persimmons

Grapes

Pears

OTHER

Ginger

Pecans

Turmeric

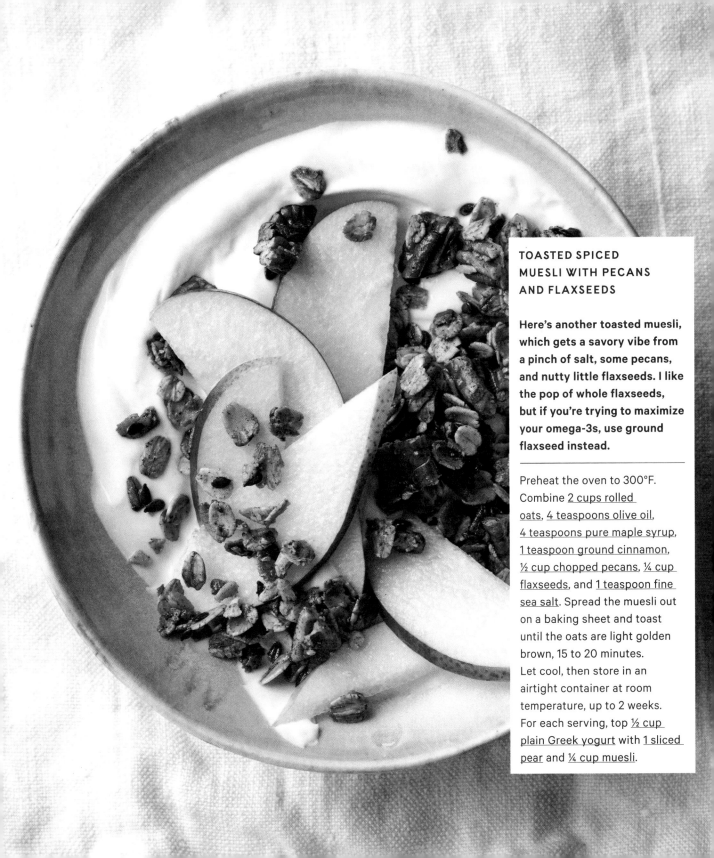

TOASTED SPICED MUESLI WITH PECANS AND FLAXSEEDS

Here's another toasted muesli, which gets a savory vibe from a pinch of salt, some pecans, and nutty little flaxseeds. I like the pop of whole flaxseeds, but if you're trying to maximize your omega-3s, use ground flaxseed instead.

Preheat the oven to 300°F. Combine 2 cups rolled oats, 4 teaspoons olive oil, 4 teaspoons pure maple syrup, 1 teaspoon ground cinnamon, ½ cup chopped pecans, ¼ cup flaxseeds, and 1 teaspoon fine sea salt. Spread the muesli out on a baking sheet and toast until the oats are light golden brown, 15 to 20 minutes. Let cool, then store in an airtight container at room temperature, up to 2 weeks. For each serving, top ½ cup plain Greek yogurt with 1 sliced pear and ¼ cup muesli.

MORNING BULGUR WITH DRIED APRICOTS AND PISTACHIOS

12 TO 15 MINUTES	MAKES 1 SERVING

- ⅓ cup medium bulgur wheat
- Pinch of fine sea salt
- 1 tablespoon chopped pistachios
- 1 teaspoon orange zest
- ⅓ cup almond milk
- 1 teaspoon honey (optional)
- ¼ cup sliced dried apricots

Bulgur is the cracked whole wheat that is the quick-cooking building block of tabbouleh, but it tastes so good in a sweeter mode, too. You can find it in the bulk section of health food stores and online from bobsredmill.com. Scented with orange and sweetened with tangy dried apricots, it's perfect for a warming (but not too heavy) breakfast.

In a small saucepan, combine the bulgur, ⅔ cup water, salt, ½ tablespoon of the pistachios, and the orange zest. Bring to a boil over medium-high heat, then reduce the heat to a very gentle simmer. Cook until the bulgur is tender, 10 to 12 minutes. Stir in the almond milk and the honey, if using. Serve topped with apricots and the remaining ½ tablespoon of pistachios.

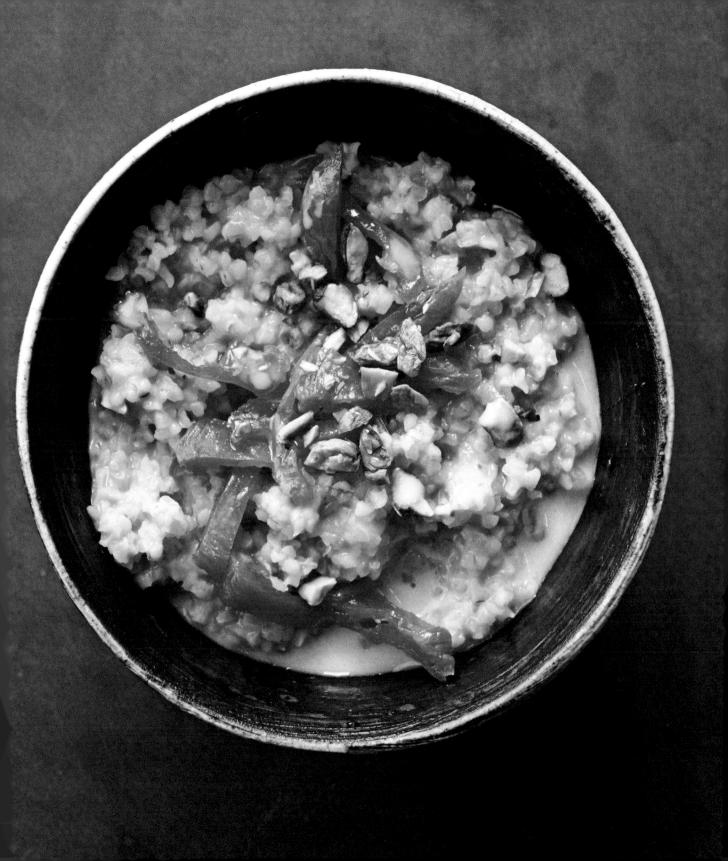

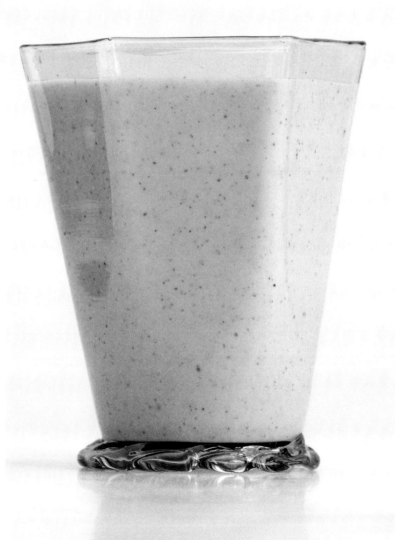

MANGO-ALMOND LASSI WITH CARDAMOM

I love the idea of a lassi, the soothing Indian yogurt drink that can be salty or sweet, but too often when I order one to go with a curry, it ends up way too sweet and heavy for the meal. Here I take the concept and make a whole breakfast out of it, with less sugar, more fruit, and some almond butter blended in to make the shake satisfying until lunch.

In a blender, combine 1 cup peeled, diced fresh mango, 1 tablespoon almond butter, ½ cup plain kefir (or ⅔ cup plain Greek yogurt mixed with 4 tablespoons water), 1 pinch ground cardamom, 1 teaspoon agave syrup, an optional pinch of salt, and ½ cup of ice. Blend on high until very smooth.

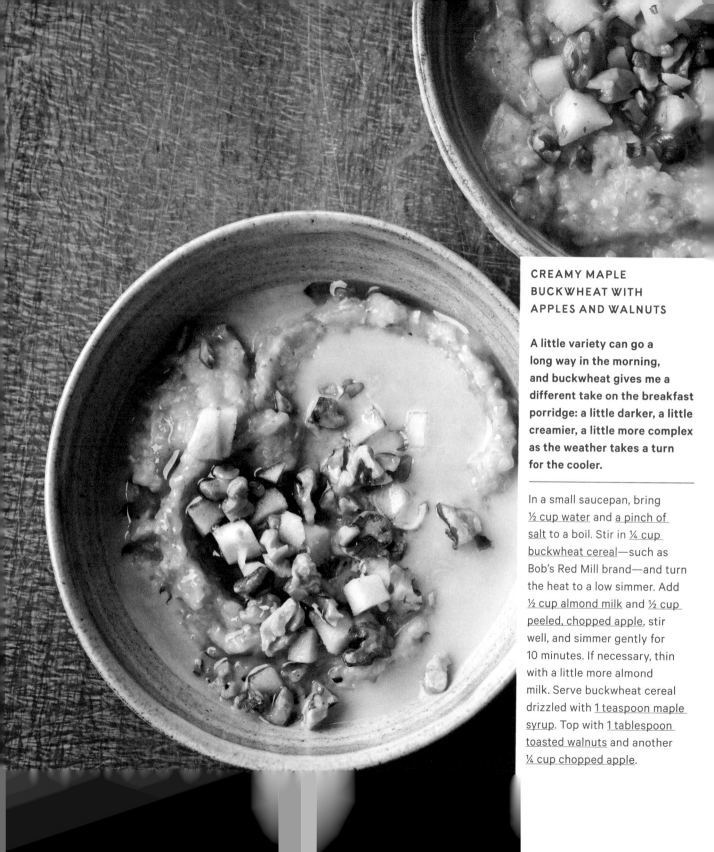

CREAMY MAPLE BUCKWHEAT WITH APPLES AND WALNUTS

A little variety can go a long way in the morning, and buckwheat gives me a different take on the breakfast porridge: a little darker, a little creamier, a little more complex as the weather takes a turn for the cooler.

In a small saucepan, bring ½ cup water and a pinch of salt to a boil. Stir in ¼ cup buckwheat cereal—such as Bob's Red Mill brand—and turn the heat to a low simmer. Add ½ cup almond milk and ½ cup peeled, chopped apple, stir well, and simmer gently for 10 minutes. If necessary, thin with a little more almond milk. Serve buckwheat cereal drizzled with 1 teaspoon maple syrup. Top with 1 tablespoon toasted walnuts and another ¼ cup chopped apple.

FRIED EGG WITH TANGY TOMATO RELISH AND SAUTÉED SPROUTS

5 MINUTES	MAKES 1 SERVING

- 2 teaspoons olive oil
- 1 or 2 large eggs
- Fine sea salt and freshly ground black pepper
- Red pepper flakes, such as Aleppo or Marash
- 1 cup pea, radish, or mung bean sprouts
- 1 tablespoon Tangy Tomato Relish (page 190)

Sprouts add a bit of crunch and greenery to your morning meal with minimal prep. Markets near me have taken to carrying fresh pea sprouts all year round, and I love their ultra-green color and nutty taste. Other sprouts will do well, too, especially those with a little bite (such as radish or broccoli sprouts) or a hearty texture (such as mung bean sprouts). If you need a more substantial breakfast, feel free to fry an extra egg for yourself.

Have a warm plate ready.

Place a nonstick pan over medium-high heat. Heat 1 teaspoon of the oil, then pour the egg(s) into the pan, season with salt, black pepper, and red pepper flakes, and let bubble and crisp a bit on the edges, about 1½ minutes. Add 2 teaspoons water and cover with a lid. Cook until the yolk is the desired firmness; a runny yolk with well-set whites takes about 1 minute. Wipe out the pan.

Heat the remaining 1 teaspoon olive oil in the skillet over medium-high heat. Add the sprouts, season with salt, and stir-fry until warm and slightly wilted, about 1 minute. Serve the egg(s) with the sautéed sprouts and tomato relish alongside.

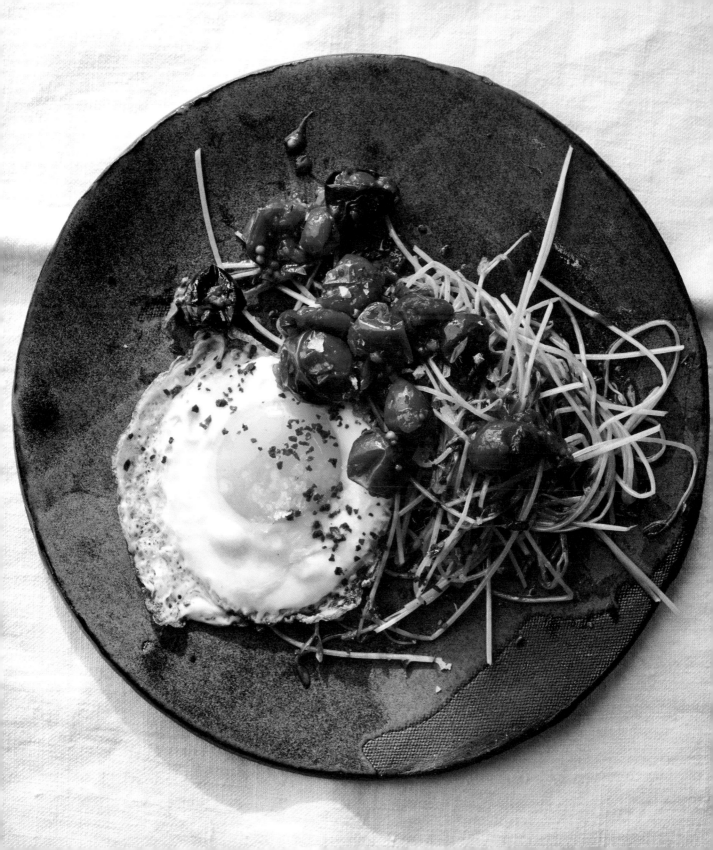

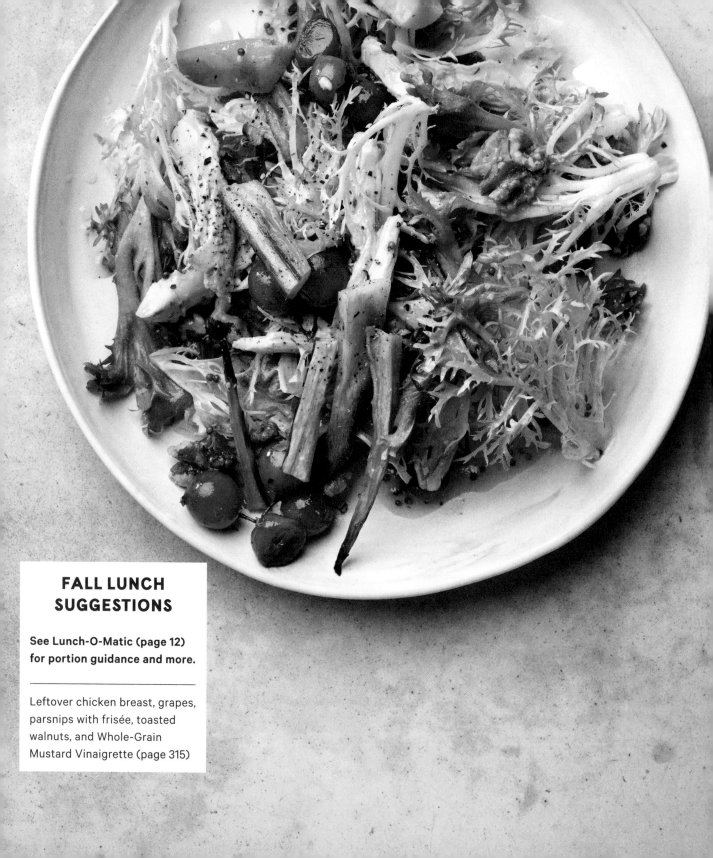

FALL LUNCH SUGGESTIONS

See Lunch-O-Matic (page 12) for portion guidance and more.

Leftover chicken breast, grapes, parsnips with frisée, toasted walnuts, and Whole-Grain Mustard Vinaigrette (page 315)

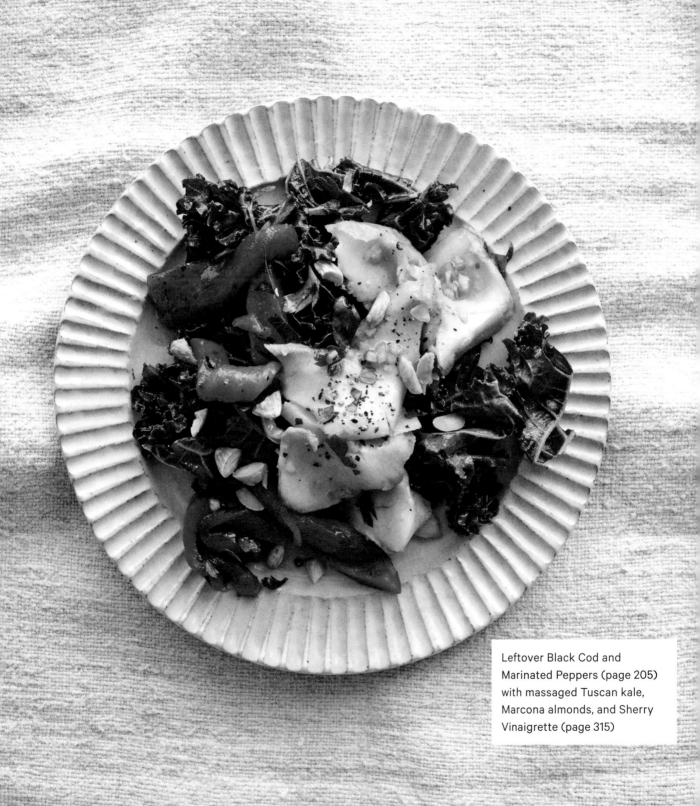

Leftover Black Cod and
Marinated Peppers (page 205)
with massaged Tuscan kale,
Marcona almonds, and Sherry
Vinaigrette (page 315)

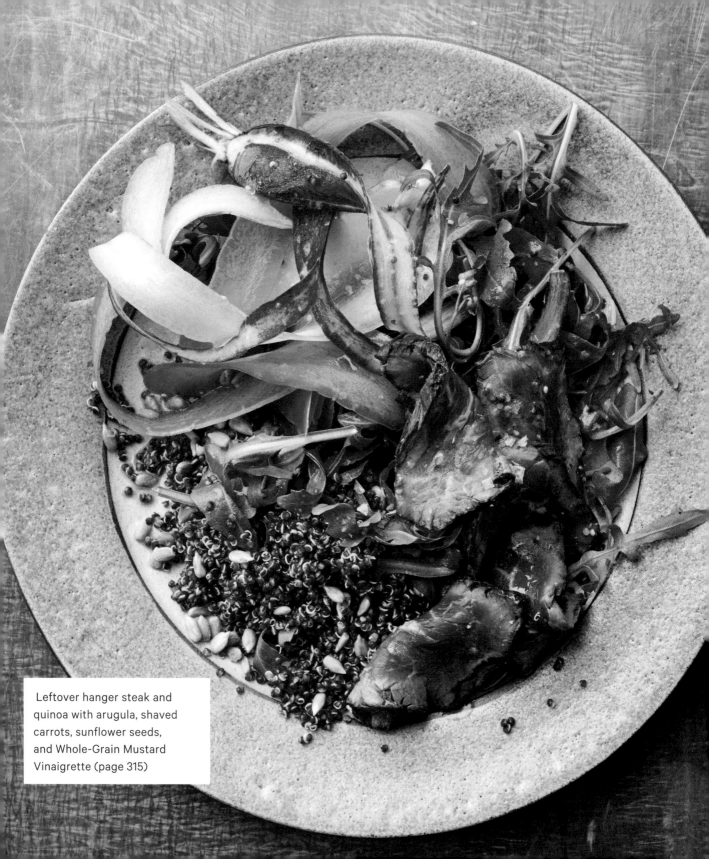

Leftover hanger steak and quinoa with arugula, shaved carrots, sunflower seeds, and Whole-Grain Mustard Vinaigrette (page 315)

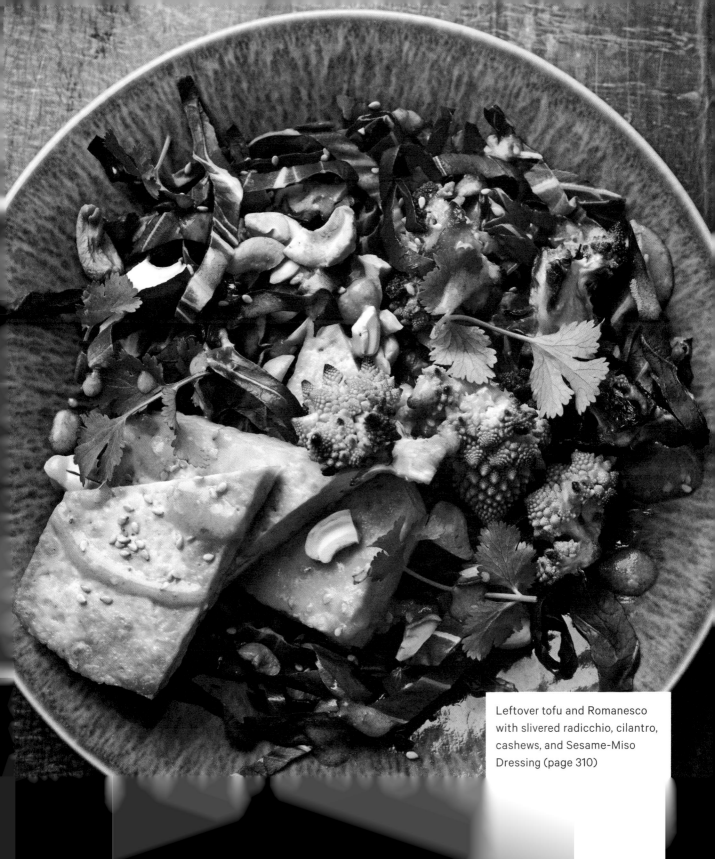

Leftover tofu and Romanesco with slivered radicchio, cilantro, cashews, and Sesame-Miso Dressing (page 310)

ROASTED PORK TENDERLOIN WITH APPLE AND MUSHROOM SAUTÉ

60 MINUTES (30 ACTIVE)	4 SERVINGS AND 1 LUNCH THE NEXT DAY

- 1¼-pound pork tenderloin, trimmed of excess external fat or membrane
- Fine sea salt and freshly ground black pepper
- 2 tablespoons vegetable oil
- 1 medium Honeycrisp or Braeburn apple, cored and cut into ¾-inch wedges
- 8 ounces cremini (baby bella) or other mushrooms, trimmed and quartered
- 1 garlic clove, finely chopped
- 1 teaspoon chopped fresh sage leaves

This is a fall dish from central casting. With the succulence of caramelized apples, the gentle tenderness of pork tenderloin, and the earthiness of sage-sautéed mushrooms, it's the kind of thing you want to eat after a day outside in the crisp air. Feel free to play around with the mix of mushrooms. Good old cremini provide abundant, meaty flavor at any time of the year, but sometimes fall brings a glut of wild finds such as chanterelles or porcini, whose distinct flavors are always welcome in my skillet.

Remove the tenderloin from the refrigerator about 30 minutes before cooking and season it generously with salt and pepper. Preheat the oven to 350°F.

Heat 1 tablespoon of the oil over medium-high heat in a large ovenproof skillet. Add the pork and apple wedges and cook, turning the pork and apples occasionally, until the pork and apples are browned, about 12 minutes. Transfer the skillet to the oven and roast until an instant-read thermometer inserted into the center of the thickest part of the pork registers 140°F, 5 to 10 minutes. Transfer the pork and apples to a plate along with any juices and let rest at least 10 minutes until slicing. Return the skillet to the stovetop.

Heat the remaining 1 tablespoon oil in the skillet over medium-high heat. Add the mushrooms and season with salt and pepper. Cook, tossing occasionally, until the mushrooms are browned and tender, about 5 minutes. Add the garlic, sage, and ½ cup water and cook, stirring and scraping up any browned bits from the bottom of the skillet, until the liquid has almost completely evaporated, about 2 minutes. Add the apples and any accumulated juices to the skillet and toss to combine.

Slice the pork across the grain into ½-inch medallions and serve with the mushrooms, apples, and pan juices.

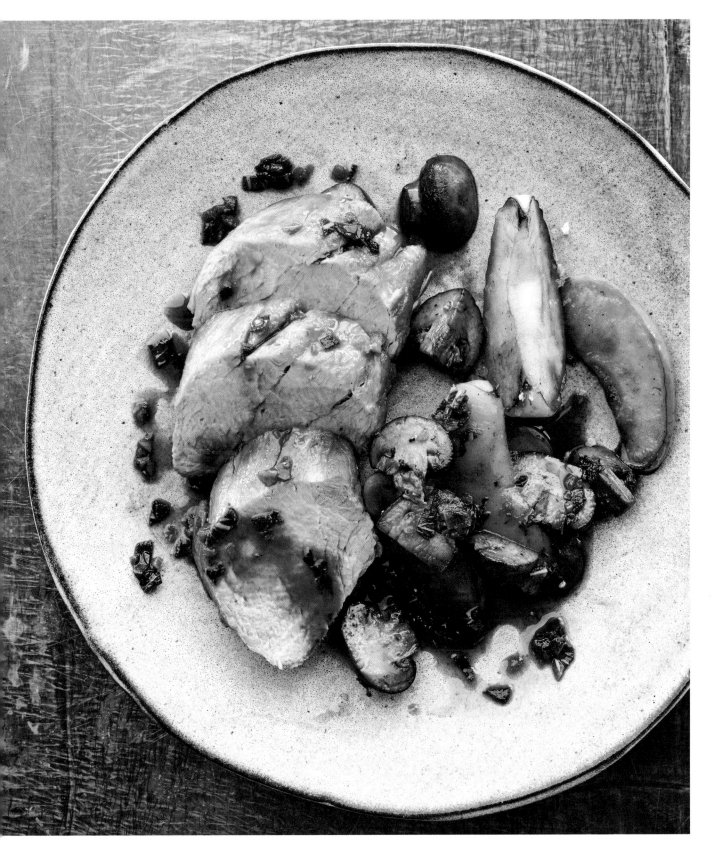

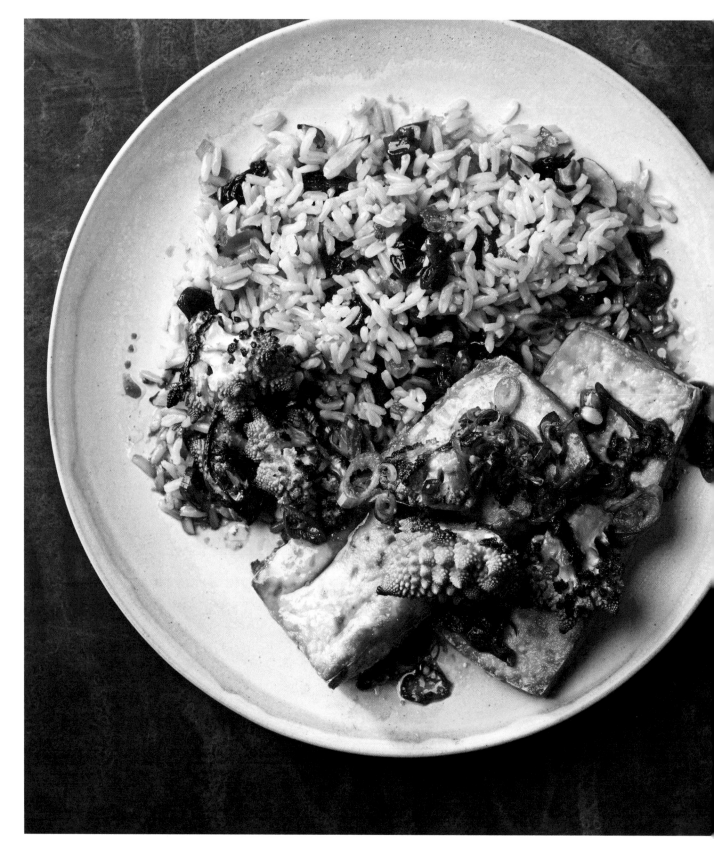

OVEN-ROASTED TOFU AND ROMANESCO WITH GINGER-SCALLION SAUCE

30 MINUTES (15 ACTIVE)	4 SERVINGS AND 1 LUNCH THE NEXT DAY

- 1 package extra-firm tofu, drained and cut into 5 lengthwise slabs (each will be about ¾ inch thick)
- 2 tablespoons plus 2 teaspoons softened coconut oil or neutral oil, such as canola or grapeseed
- Fine sea salt and freshly ground black pepper to taste
- 1 large head (2½ to 3 pounds) Romanesco or purple cauliflower, cut into ½-inch pieces
- 1 cup thinly sliced scallions, white and dark green parts (about 1½ bunches)
- 2 teaspoons finely grated peeled fresh ginger
- 1 small Thai chile, thinly sliced on the diagonal
- 1 tablespoon light soy sauce
- 2 tablespoons sherry vinegar or rice vinegar
- Flaky sea salt, for serving
- 8 fresh cilantro sprigs, for garnish (optional)

A supergroup of easy-to-find grocery ingredients, ginger, scallions, and soy sauce have the charisma and punch to wake up even the simplest ingredients. Here they turn their charms on crisp-roasted tofu and Romanesco, the pointy green cousin of cauliflower (feel free to substitute cauliflower). You could just as easily make extra dressing and toss it with soba noodles or use it to garnish thin-sliced flank steak.

Preheat the oven to 425°F.

Press the excess water out of the tofu: Place a double layer of paper towels on a large plate, spread the tofu out on it, and place another double layer on top. Weight the tofu down with another large plate (or several) for at least 15 minutes before cooking.

Brush both sides of the pressed tofu with 2 teaspoons of the oil and season with fine sea salt and pepper. Arrange in a single layer on a baking sheet. Roast until lightly browned on the surface and around the edges, about 15 minutes.

Toss the Romanesco with 2 tablespoons of the coconut oil and season to taste with fine sea salt and pepper. Arrange in a single layer on another baking sheet and roast until lightly browned and crispy, about 18 minutes. If you roast it at the same time as the tofu, rotate the pan location at least once during cooking.

In a small bowl, whisk together the scallions, ginger, chile, soy sauce, and vinegar.

Toss the roasted Romanesco with 1 tablespoon of the dressing.

Serve the roasted tofu with the Romanesco and spoon ginger-scallion dressing on top. Sprinkle with flaky sea salt and garnish with cilantro, if desired.

OVEN-ROASTED CHICKEN WITH GRAPES

16 MINUTES (8 ACTIVE)	4 SERVINGS AND 1 LUNCH THE NEXT DAY

- 2 pounds skin-on, bone-in chicken breasts
- ½ teaspoon five-spice powder or ¼ teaspoon ground cinnamon
- Fine sea salt and freshly ground black pepper
- 2 teaspoons olive oil
- 6 shallots, quartered
- 6 sprigs fresh thyme
- 1 large (12-ounce) bunch of red grapes on the stem
- 1 tablespoon white wine vinegar

Five-spice powder, the Chinese mixture that most typically contains star anise, fennel, cinnamon, cloves, and Sichuan peppercorns, is a big infatuation of mine. Its sweet-spicy aroma somehow conveys a rich meatiness to the ingredients it touches, even when I sprinkle it on vegetables or tofu. It also plays wonderfully off fruit, such as stem-on grapes tossed in the oven alongside chicken breasts to concentrate their sweet-tart juices. The method works wonderfully with plums, too.

Preheat the oven to 425°F.

Season the chicken breasts on both sides with the five-spice powder and sprinkle with salt and pepper.

In a large ovenproof skillet, heat the oil over medium-high heat. Blot the chicken breasts with paper towels and add them to the pan skin side down; add the shallots. Cook the chicken, undisturbed, until browned and crisp, about 5 minutes; turn the shallots frequently to brown on all sides while the chicken cooks. Turn the breasts over and add the thyme and grapes to the pan. Add the vinegar and ¼ cup of water to deglaze the skillet. Season with more salt and pepper.

Transfer the pan to the oven and roast until the chicken is cooked through and the grapes just start to wrinkle, about 8 minutes. Serve the chicken with the roasted grapes and shallots alongside and any pan juices spooned on top.

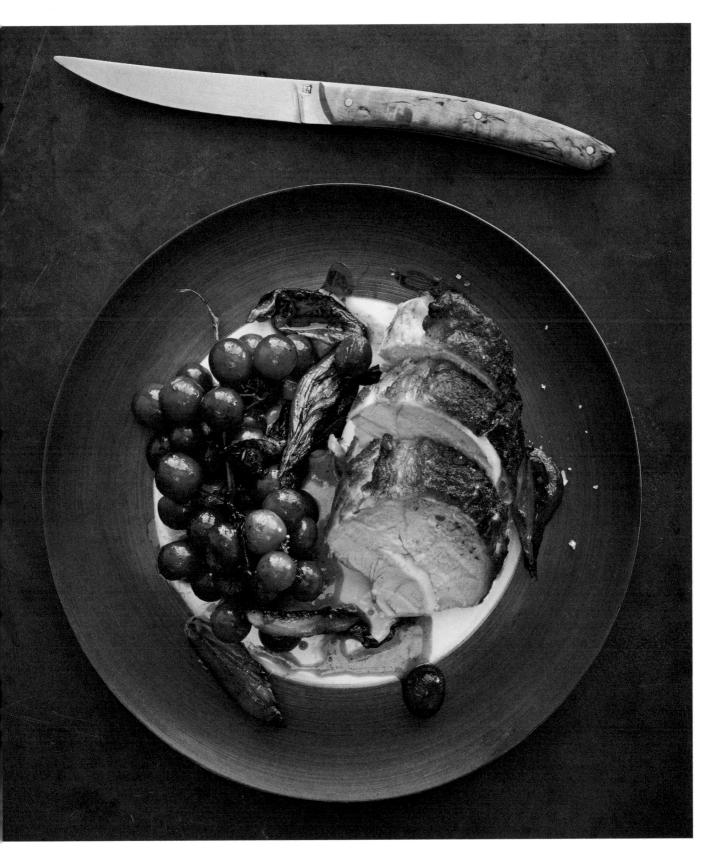

HANGER STEAK WITH TANGY TOMATO RELISH

38 MINUTES (8 ACTIVE) | **4 SERVINGS AND 1 LUNCH THE NEXT DAY**

- 1¼ pounds hanger steak (about 2 pieces), center membrane removed, or flank steak
- Fine sea salt and freshly ground black pepper to taste
- 2 teaspoons canola or vegetable oil
- Flaky sea salt (optional)
- Fresh flat-leaf parsley leaves, for garnish
- Tangy Tomato Relish (page 190)

Hanger steak is the king of what I call weeknight steaks, casual cuts of leanish meat that deliver delicious flavor without a lot of expense or fuss. The skinny strip of flesh tastes best cooked hard and fast, for a crispy char on the outside, and left nice and pink inside. Slice it with a significant slant across the grain for the best eating texture. If you can find a grass-finished hanger steak, you'll get leaner meat and a higher proportion of healthy lipids, such as omega-3s and CLAs. The bad news: hanger steak—or onglet, as it is sometimes known—can be hard to find. Even my regular butcher runs out somewhat frequently. Don't fret—just substitute flank steak.

Season the hanger steak with fine sea salt and pepper. Let steak sit at room temperature for at least 20 minutes before cooking.

Heat the oil in a heavy 9- or 10-inch skillet over high heat. Working in batches if necessary, add the steak to the pan and cook, turning once, until browned on both sides and an instant-read thermometer registers 130°F for medium-rare, 7 to 8 minutes total.

Let the steak rest at least 10 minutes, then slice it on a diagonal. Season with flaky sea salt, if desired, and serve with parsley leaves and tomato relish.

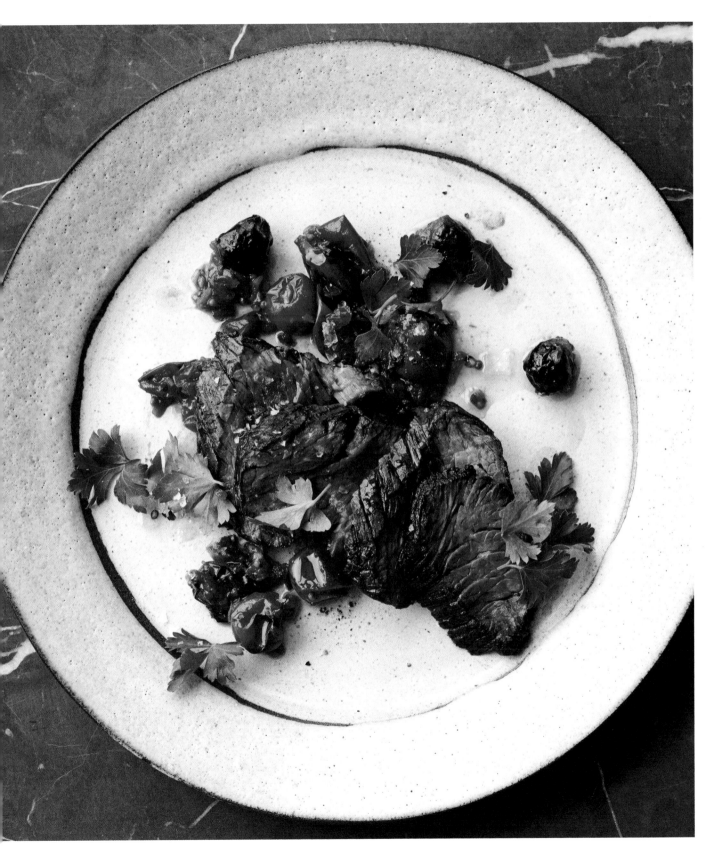

TANGY TOMATO RELISH

Pictured on page 189

30 MINUTES (10 MINUTES ACTIVE)	MAKES 3 CUPS

- 2 (14-ounce cans) cherry tomatoes, drained, or 3 cups fresh
- 2 tablespoons olive oil
- Fine sea salt and freshly ground black pepper to taste
- 1 teaspoon yellow mustard seeds
- 1 medium red onion, chopped
- 2 garlic cloves, minced
- ⅛ teaspoon red pepper flakes, such as Aleppo or Marash
- 1½ tablespoons minced peeled fresh ginger
- ¼ cup fresh orange juice
- 1 tablespoon Worcestershire sauce

I once worked for a Spanish chef who, despite his otherwise fervent nationalism, had a surprising and amusing affection for what he called "leaperrins," or Worcestershire sauce to you and me. I can't really blame him; I've been using the stuff with abandon since I was a kid. In this pairing, it gives a little depth to a tangy roasted cherry tomato relish. You may want to roast some extra cherry tomatoes while you're at it: they make a great garnish for salads and grain dishes. If you use fresh cherry tomatoes instead of skinned canned ones, you will have a more rustic texture to your relish.

Preheat the oven to 425°F.

Toss the tomatoes with 1 tablespoon of the olive oil and spread them in a single layer in a baking dish. Season with salt and black pepper to taste and roast until the tomatoes are crinkled and browned and any liquid in the pan is reduced, 18 to 20 minutes. Let cool.

In a wide nonreactive saucepan, heat the remaining 1 tablespoon oil over medium-high heat. Add the mustard seeds and cook until they pop, about 30 seconds. Add the onion, garlic, red pepper flakes, ginger, and a pinch of salt. Cook, stirring frequently, until the onion has softened, about 3 minutes. Add the roasted tomatoes and stir to combine, but take care to keep the tomatoes intact. Add the orange juice and Worcestershire sauce. Cook, stirring gently, until the juices have thickened to a jammy consistency, about 5 minutes. Taste and season with salt and black pepper. Store in an airtight container in the refrigerator for up to a week.

BROWN BASMATI RICE WITH SOUR CHERRIES AND ALMONDS *Pictured on page 184*

48 MINUTES (8 ACTIVE)	4 SERVINGS AND 1 LUNCH THE NEXT DAY

- 1¼ cups brown basmati rice (or 3½ cups previously cooked brown basmati rice)
- Fine sea salt to taste
- 1 cup chopped dried sour cherries
- ½ cup boiling water
- ¼ cup sliced almonds
- 2 tablespoons olive or coconut oil
- ½ cup chopped onion
- 1 garlic clove, chopped
- ¼ teaspoon ground cinnamon

Brown basmati rice has a more evocative fragrance than standard brown rice, and it marries well with tangy bits of dried fruit. Switching white rice for brown is a nice way to add some fiber to your meal, but do note that it will take a bit longer to pull off. Whenever I cook it, I make extra to keep around for another meal. If you make a double batch of rice beforehand, spread it out on a sheet pan to cool. When it's at room temperature, place it in an airtight container and chill or freeze.

In a medium saucepan, bring the rice, salt, and 2½ cups water to a boil over medium-high heat. Turn the heat to a low simmer, cover the pan, and cook until the rice is tender, 40 minutes. Let it sit, covered, for 10 minutes more, then fluff the rice with a fork.

While the rice is cooking, place the cherries in a small bowl and pour the boiling water over them. Let sit for at least 10 minutes.

In a large dry skillet, toast the almonds over medium-high heat, tossing frequently until lightly colored, about 2 minutes. Reserve.

In a wide skillet or saucepan, heat the oil over medium-high heat. Add the onion, season with a pinch of salt, and cook, stirring frequently, until the onion is translucent and slightly browned on the edges, 3 to 4 minutes. Stir in the garlic and cinnamon and cook for 30 seconds. Add the rice, cherries, and their liquid and stir, using a wooden spoon to break up any clumps in the rice. Cook, tossing frequently, until the water is absorbed, the rice sizzles, and the grains are nicely separated. Toss in the toasted almonds and adjust the seasoning with salt and pepper to taste.

CHICKPEA AND EGGPLANT CURRY WITH MINT CHUTNEY

35 MINUTES (20 ACTIVE)	4 SERVINGS AND 1 LUNCH THE NEXT DAY

- 2 tablespoons coconut or canola oil
- 1 teaspoon cumin seeds
- 1 teaspoon mustard seeds
- 3 garlic cloves, chopped
- 1 tablespoon minced ginger
- 1 medium onion, chopped
- Fine sea salt to taste
- 1 teaspoon ground turmeric
- Pinch of ground cayenne pepper
- 2 large tomatoes, grated on a large grate, with juices reserved
- 1¼ pounds eggplant, cut into ½-inch cubes (about 5 cups)
- 15-ounce can chickpeas, drained and rinsed, or 1¼ cups drained cooked chickpeas
- 4 teaspoons minced jalapeño
- 1 shallot, minced
- 1 tablespoon lime juice, plus more to taste
- 1 teaspoon honey
- 2 tablespoons unsweetened flaked coconut
- 1 cup roughly chopped fresh mint leaves
- ¼ cup roughly chopped fresh cilantro leaves
- Freshly ground black pepper to taste
- Plain yogurt, for garnish

Maybe there's something in the warm yellow tint in autumn sunlight, but fall makes me crave golden curries, especially vegetarian ones. The ingredient list for a curry can be a little daunting with all those spices, but the technique isn't very far from a pasta sauce: you just toast the whole spices and then move on to a sort of *sofrito* of onion, garlic, and ginger. From that flavor base, you add tomatoes and whatever veggies you desire. At the end, a quick chutney, really just a rough chopped blend of herbs and coconut, gives the stew a bright pop of flavor (the way a few torn basil leaves make that tomato sauce sing).

In a large covered skillet or Dutch oven, heat the oil over medium-high heat. Add the cumin and mustard seeds and stir for 30 seconds, then add the garlic and the ginger. Stir constantly until the garlic just begins to brown, 1 minute, then stir in the onion and a generous pinch of salt. Cook, stirring frequently, until the onion is tender, about 5 minutes. Stir in the turmeric and cayenne. Pour in the grated tomatoes and their juices, scraping up any browned bits with a wooden spoon. Add the eggplant, chickpeas, ¼ cup water, and a pinch of salt, stir well, and reduce the heat to medium-low. Cover the pan and simmer until the eggplant is tender, about 15 minutes.

Remove from the heat and add the jalapeño, shallot, lime juice, and honey. Fold in the coconut, mint, and cilantro. Season to taste with salt, black pepper, and more lime juice.

Top with a dollop of yogurt.

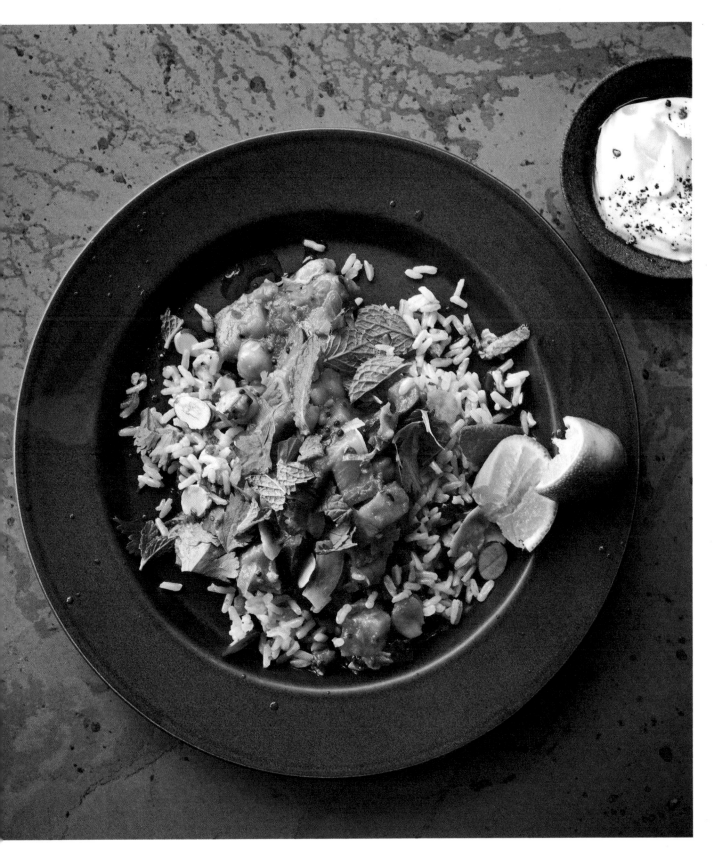

PAN-SEARED BLACK COD

15 TO 20 MINUTES (5 ACTIVE)	4 SERVINGS AND 1 LUNCH THE NEXT DAY

- 1½ pounds skin-on black cod fillet, cut into 5 portions
- Fine sea salt and freshly ground black pepper to taste
- 1 tablespoon olive oil
- Green Lentils with Thyme (recipe follows)

Black cod, also known as sable, is the fish for lovers of pork belly, brisket, and other supple, voluptuous meats. It's filled with good-for-you fish oils, and it's responsibly fished in the north Pacific. It's hard to overcook, but there are two tricks to keep the seriously flaky fish from falling apart: Cook it with its skin on (even if you remove it when you eat it). Also, salt the fish 10 to 20 minutes before cooking it to allow it to firm up a bit.

If you can't find black cod, king salmon or mackerel will give you a similar lush texture.

Season the black cod with salt and freshly ground black pepper to taste. Let it rest at room temperature for 10 to 15 minutes.

In a large skillet, heat the oil over medium-high heat. Place the cod in the pan, skin side down, and cook until browned and crisp, about 4 minutes. Gently turn the fish over and cook until just opaque at the center, about 1 minute more.

Serve the fish, skin side up, with the green lentils.

GREEN LENTILS WITH THYME

Use kitchen twine to tie together a bundle of 8 fresh thyme sprigs, 6 fresh parsley sprigs, and 1 bay leaf. Heat 2 tablespoons olive oil in a 3- or 4-quart saucepan over medium heat. Add in 1 finely chopped onion and a small dried chile; cook until the onion is fragrant and softened, about 3 minutes. Stir in 1¼ cup green lentils, and cook for 1 minute. Pour in 3 cups boiling water and 1 teaspoon fine sea salt. Reduce the heat to a low simmer, cover the pan and cook, stirring occasionally, until the lentils are tender, but still retain their shape, about 30 to 35 minutes. Sprinkle in 1¼ teaspoons fresh thyme leaves and season to taste with additional salt and black pepper. Drizzle with an additional tablespoon of olive oil and garnish with pea sprouts, if desired.

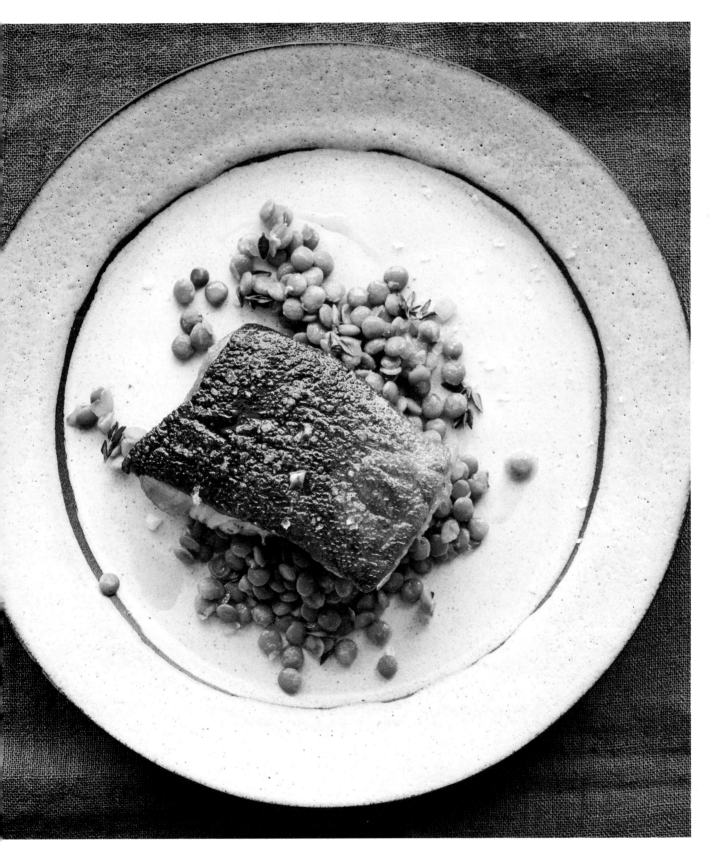

BUFFALO PATTIES WITH TANGY TOMATO RELISH, AVOCADO, AND BUTTER LETTUCE

12 TO 15 MINUTES	4 SERVINGS

- 1 pound ground bison or lean grass-fed beef
- 1 large garlic clove, minced
- ½ teaspoon ancho chili powder
- 1 tablespoon olive oil
- Fine sea salt and freshly ground black pepper to taste
- 2 teaspoons neutral oil, such as canola or grapeseed
- 1 ripe avocado, pitted, peeled, and cut into eighths
- Flaky sea salt to finish
- 1 head butter lettuce, well washed and dried
- Tangy Tomato Relish (page 190)

Bison started showing up in my local grocery not too long ago, and I started playing around with it; I like to substitute it for beef from time to time, since the lean, protein-packed meat delivers a little wildness in taste without tipping over into full-on gaminess. It crisps up beautifully in these little patties, which I serve with lettuce wraps and avocado, plus tart tomato relish. You do want to make sure not to overcook bison, since its mineraly taste is best suited to medium-rare.

In a large bowl, gently mix the ground meat with the garlic, chili powder, olive oil, and fine sea salt and pepper. Divide the meat into 8 portions and gently shape them into patties about ½ inch thick.

Heat a grill pan, griddle, or heavy-bottomed skillet over medium-high heat. Add the neutral oil, and using tongs to grip a folded paper towel, thoroughly coat the cooking surface.

Working in batches if necessary, add the patties and cook the burgers until browned on one side, 1½ to 2 minutes. Flip the burgers and cook them to the desired doneness, 2½ to 3 minutes total for medium-rare.

Top with the avocado slices and sprinkle with flaky sea salt. Serve each burger with some lettuce and tomato relish.

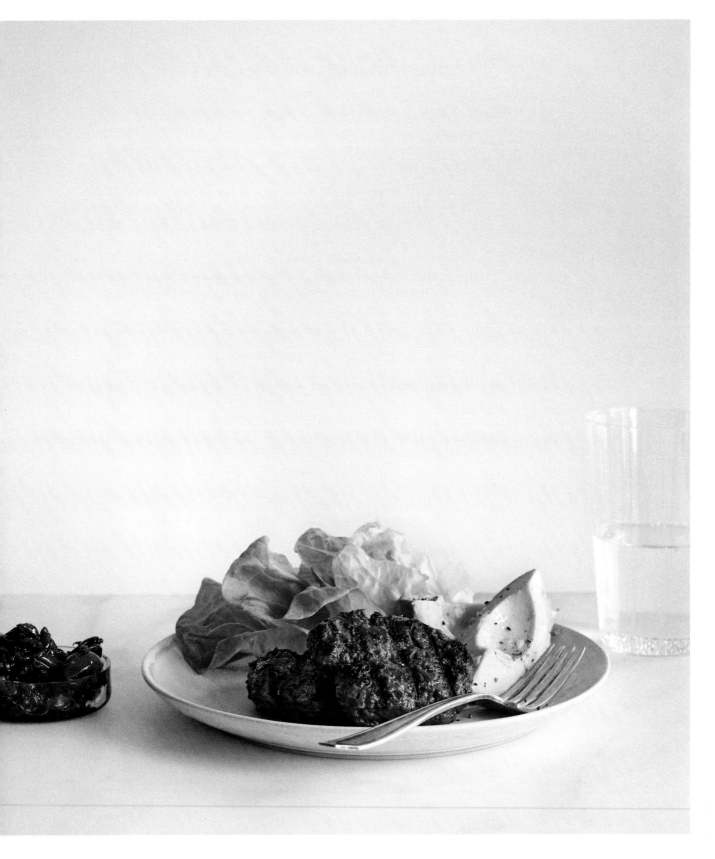

CURRIED MUSSELS WITH LEEKS

15 MINUTES	4 SERVINGS

- 2½ pounds mussels
- 1 tablespoon vegetable oil
- 1 large leek (white and light green parts, well rinsed), cut crosswise into ¼-inch slices
- Fine sea salt and freshly ground black pepper to taste
- 2 garlic cloves, sliced
- 1½ teaspoons Madras curry powder
- ½ cup canned coconut milk
- 2 tablespoons roughly chopped fresh cilantro leaves

Gorgeous black-shelled mussels contrast so elegantly with a spiced, pale yellow stock. The only trick is careful handling of your mussels. Purchase them within a couple days of cooking, and store them in the fridge in a strainer set above a big bowl, with a clean damp kitchen towel on top and a handful of ice on top of the towel. Wait to clean them shortly before cooking; it doesn't take long, and once you start cooking, you'll be impressed with how quickly this elegant dish comes together.

Clean the mussels under running water. Discard any broken shells or mussels that will not close quickly when gently squeezed. Using a clean kitchen towel, pinch and pull away any stringy beards from the mussels.

Heat the oil in a large heavy-bottomed pot over medium-high heat. Add the leek slices, season them with salt and pepper, and cook, stirring often, until softened, about 5 minutes. Add the garlic and curry powder and cook, stirring, until fragrant, about 1 minute. Add the mussels, coconut milk, and ½ cup water. Bring to a boil, reduce the heat to low, cover, and cook until the mussels have opened, about 5 minutes (discard any mussels that have not opened).

Serve the mussels topped with cilantro.

ROASTED YUKON GOLD POTATOES

Preheat the oven to 425°F. Cut 4 medium Yukon Gold potatoes into wedges, leaving the skins on for extra flavor, texture, and fiber. Toss them with 1 tablespoon olive oil, salt, and pepper, and lay them in a single layer on a baking sheet. Roast, turning once, until browned and crisp, about 25 to 28 minutes.

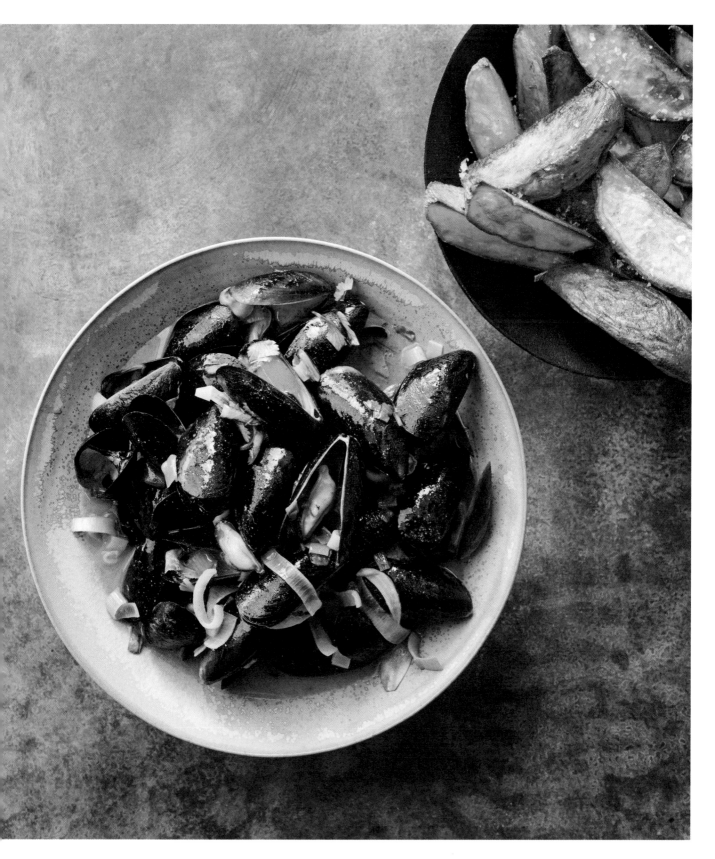

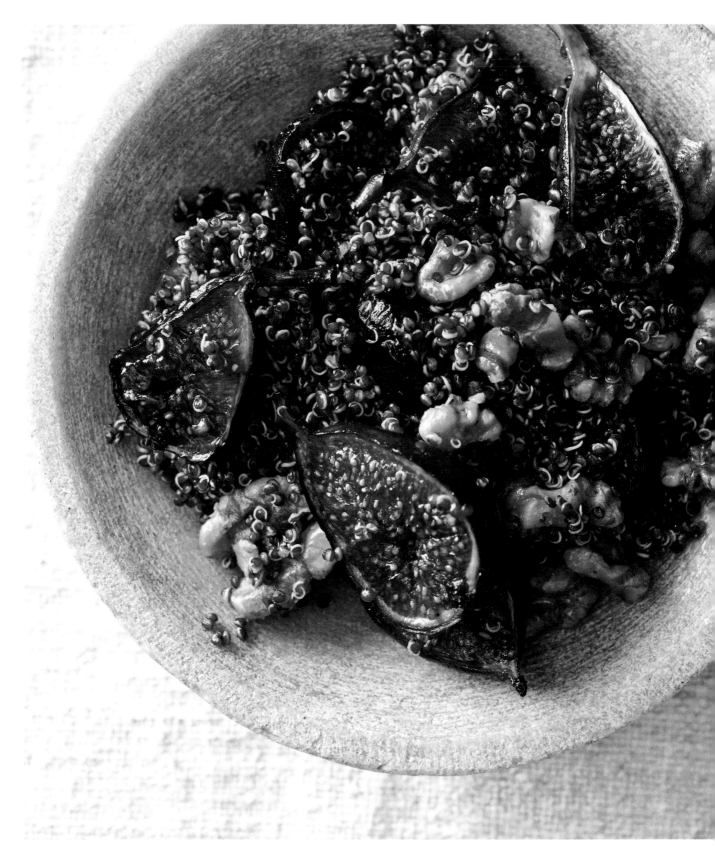

RED QUINOA WITH ROASTED FIGS AND WALNUTS

20 TO 25 MINUTES	4 SERVINGS AND 1 LUNCH THE NEXT DAY

- 8 ounces ripe figs (any variety), halved
- 1 tablespoon plus 2 teaspoons olive oil
- 2 tablespoons balsamic vinegar
- Fine sea salt and freshly ground black pepper to taste
- 1¼ cups red, white, or black quinoa
- ½ cup chopped walnuts
- ½ cup sliced scallions, white, light green, and dark green parts finely sliced and middle section discarded or saved for stock

Though they come from completely different food cultures, figs and quinoa both have little round, bursting seeds that tie together this simple pilaf. To pick the perfect figs for roasting, wait until they're heavy for their size and just a bit yielding to your touch: one or two figs in the container will likely have split open a bit. If you can't find good fresh figs, then use about 4 ounces of dried figs. (In this case skip the roasting; instead, you can plump them in simmering water for 10 minutes before tossing with the oil and balsamic.)

Preheat the oven to 425°F.

Toss the figs with the 1 tablespoon oil and 1 tablespoon of the balsamic vinegar. Arrange the figs in a single layer in a baking dish and season lightly with the salt and pepper. Roast until the figs are juicy and glazed, 15 to 18 minutes.

Meanwhile, bring a large pot of salted water to a boil. Stir in the quinoa and cook for 10 minutes. Drain and toss in a large bowl with the remaining 2 teaspoons oil and the remaining 1 tablespoon balsamic vinegar.

Arrange the walnuts on a baking sheet or in an ovenproof skillet. Toast them lightly in the oven for 2 to 3 minutes, keeping a careful eye on them to avoid burning.

Add the scallions and walnuts to the bowl with the quinoa and toss to combine. Fold in the roasted figs, making sure to scrape in any fig juices that have collected in the baking dish. Taste and add more salt and pepper, if desired.

CLAMS WITH WHITE BEANS AND GREMOLATA

8 TO 10 MINUTES	4 SERVINGS

- 2 pounds small hard-shell clams, such as Manila or littleneck, scrubbed and soaked in clean water for 15 minutes
- 1 cup finely chopped fresh flat-leaf parsley leaves
- 2 garlic cloves, finely minced
- 1 tablespoon finely grated lemon peel
- 2 tablespoons olive oil
- Pinch of hot red pepper, preferably Aleppo or Marash
- 2 (15-ounce) cans cannellini beans, drained and rinsed, or 3 cups drained cooked cannellini beans
- ¾ cup homemade chicken stock (see page 301) or low-sodium canned

Cooking in a Basque/Spanish restaurant made me appreciate the beauty of seafood (squid, mussels, clams) simmered with beans. The beans are thirsty for all the juices that the shellfish release during cooking, so no delicious essence gets lost to the pan. If you have time, cook your own cannellini beans as described on page 303. If not, choose your favorite canned bean brand. Naturally, if you have access to good jarred Spanish white beans such as pochas (spanishtable.com), I urge you to try them here!

Sort through the clams and discard any with broken shells or that do not remain closed when pinched shut. Lift them out of the soaking water, rinse, and set aside.

Mix together the parsley, half the garlic, and the lemon peel. Set aside.

In a wide covered saucepan or Dutch oven, heat the oil over medium-high heat. Stir in the remaining garlic and the red pepper flakes, and then add the clams to the pan. Stir well to coat, then add the beans and stock. Cover and cook until the clams open, 4 to 6 minutes (discard any that do not open). Stir the parsley mixture into the clams and serve each bowl with beans and a bit of stock.

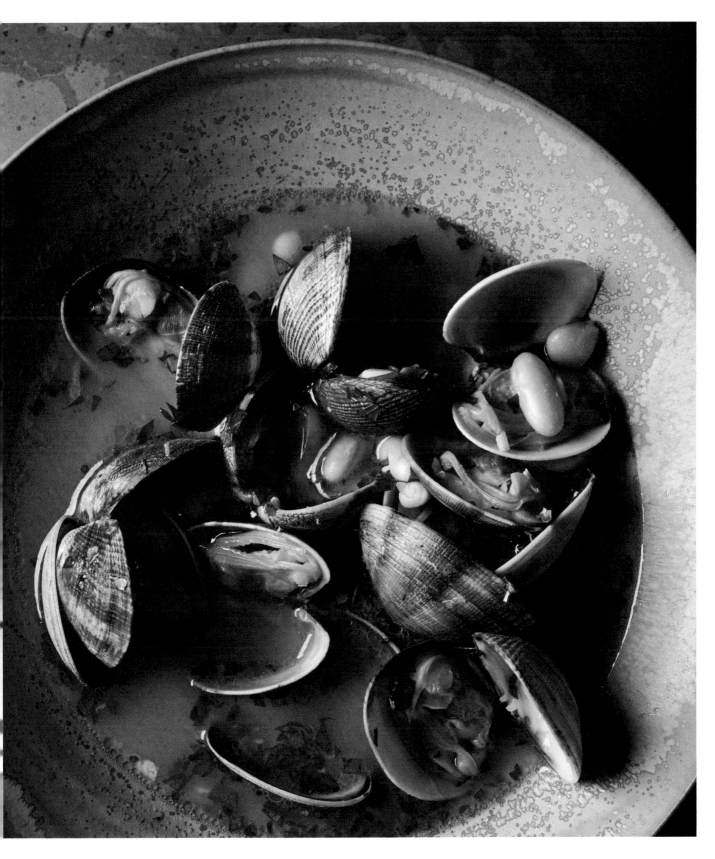

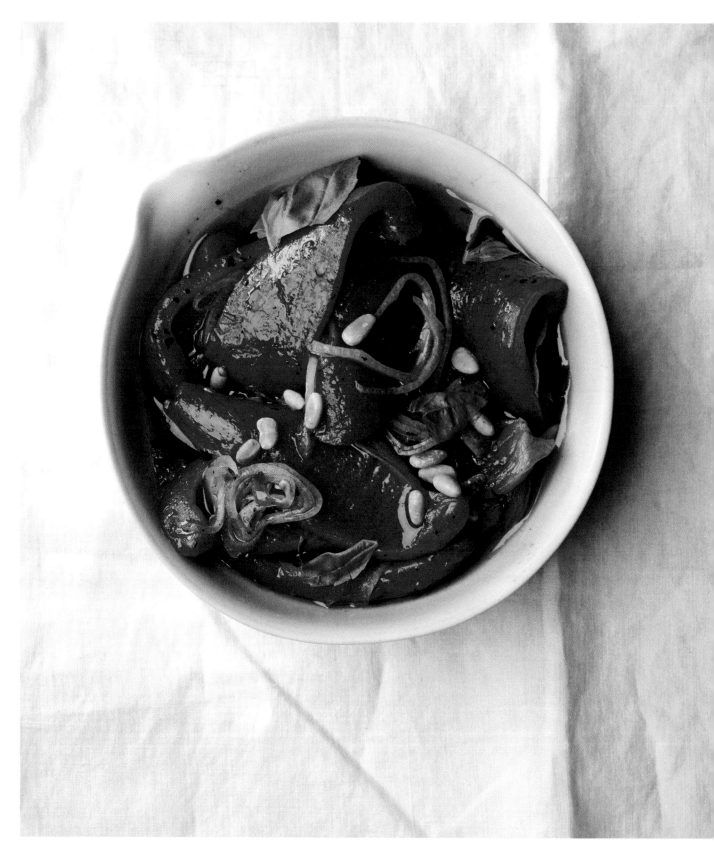

MARINATED PEPPERS

| 40 MINUTES (10 ACTIVE) | 2¼ CUPS |

- 4 large red bell peppers
- 2 tablespoons pine nuts
- 1 shallot, sliced
- 1 small garlic clove, grated
- 1 tablespoon sherry vinegar
- 3 tablespoons olive oil
- Flaky sea salt and freshly ground black pepper to taste
- ¼ cup torn fresh basil or flat-leaf parsley leaves, for garnish

Bell peppers are sometimes seen as a hack ingredient, thrown willy-nilly into dishes for a jolt of color and a simple bit of sweetness. But I'm all for an ingredient that can be found at any grocery and brings big flavor to a simple meal. Licked with the heat of a sizzling grill or a red-hot broiler, your peppers soften, sweeten, and develop just an edge of bitterness. A quick marinade of vinegar, garlic, and oil fends off any cloyingness.

Set an oven rack in the top third of the oven and preheat the broiler.

Place the bell peppers on a baking sheet and broil, turning occasionally, until they are browned and blistered all over, 18 to 20 minutes. Transfer the peppers to a medium bowl, cover, and let steam until cool enough to handle, about 15 minutes (this will help loosen the skins).

Meanwhile, in a small dry skillet, toast the pine nuts over medium-low heat, tossing often, until golden brown, 2 to 4 minutes. Remove from the pan and reserve.

In a medium bowl, whisk together the shallot, garlic, and vinegar.

When the peppers are cool enough to handle, remove the skins, stems, and seeds. Cut them into 1½-inch-wide strips and arrange them on a large shallow plate.

Whisk the oil into the shallot mixture and pour the dressing over the peppers. Season with the flaky sea salt and black pepper and garnish with the basil and toasted pine nuts.

BLACK-EYED PEAS WITH ROASTED TOMATOES AND CHIVES

25 TO 30 MINUTES	4 SERVINGS AND 1 LUNCH THE NEXT DAY

- 1 (14-ounce) can cherry tomatoes, drained, or 1 pint fresh
- 3 tablespoons olive oil
- Fine sea salt and freshly ground black pepper to taste
- 3 garlic cloves, sliced
- 2 cups frozen black-eyed peas
- ½ cup 1-inch-cut chives
- Lemon wedges, for serving

Black-eyed peas tend to be quarantined to New Year's Day. If a little hoppin' John is lucky, why shouldn't we eat black-eyed peas throughout the year? Though I'm usually a big fan of cooking up dried beans, I prefer frozen or fresh black-eyed peas—they hold on to a special herbaceous note. The recipe here calls for frozen, but if you can find shelled black-eyed peas in the refrigerated section of the grocery store, they're delicious, and unlike dried, they require no soaking. To prepare, bring 2½ cups of salted water to a boil. Add the tub of black-eyed peas, reduce the heat to a vigorous simmer, and cook for 8 to 10 minutes, or until tender. Drain and then use them in the recipe, skipping the water. Another quick note: if you've got great cherry tomatoes in your garden or at the market, feel free to roast them instead of using canned.

Preheat the oven to 425°F.

Toss the tomatoes with 1 tablespoon of the oil and season with salt and pepper. Arrange in a small baking dish and roast until the tomatoes are crinkled and browned and any remaining liquid is reduced, 15 to 18 minutes.

In a large deep skillet or wide saucepan, heat the remaining 2 tablespoons oil over medium heat. Add the garlic and stir for 30 seconds. Add the black-eyed peas and ½ cup water, cover, and cook until the beans are tender, about 4 minutes. Remove the lid and gently stir until the liquid reduces, about 5 minutes. Season with a pinch of salt, toss in the tomatoes and half the chives, and stir to combine.

Serve topped with the remaining chives and a lemon wedge for squeezing over the dish.

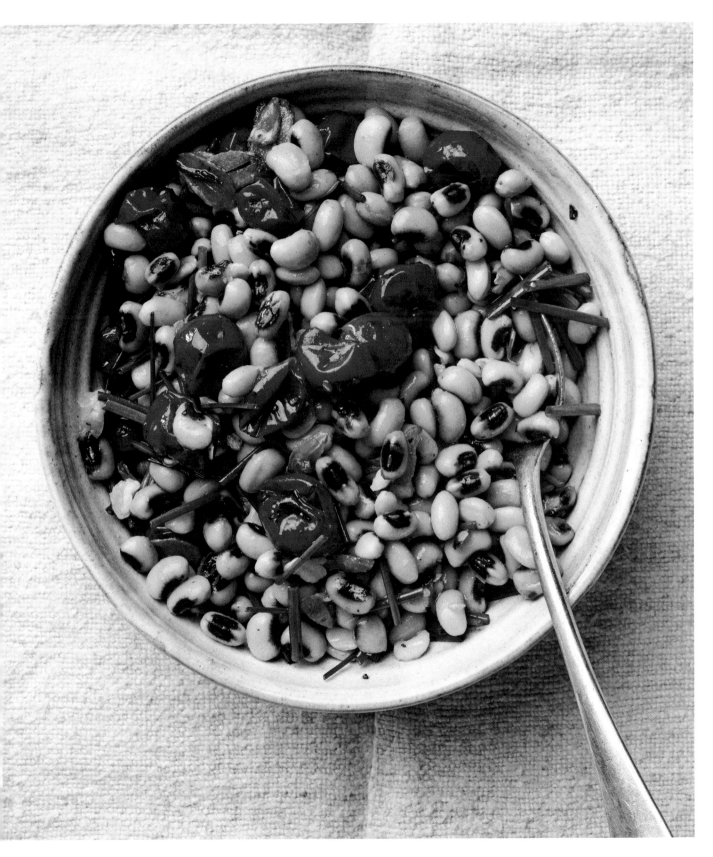

OVEN-CRISPED PARSNIPS WITH KALE

30 MINUTES (5 ACTIVE)	4 SERVINGS AND 1 LUNCH THE NEXT DAY

- 1½ pounds parsnips, peeled and quartered lengthwise
- 3 tablespoons olive oil
- Fine sea salt to taste
- 8 ounces well-washed lacinato kale (1 bunch)
- 1 garlic clove, grated

This recipe shows just how differently vegetables can react to heat. The kale, which you can grill outside or atop a grill pan, gets crisp-edged and crackly in spots, while the roasted parsnips become tender, sweet, and dappled with brown spots. They make for a lovely contrast in textures and flavors.

Preheat the oven to 425°F and preheat a grill (or a grill pan) to medium-high heat.

Toss the parsnips with 1½ tablespoons of the oil and a pinch of salt. Arrange them on a baking sheet, transfer to the oven, and roast, turning once, until browned in spots, 20 to 25 minutes.

Rub the kale with the remaining 1½ tablespoons oil and sprinkle with a pinch of salt. Grill (or cook in the grill pan) until charred and slightly wilted, turning often, about 2 minutes.

While the parsnips are still hot, place them in a large bowl and toss with the garlic. Add the kale and toss again. Season to taste with more salt, if desired.

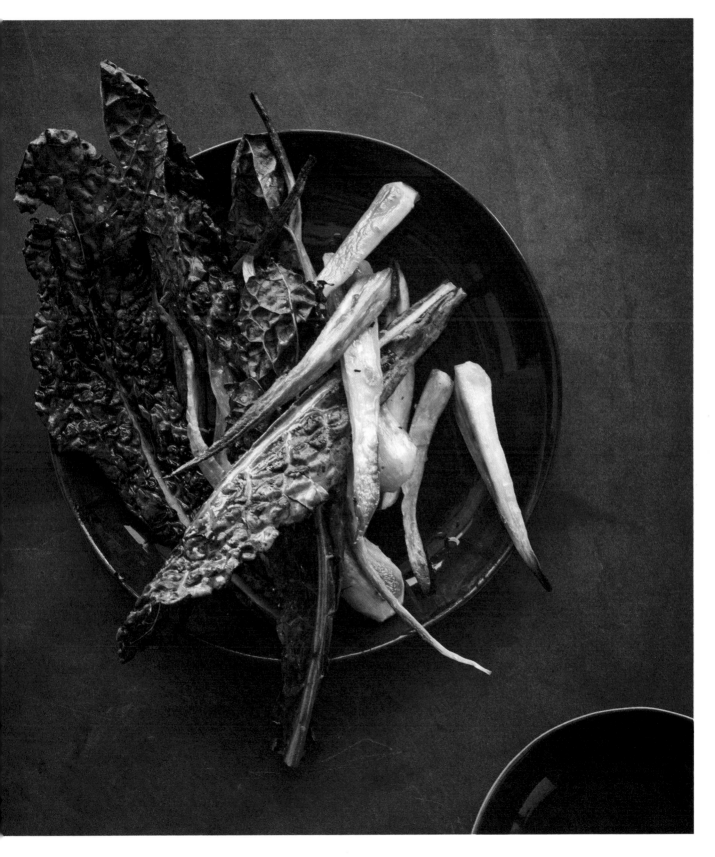

STUFFED POBLANO CHILES WITH RED RICE, DELICATA SQUASH, AND QUESO FRESCO

80 MINUTES (40 ACTIVE)	4 SERVINGS AND 1 LUNCH THE NEXT DAY

- 1¼ cups Bhutanese red rice
- Fine sea salt
- 1 small Delicata squash, halved lengthwise, seeded, and cut into ¼-inch semicircles (or smaller pieces if the squash is large; the pieces need to fit into the peppers)
- 1 tablespoon plus 2 teaspoons olive oil
- Freshly ground black pepper to taste
- 2 tablespoons pepitas (pumpkin seeds), toasted (see page 306)
- 2 cups tomato puree
- 1 large onion, chopped
- 2 garlic cloves, 1 whole, 1 chopped
- 6 fresh cilantro sprigs
- 1 teaspoon ground cumin
- ¼ cup crumbled queso fresco or fresh chèvre
- ¼ cup chopped fresh cilantro
- 5 large poblano (pasilla) chiles, halved lengthwise, cored, and seeded

Traditional *chiles rellenos* are fantastic, but labor-intensive and rich. This version is packed with chewy brown rice, slightly sweet squash, and crunchy pumpkin seeds. It's simple and wholesome at once.

Preheat the oven to 400°F.

Place the rice and 1¾ cups plus 2 tablespoons lightly salted water in a small saucepan with a lid. Bring to a boil over high heat, then reduce the heat and let the rice simmer gently, covered, for 25 minutes. Lift the lid, fluff the rice with a fork, and let it sit for at least 5 minutes. (You can cook the rice up to 2 to 3 days in advance; cool the rice and store it in an airtight container in the refrigerator.)

Toss the squash with 1 tablespoon of the oil and season with salt and black pepper. Arrange in a single layer on a baking sheet and roast until tender, 18 to 20 minutes. Turn the oven down to 350°F.

In a blender, combine the tomato puree, half the onion, 1 garlic clove, and cilantro sprigs. Whiz until smooth and season to taste.

In a sauté pan, heat the remaining 2 teaspoons oil and the remaining onion. Cook, stirring frequently, until the onion is softened, about 3 minutes. Add the remaining garlic, chopped, and the cumin and cook until fragrant, about 1 minute. Stir in the rice and set aside to cool.

Stir ½ cup of the tomato mixture into the cooled rice mixture. Toss in the roasted squash, queso fresco, and chopped cilantro and season to taste with salt and black pepper.

Place the pepper halves in a large baking dish, skin side down. Fill each pepper half with about ¼ cup of the rice mixture. Combine the remaining tomato mixture with ½ cup water and pour it around the stuffed peppers. Cover the dish tightly with aluminum foil and roast until the peppers are tender, about 30 minutes. Remove the foil and let the stuffing brown on top a bit, 5 to 6 minutes more.

Serve topped with the toasted pepitas.

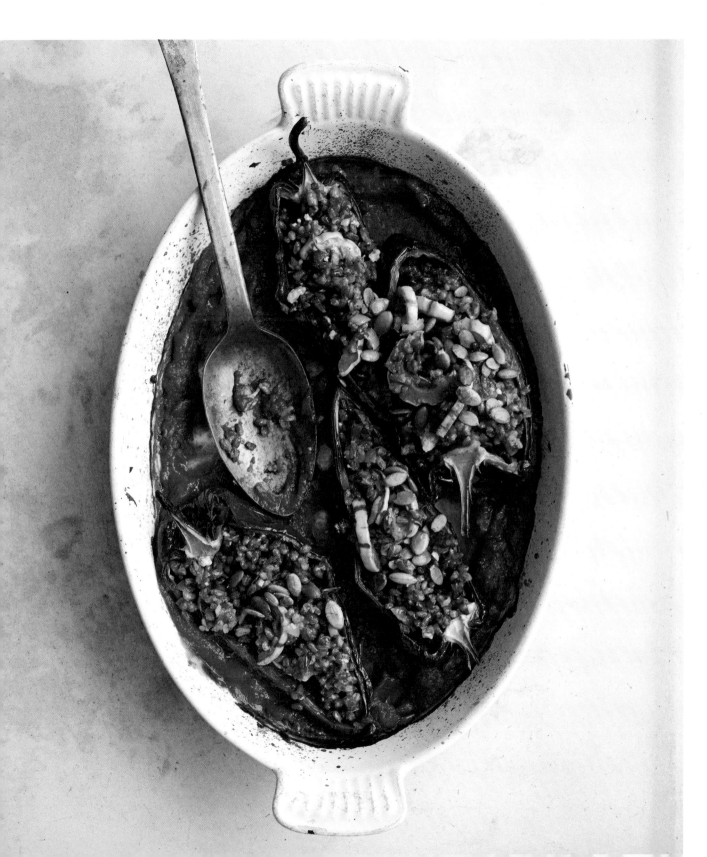

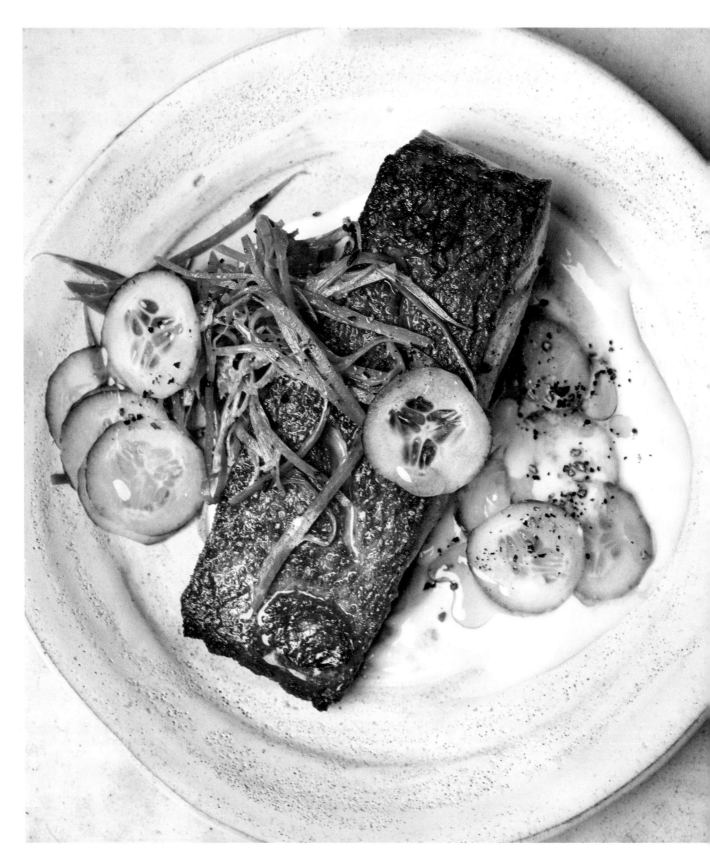

SALMON WITH CUCUMBER-YOGURT SAUCE AND CARROT SALAD

12 TO 15 MINUTES	4 SERVINGS AND 1 LUNCH THE NEXT DAY

- 1¼ pounds salmon, preferably wild-caught sockeye or king, skin on and cut into 5 fillets
- Fine sea salt and freshly ground black pepper

Cucumber-yogurt sauce

- ½ cup plain Greek yogurt
- 1 small garlic clove, grated
- 1 tablespoon lemon zest
- 1 tablespoon freshly squeezed lemon juice
- 1 cucumber, peeled and thinly sliced
- Fine sea salt and freshly ground black pepper to taste

Carrot salad

- ½ teaspoon cumin seeds
- ¼ teaspoon ground turmeric
- 1 large carrot, shredded
- 1½ tablespoons chopped fresh cilantro
- 1 tablespoon freshly squeezed lemon juice, plus more to taste
- 1 tablespoon extra-virgin olive oil, plus more for garnish
- Fine sea salt and freshly ground black pepper

- 1 tablespoon neutral oil, such as canola or grapeseed
- Flaky sea salt to finish

In September and October, I'll eat outside as often as I can, because I know I'll soon be forced by weather and darkness to start my late-fall house arrest. This dish captures a little of that in-between mood: the crisp-skinned salmon is warmed up with spices and the sweetness of carrots, but it's cooled at the same time with one of the most refreshing combinations of all time, cucumbers and yogurt.

Season the fish with fine sea salt and pepper.

To make the cucumber-yogurt sauce, in a medium bowl, combine the yogurt, garlic, lemon zest, and lemon juice. (The garlic-yogurt sauce can be made up to 1 day ahead and stored in an airtight container in the refrigerator.) Fold in the cucumber and season to taste with fine sea salt and black pepper.

To make the carrot salad, in a small dry skillet, toast the cumin seeds lightly over medium heat, about 1 minute. Add the turmeric for the last 15 to 20 seconds and toast until fragrant. In a medium bowl, combine the toasted spices, carrot, cilantro, lemon juice, and olive oil. Toss and season with fine sea salt, pepper, and additional lemon juice to taste. (The carrot salad can be made up to 8 hours in advance and kept in an airtight container in the refrigerator.)

To prepare the salmon, heat the neutral oil in a large ovenproof skillet over medium-high heat. Place the salmon fillets in skin side down. Cook, undisturbed, until the salmon skin is crisped and browned, 3 to 4 minutes. Gently turn the fillets and cook until the salmon is just opaque at the center, 1 to 2 minutes for medium-rare.

On each plate, place a salmon fillet skin side up and serve with the cucumber-yogurt sauce and the carrot salad. Drizzle on a bit of the neutral oil and sprinkle with flaky sea salt.

YOGURT CHICKEN WITH GINGER-CORIANDER CHUTNEY

40 TO 45 MINUTES (8 ACTIVE)	4 SERVINGS AND 1 LUNCH THE NEXT DAY

Chicken

- 1 garlic clove, grated
- 1 cup plain Greek yogurt
- 2 tablespoons olive oil, plus more for brushing
- ¼ teaspoon hot paprika or ground cayenne pepper
- Fine sea salt to taste
- 1½ pounds skinless, boneless chicken thighs, trimmed of fat and gristle, each cut into 2 or 3 pieces

Chutney

- 1 bunch fresh cilantro, chopped
- 1 serrano chile, seeded and minced
- ¼ cup unsweetened organic flaked coconut
- 1½ tablespoons fresh lemon juice
- 1 tablespoon chopped peeled fresh ginger
- Fine sea salt to taste

Yogurt is a big part of my kitchen arsenal. When used as a marinade, it does a few interesting things: it has a tenderizing effect; paired with olive oil, it coats the meat to allow for browning even when the skin has been removed; and of course, it adds great tangy flavor. For these reasons, this marinade can work very well for fish, lamb, or even tofu.

To prepare the chicken, whisk together the garlic, yogurt, 2 tablespoons of the oil, the paprika, and salt in a large bowl. Add the chicken and toss to coat with the marinade. Cover and chill for at least 20 minutes and up to 1 day.

To make the chutney, puree the cilantro, serrano chile, coconut, lemon juice, ginger, salt, and ¼ cup water in a blender or food processor until smooth. Set aside.

Place one rack in the middle of the oven and another in the top third and preheat the oven to 425°F. Lightly brush a rimmed baking sheet with oil.

Remove the chicken from the marinade and shake off the excess. Place the chicken in a single layer on the prepared sheet and bake on the middle rack until cooked through, 10 to 15 minutes. Turn on the broiler and move the chicken to the upper rack. Broil until the tops of the chicken pieces are browned in spots, about 3 minutes.

Serve the chicken with the chutney.

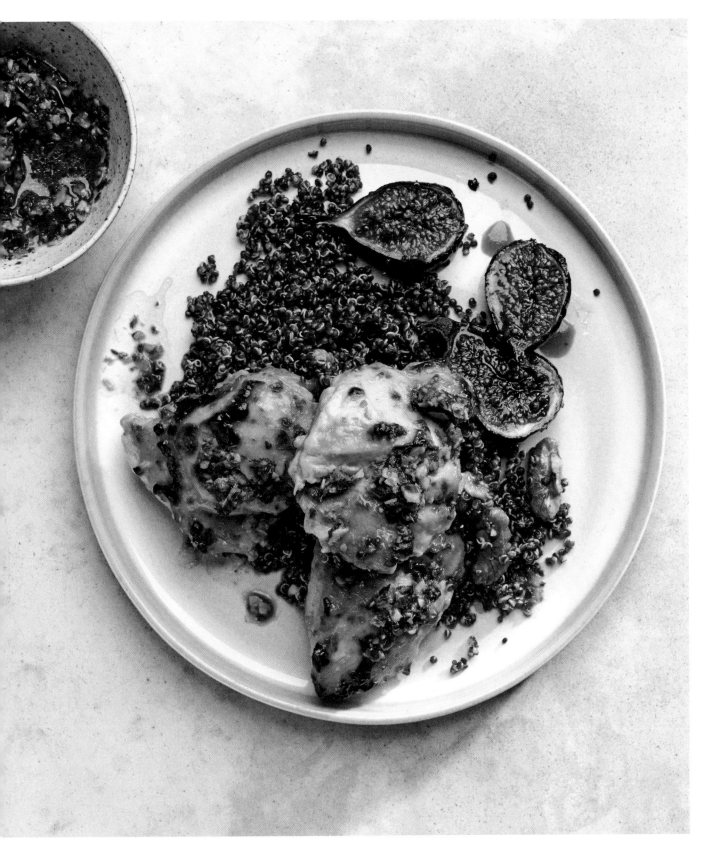

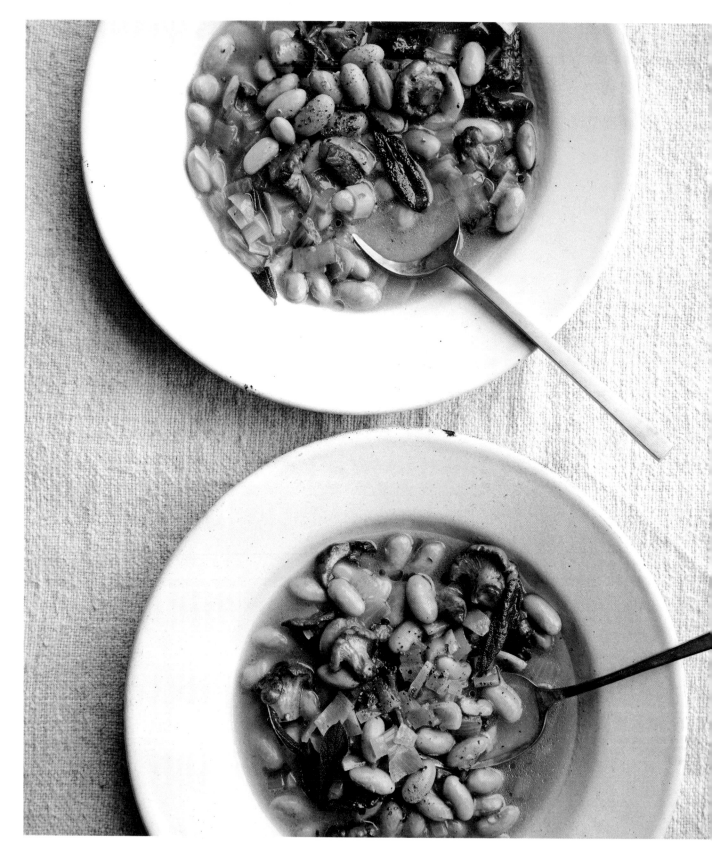

CRANBERRY BEAN RAGOUT WITH CHANTERELLES AND SAGE

35 TO 40 MINUTES	4 SERVINGS AND 1 LUNCH THE NEXT DAY

- 2 cups shelled fresh cranberry beans (about 12 ounces) or 2 pounds in shell
- 2 or 3 fresh thyme sprigs
- 1 large onion, half peeled and left uncut and half chopped
- 2 whole garlic cloves
- 1 large leek (white and light green parts), cut into ¼-inch slices and rinsed (about 1 cup), green stalk reserved
- Fine sea salt
- 3 tablespoons olive oil
- 20 fresh sage leaves (from about 4 stalks)
- 12 ounces chanterelles, cut into ½-inch wedges
- 1 garlic clove, minced
- ¾ cup homemade chicken stock (see page 301), low-sodium canned, or water
- Freshly ground black pepper

Fresh shelling beans are firm and flavorful and don't require any presoaking. Like so many seasonal things, however, they can be elusive. But don't worry; you can make this savory ragout with dried beans, or you could sub in canned beans: borlotti, cannellini, or butter beans. As for the chanterelles, look for them to drop in price dramatically in midautumn. If they're not showing up in your market, I would double up on the leeks instead.

In a 2- or 3-quart saucepan, combine the beans, thyme, the uncut onion half, whole garlic cloves, and reserved leek stalk. Add enough water to cover everything by 2 inches and bring to a boil over medium-high heat. Season with salt and turn the heat down to a lively simmer. Cook until the beans are tender, 20 to 30 minutes. Drain the beans, discard the cooking liquid, and pluck out the onion, leek stalk, thyme, and garlic. Set the beans aside.

Meanwhile, in a small saucepan, heat 2 tablespoons of the oil over medium heat. Have ready a slotted spoon or tongs and a plate lined with paper towels. Add 1 sage leaf to the pan; if it bubbles vigorously, the heat is correct. Place a single layer of sage leaves in the oil and cook, turning once, until the bubbling subsides and the leaves darken a bit, 30 to 45 seconds. Transfer to the paper towels to drain. Repeat with the remaining sage leaves, then turn off the heat. Reserve the sage oil.

In a wide, deep skillet or saucepan, heat the remaining 1 tablespoon oil and the sage oil over medium-high heat. Add the chanterelles and cook them undisturbed until browned on one side, 3 to 4 minutes. Season with a pinch of salt and stir. Cook for another 2 to 3 minutes, or until the chanterelles are nicely browned. Stir in the minced garlic and cook for 15 seconds, then add the sliced leeks, chopped onion, and 2 tablespoons of the stock. Turn the heat down to medium-low, cover, and cook for 3 to 4 minutes, until the leeks wilt. Uncover and cook for 4 to 5 minutes, until the onion is softened. Add the reserved beans and the remaining stock or water. Season to taste with salt and freshly ground pepper. Cook until the stock has thickened and the flavors have melded nicely, about 5 minutes.

Serve topped with fried sage leaves.

SAUCY BRAISED CHICKEN THIGHS WITH FENNEL AND LEMON

50 TO 55 MINUTES	4 SERVINGS AND 1 LUNCH THE NEXT DAY

- 5 boneless chicken thighs (1½ pounds)
- Fine sea salt and freshly ground black pepper to taste
- 2 tablespoons olive oil, plus more if needed
- 2 fennel bulbs, trimmed, core intact, cut into ½-inch-thick wedges
- 2 teaspoons fennel seeds
- 2 garlic cloves, sliced thinly
- 1 cup homemade chicken stock (see page 301) or low-sodium canned
- 1 lemon, sliced thinly crosswise
- ¼ cup fresh flat-leaf parsley leaves, chopped, for garnish

Friends often ask me what kind of pots to get, and one I urge upon everyone is a covered braising pan, which is the ideal pot for a stewy, aromatic dish like this. I've got a turquoise enameled beauty, which I can fire up on the stovetop for browning all the chicken and vegetables, then tuck it into the oven for some mellow braising heat. When the meal is cooked, I throw some herbs on top and serve straight from the attractive pan. No matter what pan you use, the combination of sweetly caramelized fennel, rich chicken thighs, and lemon is hard to resist.

Preheat the oven to 425°F.

Season the chicken thighs with salt and pepper.

In a large deep-sided ovenproof skillet or wide saucepan, heat 1 tablespoon of the oil over medium-high heat. Add half the fennel wedges and cook until brown on one side, about 3 minutes; flip, add a pinch of salt, cook 2 more minutes, and remove from the pan, adding more olive oil if needed. Repeat to cook the remaining fennel. Wipe out the pan.

Add the fennel seeds and toast until fragrant, about 1 minute. Set aside.

Heat the remaining 1 tablespoon oil over medium heat. Pat the chicken thighs dry with a paper towel and add to the pan in a single layer. Cook until browned, about 4 minutes. Turn the chicken over, sprinkle the garlic slices onto the surface of the pan between the chicken pieces, and cook until fragrant, about 30 seconds. Add the stock and toasted fennel seeds and tuck the fennel pieces and lemon slices around the chicken.

When the stock comes to a boil, about 3 minutes, transfer the pan to the oven. Cook until the chicken is cooked through, the pan juices are thickened, and the fennel is glazed, 22 to 25 minutes. Serve topped with parsley.

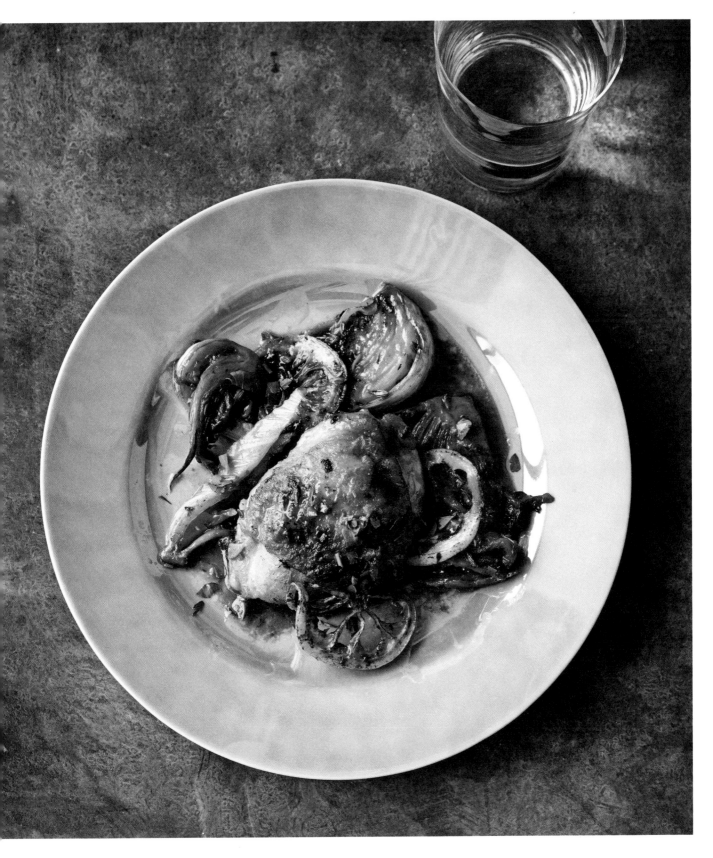

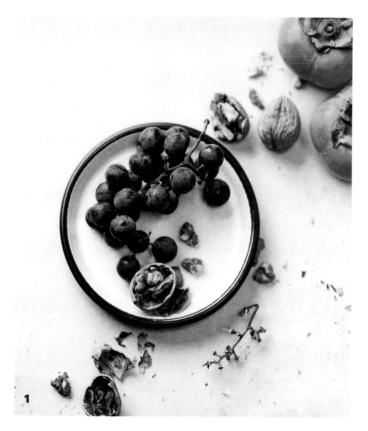

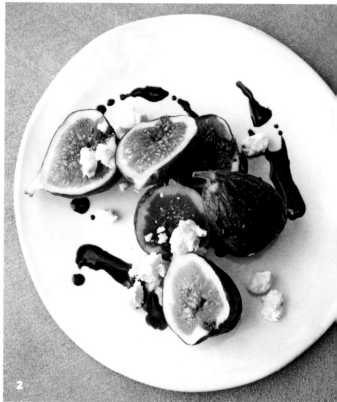

FALL DESSERTS

Here are some suggested fall desserts with approximate portions for a single serving.

1. Fuyu persimmons, Concord grapes, and walnuts
1 persimmon, 1 small cluster grapes, and
3 or 4 walnut halves

2. Figs with chèvre crumbles, drizzled with balsamic
2 large figs plus 1 or 2 teaspoons chèvre

3. Pears with toasted pecans
1 pear and 5 pecan halves

**4. Apple slices with Honey-Chamomile Dressing
(page 312)**
1 apple and 1 tablespoon dressing

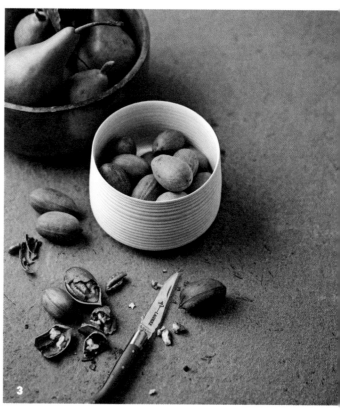

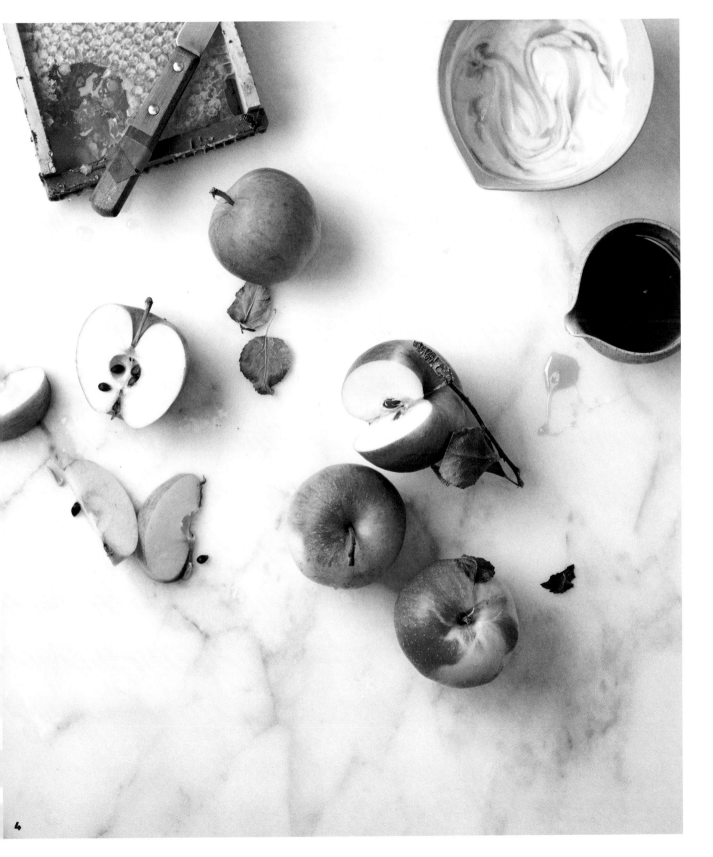

CLEANSE MENU

DAY 1

(STARTS WITH DINNER)

DINNER
Chickpea and Eggplant
Curry with Mint Chutney
(page 192)

Brown Basmati Rice with
Sour Cherries and Almonds
(page 191)

DESSERT
Pecan-Ginger Bark
(page 226)

DAY 2

BREAKFAST
Morning Bulgur with Dried
Apricots and Pistachios
(page 172)

LUNCH
Leftover curry served with a
salad of kale, cashews, late
cherry tomatoes, and Sherry
Vinaigrette (page 315)

SNACK
Red plum with cashews

DINNER
Hanger Steak with Tangy
Tomato Relish (page 188)

Red Quinoa with Roasted
Figs and Walnuts (page 201)

DESSERT
Apple slices with Honey-
Chamomile Dressing
(pictured on page 221)

DAY 3

BREAKFAST
Toasted Spiced Muesli
with Pecans and Flaxseeds
(page 171)

LUNCH
Leftover hanger steak and
quinoa with arugula, shaved
carrots, sunflower seeds,
and Whole-Grain Mustard
Vinaigrette (pictured on
page 180)

SNACK
Smoked Trout Spread
(page 321) with all-rye
crackers

DINNER
Pan-Seared Black Cod
(page 194)

Green Lentils with Thyme
(page 194)

Marinated Peppers
(page 205)

DESSERT
Figs with chèvre crumbles,
drizzled with balsamic
(pictured on page 220)

DAY 4

BREAKFAST
Fried Egg with Tangy Tomato Relish and Sautéed Sprouts (page 176)

LUNCH
Leftover black cod and marinated peppers with massaged Tuscan kale, Marcona almonds, and Sherry Vinaigrette (pictured on page 179)

SNACK
Spicy Carrot Dip (page 318) with crudités

DINNER
Roasted Pork Tenderloin with Apple and Mushroom Sauté (page 182)

Black-Eyed Peas with Roasted Tomatoes and Chives (page 206)

DESSERT
Fuyu persimmons, Concord grapes, and walnuts (pictured on page 220)

DAY 5

BREAKFAST
Creamy Maple Buckwheat with Apples and Walnuts (page 175)

LUNCH
Leftover pork with watercress and Asian pear in Sherry Vinaigrette (page 315), leftover black-eyed peas on the side

SNACK
Smoked Trout Spread (page 321) with all-rye crackers

DINNER
Oven-Roasted Chicken with Grapes (page 186)

Oven-Crisped Parsnips with Kale (page 208)

DESSERT
Pecan-Ginger Bark (page 326)

DAY 6

BREAKFAST
Mango Almond Lassi with Cardamom (page 174)

LUNCH
Leftover chicken breast, grapes, parsnips with frisée, toasted walnuts, and Whole-Grain Mustard Vinaigrette (pictured on page 178)

SNACK
Blanched cauliflower (see page 304) with Chickpea and Hazelnut Dukkah (page 322)

DINNER
Curried Mussels with Leeks (page 198)

Roasted Yukon Gold Potatoes (page 198)

DESSERT
Fuyu persimmons, Concord grapes, and walnuts (pictured on page 220)

CLEANSE MENU

DAY 7

BREAKFAST
Fried Egg with Tangy Tomato Relish and Sautéed Sprouts (page 176)

LUNCH
Canned albacore tuna with spinach, black olives, thinly sliced peperoncino peppers, and Sherry Vinaigrette (page 315)

SNACK
Spicy Carrot Dip (page 318) and crudités

DINNER
Stuffed Poblano Chiles with Red Rice, Delicata Squash, and Queso Fresco (page 210)

DESSERT
Pears with toasted pecans (pictured on page 220)

DAY 8

BREAKFAST
Toasted Spiced Muesli with Pecans and Flaxseeds (page 171)

LUNCH
Leftover poblano chile with salad of spinach, slivered shallots, and pepitas with Sherry Vinaigrette (page 315)

SNACK
Red plum with cashews

DINNER
Salmon with Cucumber-Yogurt Sauce and Carrot Salad (page 213)

Black-Eyed Peas with Roasted Tomatoes and Chives (page 206)

DESSERT
Figs with chèvre crumbles, drizzled with balsamic (pictured on page 220)

DAY 9

BREAKFAST
Morning Bulgur with Dried Apricots and Pistachios (page 172)

LUNCH
Leftover salmon with watercress, pear, butter lettuce, and Whole-Grain Mustard Vinaigrette (page 315)

SNACK
Spicy Carrot Dip (page 318) with crudités

DINNER
Yogurt Chicken with Ginger-Coriander Chutney (page 214)

Red Quinoa with Roasted Figs and Walnuts (page 201)

DESSERT
Apple slices with Honey-Chamomile Dressing (pictured on page 221)

DAY 10

BREAKFAST
Creamy Maple Buckwheat
with Apples and Walnuts
(page 175)

LUNCH
Leftover chicken with
cabbage, apples, cilantro,
avocado, and Sesame-Miso
Vinaigrette (page 310)

SNACK
Blanched cauliflower (see
page 304) with Chickpea and
Hazelnut Dukkah (page 322)

DINNER
Cranberry Bean Ragout
with Chanterelles and Sage
(page 217)

Rosemary Socca (page 122)

DESSERT
Pecan-Ginger Bark
(page 326)

DAY 11

BREAKFAST
Mango Almond Lassi with
Cardamom (page 174)

LUNCH
Leftover beans with boiled
egg, tossed with pale
chicories, and Whole-Grain
Mustard Vinaigrette
(page 315)

SNACK
Red plum with cashews

DINNER
Buffalo Patties with
Tangy Tomato Relish,
Avocado, and Butter Lettuce
(page 196)

Oven-Crisped Parsnips with
Kale (page 208)

DESSERT
Fuyu persimmons, Concord
grapes, and toasted walnuts
(pictured on page 220)

DAY 12

BREAKFAST
Fried Egg with Tangy Tomato
Relish and Sautéed Sprouts
(page 176)

LUNCH
Leftover parsnips and kale
with arugula, chickpeas,
chopped dried apricot,
dukkah (see page 322),
lemon juice, and olive oil

SNACK
Smoked Trout Spread
(page 321) with all-rye
crackers

DINNER
Oven-Roasted Tofu and
Romanesco with Ginger-
Scallion Sauce (page 185)

Brown Basmati Rice with
Sour Cherries and Almonds
(page 191)

DESSERT
Pears with toasted pecans
(pictured on page 220)

DAY 13

BREAKFAST
Toasted Spiced Muesli with
Pecans and Flaxseeds
(page 171)

LUNCH
Leftover tofu and Romanesco
with slivered radicchio,
cilantro, cashews, and
Sesame-Miso Vinaigrette
(pictured on page 181)

SNACK
Spicy Carrot Dip (page 318)
with crudités

DINNER
Saucy Braised Chicken
Thighs with Fennel and
Lemon (page 218)

Green Lentils with Thyme
(page 194)

DESSERT
Pecan-Ginger Bark
(page 326)

DAY 14

BREAKFAST
Creamy Maple Buckwheat
with Apples and Walnuts
(page 175)

LUNCH
Leftover chicken with
spinach, shaved pear, fennel,
and Whole-Grain Mustard
Vinaigrette (page 315)

SNACK
Blanched cauliflower (see
page 304) with Chickpea
and Hazelnut Dukkah (page
322)

DINNER
Clams with White Beans
and Gremolata (page 202)

Marinated Peppers
(page 305)

DESSERT
Apple slices with Honey-
Chamomile Dressing
(pictured on page 221)

SHOPPING LIST

We've put together a shopping list for you following the number of servings in our recipes; that means dinner recipes are for four people, but breakfasts, lunches, snacks, and desserts are portioned for one person. Please adjust according to your needs!

PANTRY

CANNED AND DRIED GOODS

- albacore tuna, small can
- almond milk, 1 quart
- cannellini beans, 2 (15-ounce) cans
- cherry tomatoes, 6 (14-ounce) cans (okay to substitute fresh)
- chicken stock, homemade or low-sodium canned, 2½ cups
- chickpeas, 2 (15-ounce) cans
- coconut milk
- almond butter
- black olives, small container
- Dijon mustard
- peperoncino peppers, 1 or 2
- tomato puree, 2 cups

CONDIMENTS

- soy sauce, light
- white miso
- whole-grain mustard
- Worcestershire sauce

DRIED FRUIT

- coconut, flaked, unsweetened, ¾ cup
- dried apricots, ⅔ cup
- dried sour cherries, 2 cups

FROZEN FOODS

- black-eyed peas, frozen, 4 cups

GRAINS

- all-rye crackers
- Bhutanese red rice, 1¼ cups
- brown basmati rice, 2½ cups
- buckwheat cereal (such as Bob's Red Mill Creamy buckwheat), ¾ cup
- bulgur, medium, ⅔ cup
- garbanzo flour, 1 cup
- green lentils, 2½ cups
- red quinoa, 2½ cups
- rolled oats, 2 cups

NUTS AND SEEDS

- cashews, ½ cup
- flaxseeds, ¼ cup
- hazelnuts, 1½ teaspoons
- Marcona almonds, 1 tablespoon
- pecan halves, 1¼ cups
- pepitas (pumpkin seeds), 3 tablespoons
- pine nuts, ¼ cup
- pistachios, shelled, 2 tablespoons
- roasted chickpeas or additional hazelnuts, ¼ cup
- sesame seeds, 2 tablespoons
- sliced almonds, ½ cup
- sunflower seeds, 2 tablespoons
- walnuts, 1½ cups

OILS AND VINEGARS

- balsamic vinegar
- canola, grapeseed, or vegetable oil, 16 ounces
- coconut oil (okay to substitute canola)
- extra-virgin olive oil, small bottle
- olive oil, large bottle or 34-ounce can
- rice vinegar
- sherry vinegar
- toasted sesame oil
- white wine vinegar

SPICES

- bay leaves, 2
- black peppercorns
- caraway seeds, 1 teaspoon
- cayenne pepper, ground, 1 teaspoon
- chamomile flowers, ¼ cup (or 12 chamomile tea bags)
- ancho chili powder, 1 teaspoon
- cardamom, ground, 1 teaspoon
- cinnamon, ground, 2 teaspoons
- coriander seeds, 2 tablespoons
- cumin, ground, 2 tablespoons
- cumin seeds, 4 tablespoons
- small dried chile, such as arbol or japones, 2
- fennel seeds, 2 tablespoons
- fine sea salt, container, typically 26 ounces
- five-spice powder, 1 teaspoon
- flaky sea salt, small container
- hot paprika, 1 teaspoon (can substitute ground cayenne pepper)
- Madras curry powder, 2 teaspoons
- mustard seeds, 1 tablespoon
- red pepper flakes, preferably Aleppo or Marash, ¼ cup
- turmeric, 2 teaspoons

SWEET GOODS

- agave syrup
- honey
- maple syrup
- bittersweet chocolate, 8 ounces

SHOPPING LIST

DAIRY AND OTHER REFRIGERATED ITEMS

- chèvre, 4 to 6 ounces
- eggs, large, 1 dozen
- Greek yogurt, plain, 1 quart
- plain kefir (can substitute plain Greek yogurt), 1 quart
- orange juice, 1 small container
- queso fresco or chèvre, ¼ cup
- sheep's milk yogurt, 1 small container (can substitute Greek yogurt)

MEAT AND SEAFOOD

- chicken breasts, bone in, skin on, 2 pounds
- hanger steak, 1¼ pounds
- pork tenderloin, 1¼ pounds
- black cod, skin on, 1½ pounds
- black mussels, 2½ pounds
- smoked trout, 2 fillets

PRODUCE

- apples, Honeycrisp or Braeburn, 2
- apple, Granny Smith, 1
- arugula, 3 to 4 cups
- Asian pear, 1 medium
- basil, 1 bunch
- Belgian endive, 2 heads
- carrots, 2 pounds (about 8 large)
- cauliflower, 1 head
- cherry tomatoes, 1 pint
- chiles, poblano (pasilla), 5 large
- chives, 1 small bunch
- cilantro, 1 bunch
- Concord grapes, 1 small bunch
- Delicata squash, 1 small
- dill, 1 bunch
- Japanese eggplant, 1¼ pounds
- figs, fresh, 1 pint
- flat-leaf parsley, 1 bunch
- frisée, 1 medium head
- Fuyu persimmons, 2
- garlic, 2 heads
- ginger, 1 large piece
- kale, 2 bunches
- kale, lacinato, 1 bunch
- leek, 1 large
- lemons, 3
- lime, 1
- mango, 1 medium
- lemon, Meyer, 1
- mint, 1 bunch
- mushrooms, cremini, or other, 8 ounces
- onions, 2 large, 1 medium
- onion, red, 1 medium
- orange, 1
- parsnips, 1½ pounds
- pea sprouts (or radish or mung bean), 3 cups
- pears, 2
- peppers, red bell, 4 large
- plum, 1
- red grapes, 1 large bunch, about 12 ounces
- sage, 1 small bunch
- scallions, 1 bunch
- shallots, 9
- snow peas, 1 cup (or other crudité)
- thyme, 1 bunch
- tomatoes, 2 large (about 20 ounces)
- watercress, 1 bunch
- Yukon gold potatoes, 4 medium

SHOPPING LIST

Do a quick inventory before heading out shopping for your second week—some of your dairy, produce, and sauces may be in fine shape for a second week!

DAIRY AND OTHER REFRIGERATED ITEMS

- chèvre, 2 teaspoons
- eggs, large, ½ dozen
- plain Greek yogurt, 1 quart
- orange juice, 1 small container
- plain kefir, 1 quart (can substitute plain Greek yogurt)
- sheep's milk yogurt, 1 small container (can substitute plain Greek yogurt)
- tofu, firm, 1 (14-ounce) package

MEAT AND SEAFOOD

- chicken thighs, boneless, 3 pounds (half skinless, half skin on)
- bison, ground, 1 pound (okay to substitute grass-fed beef)
- salmon, 1¼ pounds, preferably wild caught
- small hard shell clams (like littleneck or manila, 2 pounds)

PRODUCE

- apples, Braeburn or Honeycrisp, 3
- apples, Granny Smith, 2
- arugula, 3 to 4 cups
- avocados, 2
- Belgian endive, 1
- butter lettuce, 2 heads
- cabbage, 1 small head
- carrots, 7 to 8 large
- cauliflower, 1 head
- chanterelles, 12 ounces
- chile, Fresno or jalapeño, 1
- chile, Thai, 1
- chives, 1 small bunch
- cilantro, 2 bunches
- Concord grapes, 1 small cluster
- cranberry beans, 2 pounds in shell or 2 cups shelled
- cucumber, 1 medium
- fennel, 2 bulbs
- figs, 1 pint
- Fresno or jalapeño chile, 1
- frisée, 1 small head
- Fuyu persimmon, 1
- garlic, 1 head
- ginger, 1 large piece
- kale, lacinato, 1 bunch
- leek, 1 large
- lemons, 5
- lime, 1
- mangoes, 2 medium
- onions, 3 large
- onion, red, 1 medium
- orange, 1

- parsley, flat-leaf, 1 bunch
- parsnips, 1½ pounds
- pea sprouts (or radish or mung bean), 1 cup
- pears, 3
- plums, 2
- radicchio, 2 heads
- Romanesco or cauliflower, 1 large head, 2 to 3 pounds
- rosemary, ½ teaspoon minced
- sage, 1 small bunch
- scallions, 3 bunches
- serrano chile, 1
- shallots, 2
- snow peas, ½ cup (or other crudité)
- spinach, 6 to 8 cups
- thyme, 1 bunch
- watercress, 1 bunch

WIN

TER

Winter, and specifically the beginning of the year, is the most common time for all of us to test our resolve to form healthier habits. While it's not the liveliest time at the farmers' market, the quiet after the swirl of the holiday season is a good opportunity to retreat to home-cooked meals. We can hunker down with root vegetables and steamy stews and hearty grains. All that comforting food is best when set off with the bright intensity of herbs or the citrus fruits that are at their prime. Ever-available parsley is another key to freshening up your food during this time. Simple as it is, it gives rich winter meals the contrast they need.

WINTER'S KEY INGREDIENTS

VEGETABLES

Beets
Brussels sprouts
Cabbage
Celery root
Kale
Leeks
Parsley
Parsnips

FRUIT

Grapefruit
Lemons
Oranges
Pomegranates

OTHER

Barley
Dried beans
Steel-cut oats
Walnuts

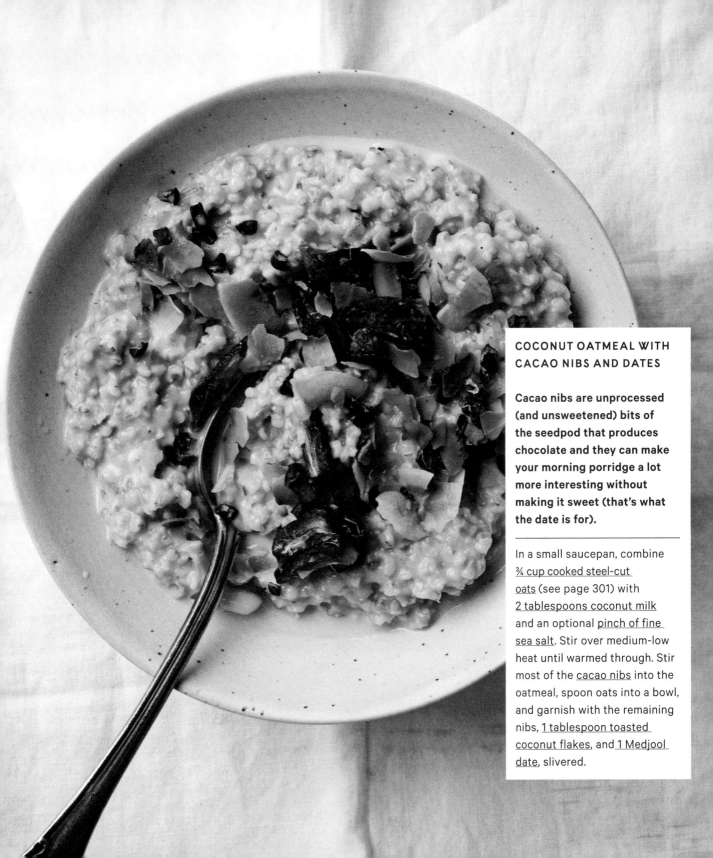

COCONUT OATMEAL WITH CACAO NIBS AND DATES

Cacao nibs are unprocessed (and unsweetened) bits of the seedpod that produces chocolate and they can make your morning porridge a lot more interesting without making it sweet (that's what the date is for).

In a small saucepan, combine ¾ cup cooked steel-cut oats (see page 301) with 2 tablespoons coconut milk and an optional pinch of fine sea salt. Stir over medium-low heat until warmed through. Stir most of the cacao nibs into the oatmeal, spoon oats into a bowl, and garnish with the remaining nibs, 1 tablespoon toasted coconut flakes, and 1 Medjool date, slivered.

SCRAMBLED EGGS WITH SMOKED SALMON, CHIVES, AND RYE CRACKER

ABOUT 5 MINUTES	MAKES 1 SERVING

- 2 large eggs, beaten
- 1 tablespoon chopped fresh chives, plus a pinch for garnish
- Fine sea salt and freshly ground black pepper
- 1 teaspoon olive oil
- 1½ ounces hot smoked salmon fillet (or canned sardine fillets)
- ¼ teaspoon za'atar (optional)
- 1 all-rye cracker

Unlike silky lox, hot-smoked salmon, which has been baked as it is smoked, falls into very satisfying flakes when it's mixed with your morning eggs. Its texture is a perfect fit, as are other hot-smoked fish such as sardines and kippers. If you are practical-minded, you may prefer to keep your rye cracker whole, as a vehicle to scoop up your eggs, but I kind of like to break mine into shards and sprinkle it atop the soft scramble.

In a medium bowl, whisk together the eggs, chives, and salt and pepper.

Heat the oil in a nonstick skillet over medium heat. Pour in the eggs; when curds start to form, gently scrape from the bottom of the pan while stirring. Add the smoked salmon, using a spatula to break it into small chunks. Cook the eggs to the desired texture and top with the za'atar, if using. Serve with a rye cracker and top with the pinch of chives.

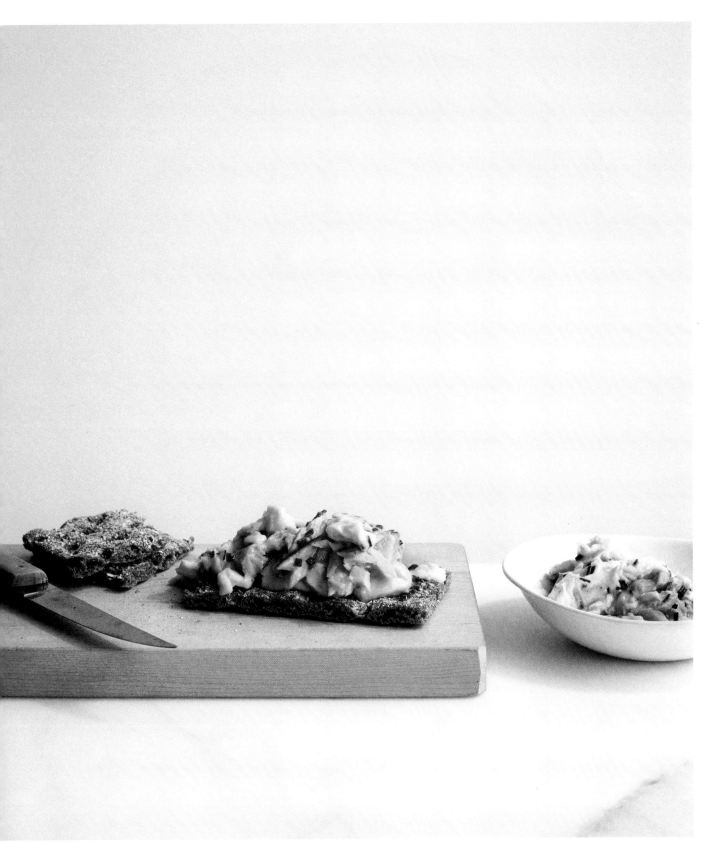

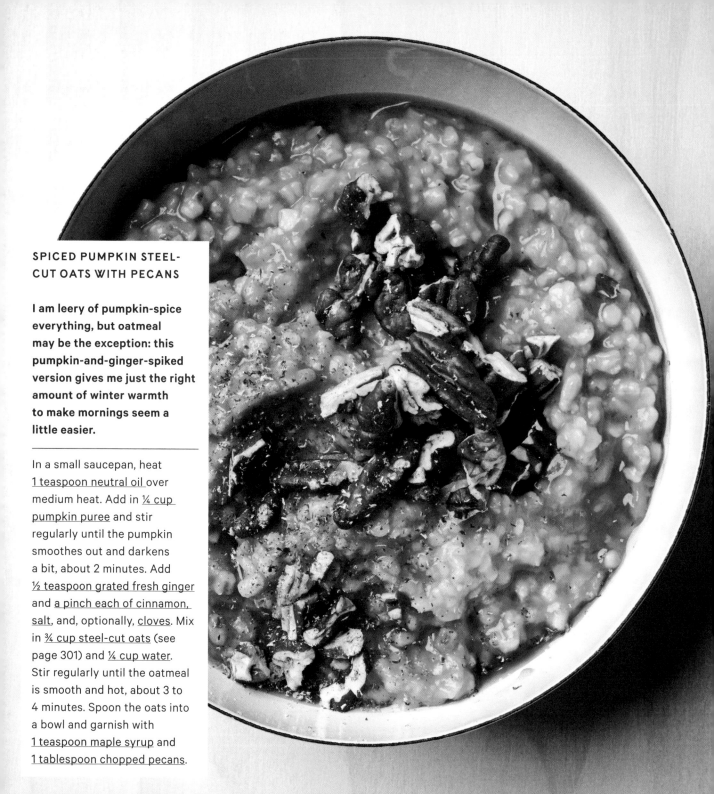

SPICED PUMPKIN STEEL-CUT OATS WITH PECANS

I am leery of pumpkin-spice everything, but oatmeal may be the exception: this pumpkin-and-ginger-spiked version gives me just the right amount of winter warmth to make mornings seem a little easier.

In a small saucepan, heat 1 teaspoon neutral oil over medium heat. Add in ¼ cup pumpkin puree and stir regularly until the pumpkin smoothes out and darkens a bit, about 2 minutes. Add ½ teaspoon grated fresh ginger and a pinch each of cinnamon, salt, and, optionally, cloves. Mix in ¾ cup steel-cut oats (see page 301) and ¼ cup water. Stir regularly until the oatmeal is smooth and hot, about 3 to 4 minutes. Spoon the oats into a bowl and garnish with 1 teaspoon maple syrup and 1 tablespoon chopped pecans.

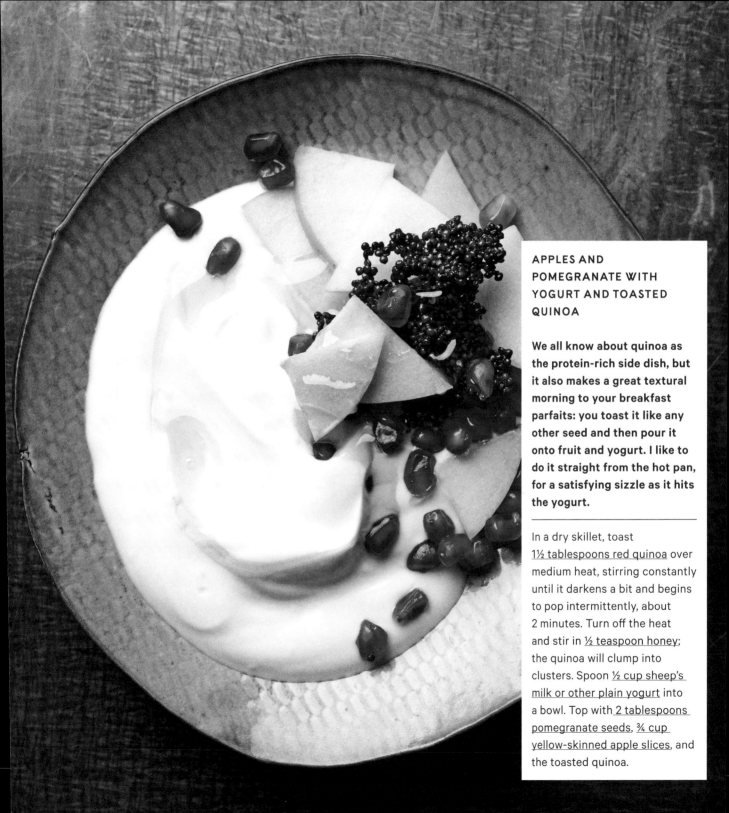

APPLES AND POMEGRANATE WITH YOGURT AND TOASTED QUINOA

We all know about quinoa as the protein-rich side dish, but it also makes a great textural morning to your breakfast parfaits: you toast it like any other seed and then pour it onto fruit and yogurt. I like to do it straight from the hot pan, for a satisfying sizzle as it hits the yogurt.

In a dry skillet, toast 1½ tablespoons red quinoa over medium heat, stirring constantly until it darkens a bit and begins to pop intermittently, about 2 minutes. Turn off the heat and stir in ½ teaspoon honey; the quinoa will clump into clusters. Spoon ½ cup sheep's milk or other plain yogurt into a bowl. Top with 2 tablespoons pomegranate seeds, ¾ cup yellow-skinned apple slices, and the toasted quinoa.

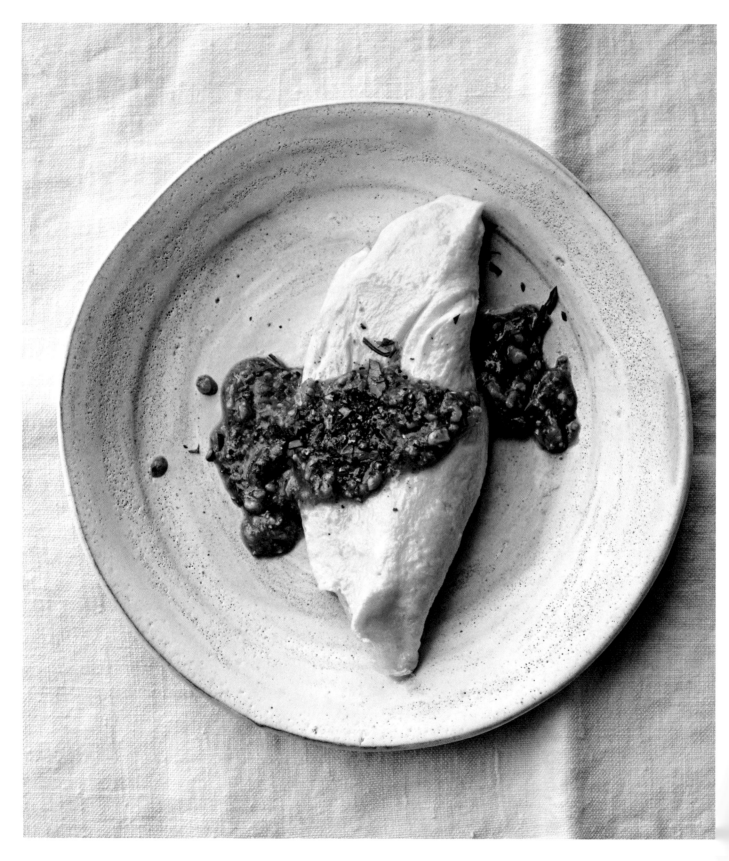

TWO-EGG OMELET WITH WALNUT PESTO

4 TO 5 MINUTES	MAKES 1 SERVING

- 2 large eggs
- Fine sea salt and freshly ground black pepper
- 1 teaspoon olive oil
- 1 to 2 tablespoons Walnut-Parsley Pesto (page 277)

The walnut pesto here may be the hardest-working item in our winter arsenal: rich with flavorful walnuts, this pantry item adds a little heft and luxury to a simple omelet.

In a medium bowl, whisk together the eggs with salt and pepper.

Have a warm plate ready. Heat the oil in an 8-inch nonstick skillet over medium heat. Pour in the eggs. Stir once or twice with a spatula. As soon as the perimeter of the eggs starts to set, use the spatula to lift the edge of the cooked egg and tilt the pan to let raw egg run underneath to the bottom of the pan. Repeat until there's no longer enough raw egg to run under the edge (60 to 90 seconds).

Lift the edge of the omelet with the spatula and fold it in half. Tip the pan and let it slide onto the plate. Season with more salt and pepper if necessary and top with the walnut pesto.

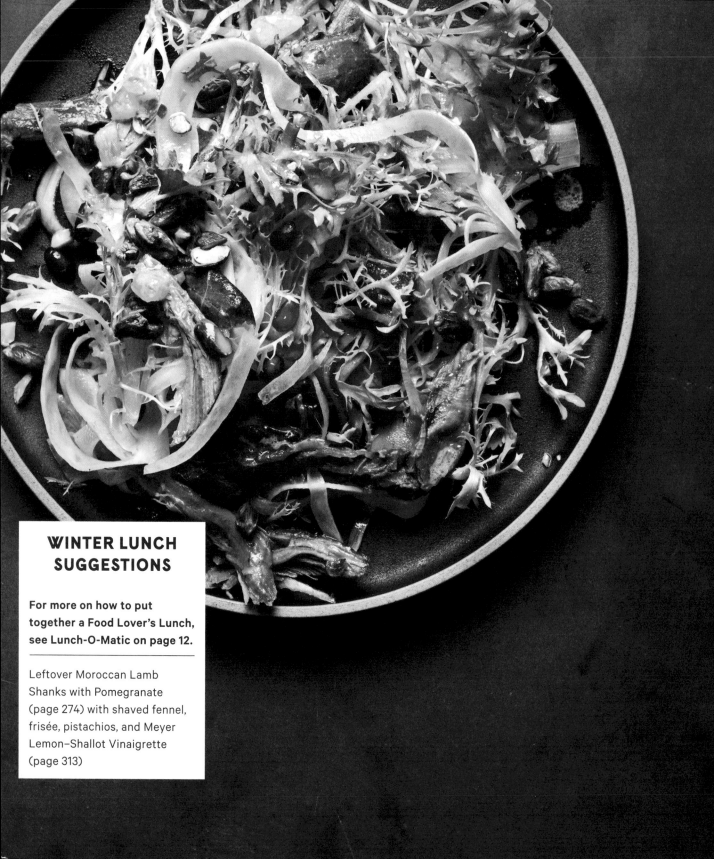

WINTER LUNCH SUGGESTIONS

For more on how to put together a Food Lover's Lunch, see Lunch-O-Matic on page 12.

Leftover Moroccan Lamb Shanks with Pomegranate (page 274) with shaved fennel, frisée, pistachios, and Meyer Lemon–Shallot Vinaigrette (page 313)

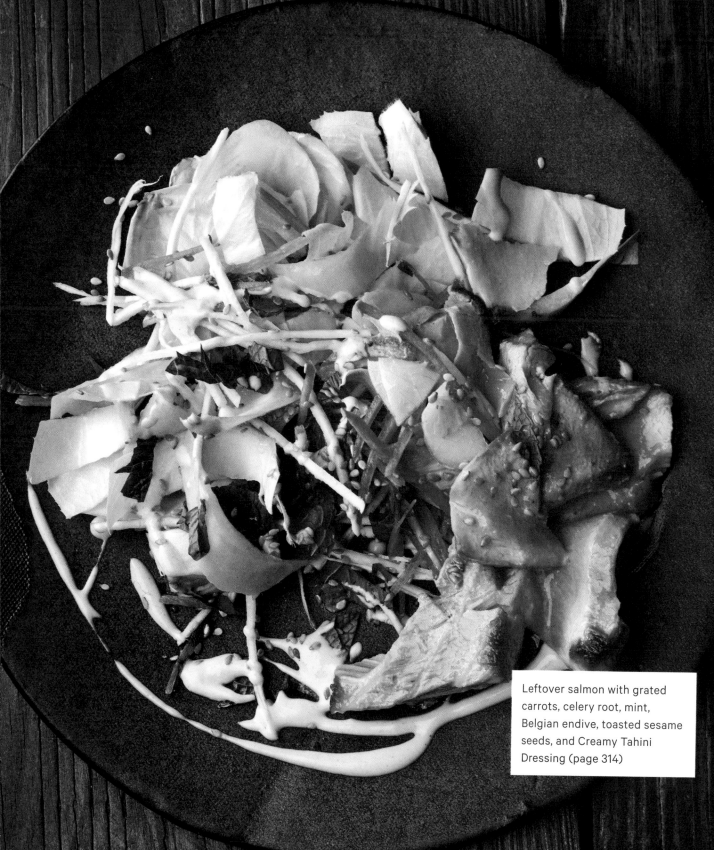

Leftover salmon with grated carrots, celery root, mint, Belgian endive, toasted sesame seeds, and Creamy Tahini Dressing (page 314)

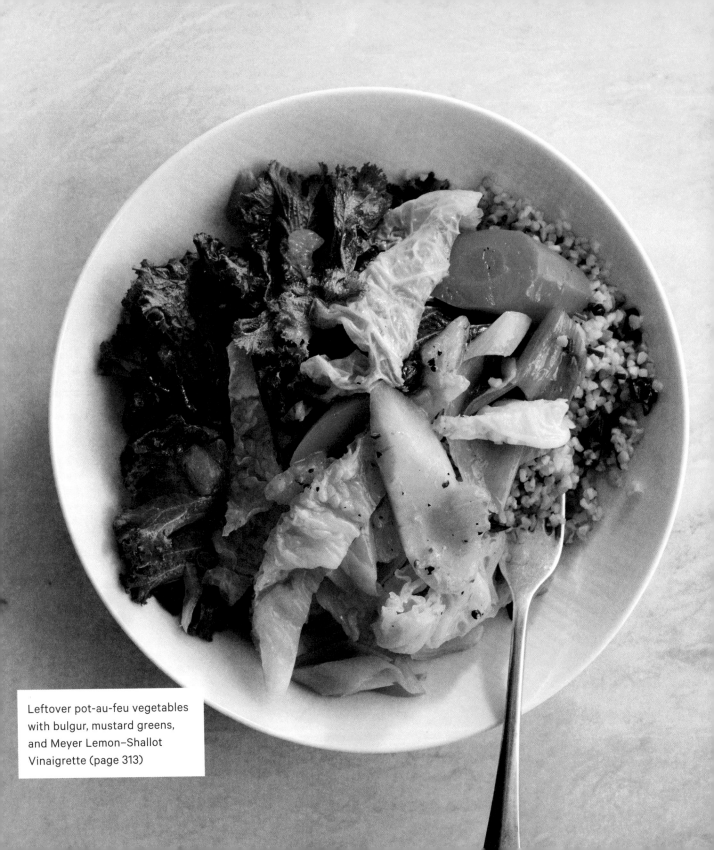

Leftover pot-au-feu vegetables with bulgur, mustard greens, and Meyer Lemon–Shallot Vinaigrette (page 313)

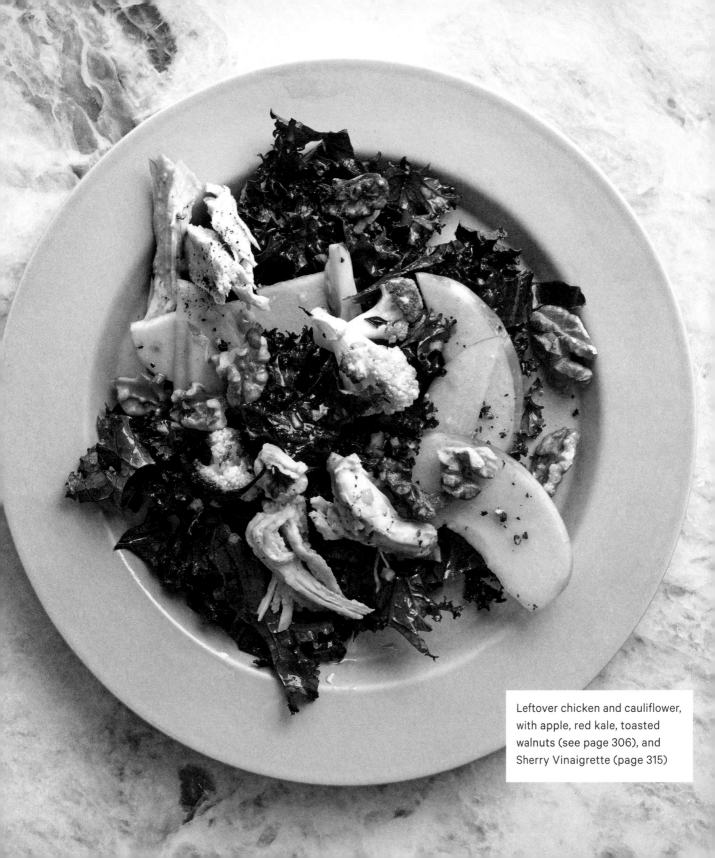

Leftover chicken and cauliflower, with apple, red kale, toasted walnuts (see page 306), and Sherry Vinaigrette (page 315)

TUNISIAN-STYLE POACHED EGGS IN RED PEPPER SAUCE

ABOUT 40 MINUTES	4 SERVINGS

- 2 tablespoons olive oil
- 1 medium red onion, chopped
- 2 garlic cloves, finely chopped
- 4 red bell peppers, cored, seeded, and cut lengthwise into ½-inch-wide strips
- Fine sea salt to taste
- 1 large tomato, cored, seeded, and grated using the large holes on a box grater
- 1 tablespoon (or more) harissa paste, such as Preserved Lemon Harissa (page 320)
- 1 teaspoon white wine vinegar or apple cider vinegar
- 4 large eggs
- Flaky sea salt, such as Maldon
- Red pepper flakes, preferably Aleppo or Marash, to taste

Breakfast for dinner is one of my favorite moves, but I'm less of a pancake person than an egg fan. Here my favorite poached eggs are dressed up with a beautiful, chunky brick-red sauce in the manner of *shakshouka*, the ubiquitous Middle Eastern dish that likely originated in Tunisia. The key to red peppers is cooking them until they're sweet and mysterious and then adding something a little aggressive to the mix; here it is the spicy North African condiment harissa, which bundles warm spice and chile heat in one package. Feel free to use homemade Preserved Lemon Harissa if you have been industrious, or stick with your favorite commercial brand.

Heat the oil in a large skillet over medium heat. Add the onion and cook, stirring often, until softened, about 5 minutes. Add the garlic and stir until fragrant, about 1 minute. Add the peppers, season with fine sea salt, and cook, stirring often, until the peppers are wilted, 5 to 8 minutes. Add the tomato, harissa, and 1 cup water; reduce the heat to medium-low and cook, stirring often and adding more water as needed, until the peppers are soft, 15 to 20 minutes. Season with fine sea salt and more harissa, if desired. Keep warm.

Meanwhile, fill a large skillet with water. Add the vinegar and a generous pinch of fine sea salt; bring to a simmer. Crack each egg into a teacup, then slide each one into the water; reduce the heat to low. Poach the eggs until the whites are set and the yolks are gently set, 3 to 4 minutes.

Divide the pepper sauce among four warm bowls and top each with an egg. Season the egg with flaky sea salt and red pepper flakes.

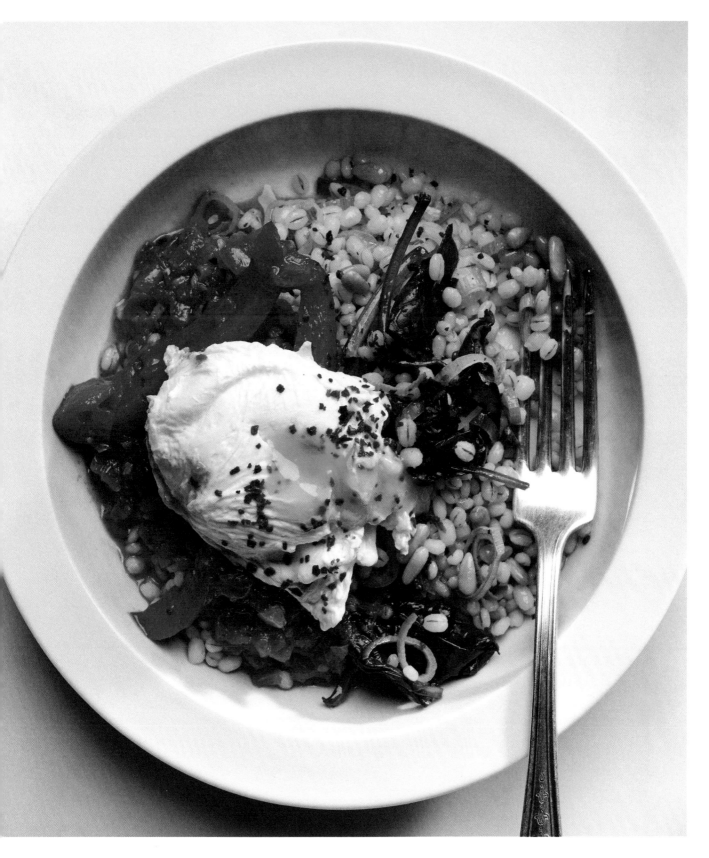

BARLEY PILAF WITH SPINACH AND PINE NUTS

Pictured on page 245

40 TO 50 MINUTES (5 ACTIVE)	4 SERVINGS AND 1 LUNCH THE NEXT DAY

- Fine sea salt
- 1 leek (white and light green parts), thinly sliced
- 12 ounces baby spinach
- 2 tablespoons olive oil
- 1 garlic clove, minced
- 1 pinch red pepper flakes, preferably Aleppo or Marash
- 3 cups cooked barley*
- 2 teaspoons finely grated lemon zest
- Freshly ground black pepper to taste
- 3 tablespoons pine nuts, toasted (see page 306)
- Lemon wedges, for garnish

To cook barley, bring a large pot of salted water to a boil. Stir in the barley, reduce the heat to a simmer, and cook until tender, 35 to 45 minutes. One cup dry barley yields a rounded 3 cups cooked.

Pearl barley takes a while to cook, but if you have it in your refrigerator or freezer, you've got a satisfying side dish that can come together quite quickly. Barley is a classic in a soup with mushrooms, of course, but I like it best when it's paired with something urgently bright and fresh tasting, like quickly sautéed spinach. A nice grating of lemon zest underscores the freshness here for a side dish that's equally appealing as a whole-grain salad the next day.

Bring a large pot of salted water to a boil. Prepare a bowl of ice water.

Add the leek to the water and cook for 1 minute. Add the spinach and as soon as it softens, about 30 seconds, use a slotted spoon or spider to remove the spinach and leek to the ice water to cool. Drain and squeeze the spinach mixture several times to remove any extra water. Coarsely chop the spinach and leek.

In a large skillet, heat the oil over medium heat. Add the garlic and red pepper flakes and stir for 20 seconds. Add in the spinach-leek mixture and a pinch of salt and toss well with the oil. Add the barley to the pan, stirring well to distribute the spinach evenly. Cook until warmed through, about 3 minutes. Toss in the lemon zest and season with salt and pepper.

Top with the toasted pine nuts and serve with lemon wedges to garnish.

ACORN SQUASH PUREE WITH CHILI OIL

63 MINUTES (8 ACTIVE)	4 SERVINGS

- 1 tablespoon olive oil
- 2 medium acorn squash, halved and seeded
- Fine sea salt and black pepper to taste
- 2 garlic cloves
- ½ teaspoon five-spice powder
- 1 teaspoon Chinese chili oil, plus more to taste

I'll take my chile peppers in as many ways as I can get them, and Chinese chili oil is a great way to go when you want an even layer of rich, mouth-coating heat. The oil is best added to finish a dish, like here, where it pairs with five-spice powder to make something special out of a simply roasted squash. Just be careful when you add your chili oil: because the hot capsaicin—the hot flavoring element in peppers—is suspended in fat, it lingers longer on your palate than vinegar-based hot sauces. Start with just a bit, then taste and build up heat from there.

Preheat the oven to 425°F.

Rub the interior of the squash with olive oil and season with salt and pepper. Place the squash cut side down on a baking sheet. Tuck the garlic cloves under a couple of the squash halves. Roast until the squash is completely tender, 45 to 55 minutes. When cool enough to handle, scoop out the squash flesh and transfer it to a medium bowl. Add the roasted garlic, five-spice powder, and chili oil and mash with a wooden spoon or potato masher into a relatively smooth puree (if you prefer it smoother still, use a food mill or a food processor). Season well with salt and pepper and add more chili oil, if desired.

MISO FLANK STEAK WITH SHIITAKE–MUSTARD GREEN ESCABECHE

50 MINUTES (25 ACTIVE)	4 SERVINGS AND 1 LUNCH THE NEXT DAY

- 2 tablespoons white miso
- ½ teaspoon grated peeled fresh ginger
- ½ teaspoon freshly ground black pepper
- 4 tablespoons neutral oil, such as canola or grapeseed
- 1¼ pounds grass-fed flank steak, large fat pieces trimmed
- 1 teaspoon yellow mustard seeds
- 1 small onion, thinly sliced
- 1 garlic clove, thinly sliced
- 1 small dried chile, such as japones or chile de arbol
- 1 (2-inch) piece fresh ginger, peeled and minced
- 8 ounces shiitake mushrooms, stems removed and mushrooms quartered if more than 2 inches across
- Fine sea salt to taste
- 1 tablespoon soy sauce
- 1 tablespoon rice vinegar
- 8 ounces mustard greens, well washed, large stems removed, leaves torn into 2-inch pieces
- Flaky sea salt to finish

Miso makes the best marinade: it's deliciously robust, its sweetness encourages a nice brown crust, and it supposedly tenderizes meat as well. A real-life trick for making fibrous cuts like flank steak easier to chew is to slice them thinly and diagonally across the grain. Here, smoky-sweet meat goes well with the sharp little garnish of vinegary mushrooms and mustard greens.

Mix the miso, grated ginger, pepper, and 1 tablespoon of the oil in a small bowl. Rub the mixture on the steak and let rest at least 15 minutes (or cover and chill overnight).

Heat 1 tablespoon of the oil in an ovenproof skillet over medium-high heat. Pat the surface of the flank steak to dry it a bit (don't worry about wiping off all the marinade, though). Cook, undisturbed, until browned, 3 to 4 minutes. Turn the steak and transfer the pan to the oven. Cook to the desired doneness, 5 to 6 minutes for medium-rare (130°F to 135°F), depending on the thickness of the meat. Let the steak rest at least 10 minutes.

Heat 1 tablespoon of the oil in a large skillet over medium heat. Add the mustard seeds and toast for 30 seconds, then stir in the onion. Cook, stirring frequently, until the onion is softened, about 4 minutes. Stir in the garlic, chile, and minced ginger and cook 1 minute. Add the mushrooms, season with the fine sea salt, and cook until browned, about 5 minutes. Pour in the soy sauce and vinegar and let the liquid reduce for about 1 minute, then remove the mushrooms to a plate.

Rinse out the pan, dry it well, and place it over medium-high heat. Heat up the remaining 1 tablespoon oil and add the mustard leaves and a pinch of fine sea salt. Cook, tossing continuously, until the greens are softened but still vivid in color, about 2 minutes. Add the mushrooms, stir to combine, and turn off the heat.

Slice the steak across the grain with an angled cut, sprinkle with flaky sea salt, and serve it with the mushrooms and mustard greens.

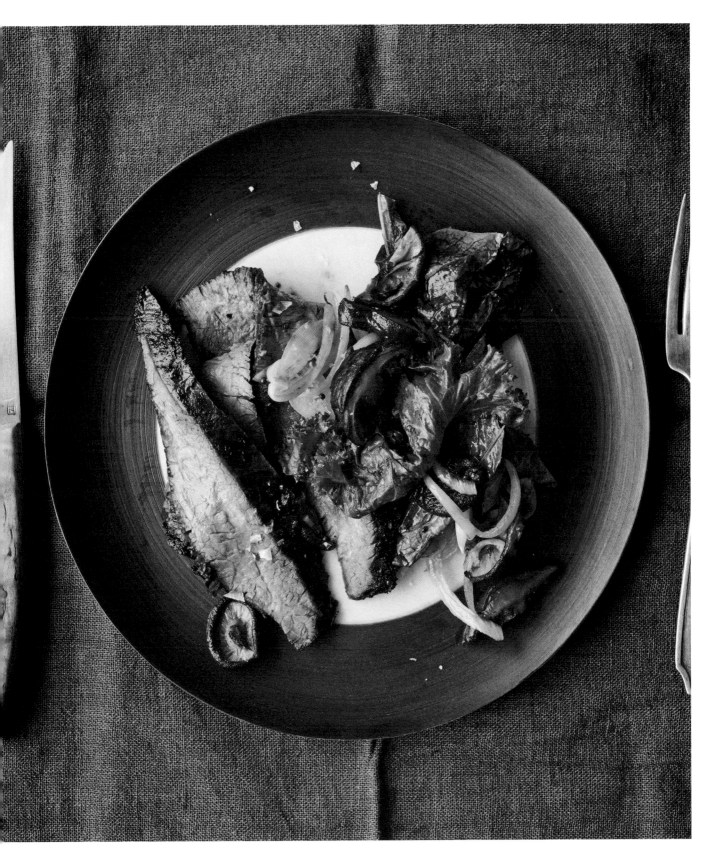

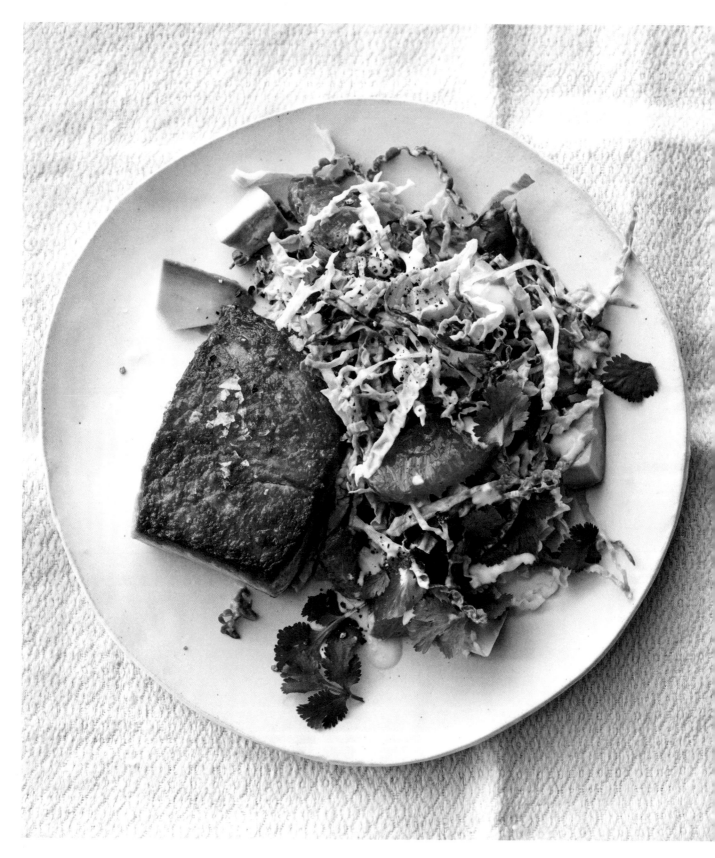

PAN-ROASTED SALMON WITH GRAPEFRUIT-CABBAGE SLAW

18 MINUTES	4 SERVINGS AND 1 LUNCH THE NEXT DAY

- 1 large pink grapefruit, cut into supremes (see page 306), juice reserved
- 1 small shallot, finely chopped
- 5 (4-ounce) salmon fillets, preferably wild-caught sockeye or king, skin on, pin bones removed
- Fine sea salt and freshly ground black pepper
- 2 tablespoons olive oil
- 1 tablespoon plain Greek yogurt
- ½ ripe avocado, cut into ½-inch dice
- ½ medium Savoy cabbage head, cored and very thinly sliced
- ¼ cup fresh cilantro leaves, for serving

This dish can help generate a little sunny feeling in the darkest days of winter. It's partly about the color story, with the pretty coral tones of the salmon and the grapefruit set against the pale green avocado. But there's also something beachy and Californian about the creamy cabbage slaw that's inspired by my favorite Baja-style taco stands. The winter might be chilly and damp, but somewhere out there, the sun is shining bright.

Combine the grapefruit juice and shallot in a small bowl; set aside.

Score the skin side of the salmon and season all over with salt and pepper.

Heat 1 tablespoon of the oil in a large nonstick skillet over medium-high heat. Place the salmon skin side down in the skillet. Cook until the skin is browned and crisp, about 5 minutes. Flip the fillets, reduce the heat to medium, and cook until the fish is barely opaque at the center of each fillet, about 4 more minutes. Set aside.

In a large bowl, whisk together the grapefruit juice–shallot mixture, yogurt, and remaining 1 tablespoon of oil. Add the grapefruit segments, avocado, and cabbage and toss gently to combine; season with salt and pepper. Top the slaw with cilantro and serve alongside the salmon.

REFRIED BLACK BEANS

ABOUT 6 MINUTES	4 SERVINGS

- 2 tablespoons neutral oil, such as canola or grapeseed
- 1 tablespoon finely chopped Fresno or jalapeño chile, plus more for garnish (about 1 whole, seeds and pith removed)
- 1 garlic clove, chopped
- 2 (15-ounce) cans black beans, drained, liquid reserved, or 3 cups cooked black beans, with ⅓ cup cooking liquid reserved
- ½ teaspoon ground ancho pepper
- ½ teaspoon ground cumin
- Fine sea salt to taste
- 1 radish, julienned, for garnish

Plain beans can be as dull as dirt, but it takes so little to make them exciting: a prickle of chile heat, a background note of cumin, and a bit of garlicky pungency. Once you've seasoned them up, you can serve them with eggs for breakfast, use them as a dip for jicama and carrots, or layer them into a veggie taco. If you've got a little time on your hands, black beans are among the quickest to cook from dry form; use the basic bean-cooking method on page 303. You can also puree any extra beans and their cooking liquid into a quick soup.

In a large skillet, preferably nonstick, heat the oil over medium-high heat. Add the 1 tablespoon of chile and the garlic and stir for 20 seconds. Pour in the beans, stir well, and season with the ancho pepper, cumin, and salt. Cook, stirring frequently, until the beans are warmed through and the liquid begins to thicken, about 5 minutes. If it gets too thick, add a bit of the reserved bean liquid. Remove from the heat and season with additional salt, if desired.

Top with the julienned radish and additional chopped chile.

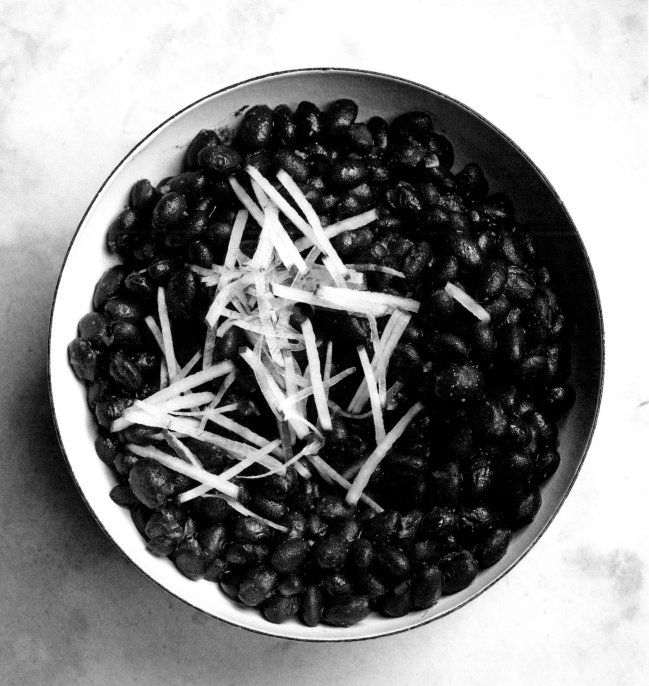

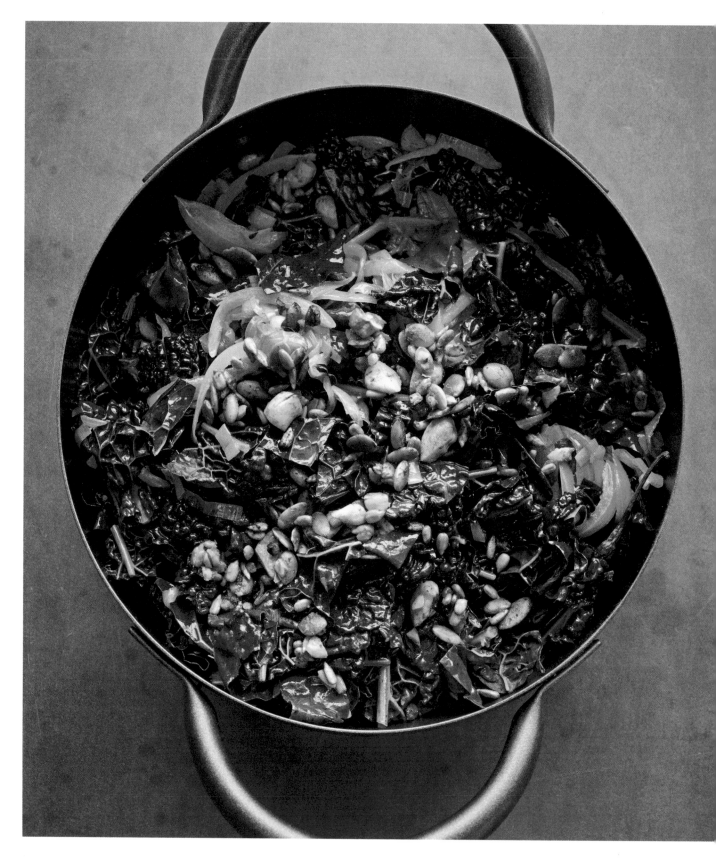

KALE SAUTÉED WITH ONIONS, LEEKS, AND TURMERIC

ABOUT 20 MINUTES	4 SERVINGS AND 1 LUNCH THE NEXT DAY

- 2 tablespoons olive oil
- 1 large leek (white and light green parts, well rinsed), thinly sliced
- 1 medium onion, thinly sliced
- 1 (2-inch) section turmeric root, peeled and julienned, or ¾ teaspoon ground turmeric
- 1 small dried chile, such as chile de arbol or japones
- Fine sea salt to taste
- 1½ pounds kale (about 3 bunches— I used a mix of frilly and lacinato), well washed, large stems removed, sliced crosswise into 2-inch ribbons
- Freshly ground black pepper to taste
- 3 tablespoons Spiced Pumpkin Seed and Cashew Crunch (page 316)

I remember some twenty years ago when Nancy Silverton, my boss at Campanile, made me seek out an exotic green in the Santa Monica farmers' market; it was cavolo nero, now more commonly known as lacinato, or dinosaur, kale. I had never eaten kale before, only plucked a curly kale garnish off the side of my brunch plate a few times. Back at the restaurant, we served it in minestrone and as a counterpoint to meaty braises, and I loved it: here was this green that was complex, and un-spinach-like in its sturdy texture, with a bit of underlying sweetness to boot. I would never have imagined decades later we would all be throwing it into smoothies, but I knew then I'd met an ingredient that would stick around in my kitchen toolbox.

Here, dark kale is paired with the brightly pungent bite of turmeric. See if you can find fresh turmeric (which grows as a rhizome like ginger, and looks similar) at the health food store; it's very pretty sliced into thin golden-orange ribbons. If not, ground turmeric is just fine.

In a large skillet or braising pan, heat the oil over medium heat. Add in the leek, onion, turmeric, chile, and 2 tablespoons water. Season with salt and stir until the onion and leek have softened, about 5 minutes. Add the kale, ¼ cup water, and more salt.

Cover the pan and cook until the kale becomes easy to stir, about 3 minutes. Remove the lid, toss well, and cook until the kale is tender but still bright green and toothsome, about 2 minutes. Season to taste with more salt and the pepper and remove the chile pod.

Serve with the pumpkin seed and cashew crunch on top.

CURRIED PORK WITH GARNET YAMS AND GREEN BEANS

3 HOURS (25 MINUTES ACTIVE)	4 SERVINGS AND 1 LUNCH THE NEXT DAY

- 2 tablespoons canola oil
- 1 pound pork shoulder, trimmed of excess external fat and cut into 2-inch chunks
- 4 cups homemade chicken stock (see page 301) or low-sodium canned, plus up to 2 more cups water or stock, if necessary
- 2 kaffir lime leaves (optional)
- 1 medium onion, chopped
- Fine sea salt
- 1½ tablespoons yellow Thai curry paste
- ¾ cup coconut milk
- 1 pound garnet yams (or other sweet potato variety), peeled and cut into 1- to 1½-inch chunks (about 4 cups)
- 4 ounces haricots verts or regular green beans, trimmed and sliced diagonally into 2-inch pieces (about 2 cups)
- 1 Fresno chile, thinly sliced, for garnish
- Fresh cilantro sprigs, for garnish
- Lime wedges, for garnish

In my day, I've pounded a few Thai curry pastes in a mortar and pestle, and it's effort well spent; the kitchen fills with wonderful fragrance and I get a little arm workout, too. But I'm also very happy to use packaged curry pastes to add a little color to my weeknight dinner. If you do use a shortcut curry, it's a good idea to layer in some fresh aromatics of your own: onion, fresh chiles, cilantro, and, if you can find them, fresh lime leaves.

Heat 1 tablespoon of the oil in a small Dutch oven over medium-high heat. Working in batches if necessary, brown the pork on all sides, about 12 minutes. Transfer the pork to a plate or platter and set aside.

Add the stock to the pot and bring to a boil, stirring and scraping up any browned bits. Reduce the heat until the liquid is at a gentle simmer. Return the pork to the pot and simmer, covered, until the pork is cooked through and tender enough to be teased into smaller pieces with a fork, from 1 hour 45 minutes to 2 hours.

Transfer the pork to a plate and shred it into smaller pieces. Use a spoon to skim off as much fat as possible from the surface of the liquid. Pour it into a measuring cup and add enough water to measure 2½ cups; set aside.

Wipe out the pot and warm the remaining 1 tablespoon of oil over medium heat. Stir in the lime leaves, if using, and onion, season with a pinch of the salt, and cook until softened, about 4 minutes. Add the curry paste and cook, stirring, until the onion is well coated. Add the stock mixture and the coconut milk to the curry paste, stirring well to dissolve the paste. Bring to a boil.

Return the pork to the pot and add the yams. Reduce the heat and simmer until the yams are almost tender at the center, about 15 minutes. Add the haricots verts, stir well, and cook, covered, for 1 or 2 minutes, or until the beans are crisp-tender and the yams are cooked through. Taste the stock and season with more salt if necessary.

Serve the stew with the Fresno chile slices, cilantro sprigs, and lime wedges as a garnish.

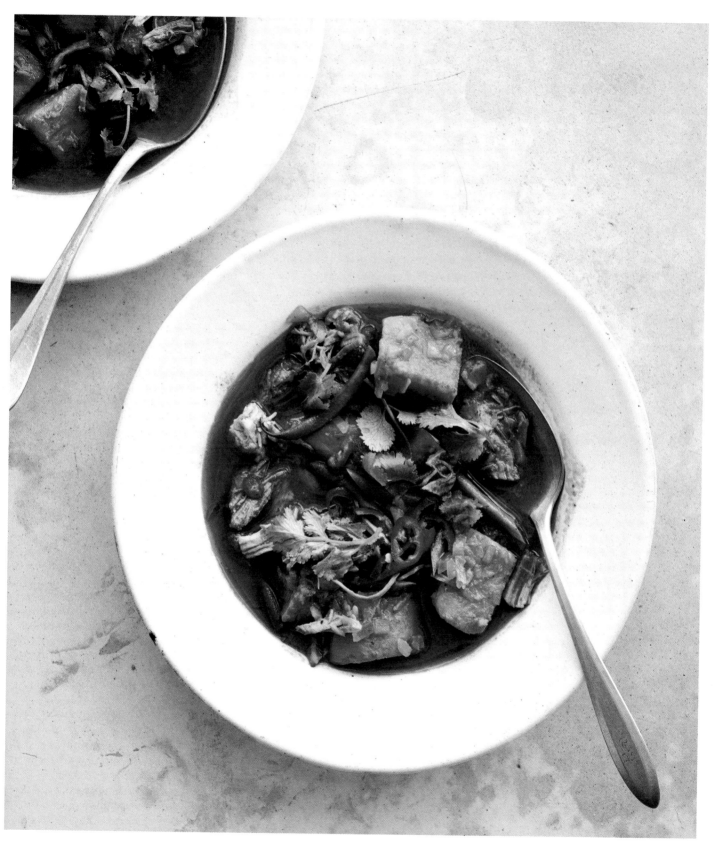

TAHINI-BROILED ROCKFISH WITH BRUSSELS SPROUT SLAW

16 TO 18 MINUTES	4 SERVINGS AND 1 LUNCH THE NEXT DAY

Brussels sprout slaw

- 1 tablespoon olive oil
- 2 tablespoons brown mustard seeds
- 2 large shallots, sliced
- Fine sea salt
- 1½ pounds Brussels sprouts, trimmed and shredded
- 2 tablespoons fresh lemon juice

Rockfish

- 1½ pounds rockfish or snapper fillets, skin removed (2 fillets)
- Fine sea salt
- 1½ tablespoons plain yogurt
- 2 tablespoons tahini
- 1 teaspoon za'atar (see page 260) or ½ teaspoon dried oregano or thyme
- ¼ teaspoon grated garlic
- 1 teaspoon olive oil
- 2 tablespoons Spiced Pumpkin Seed and Cashew Crunch (page 316) or chopped toasted walnuts (see page 306), for garnish

Sometimes a little ahead-of-time prep can make the actual cooking of a dish lightning-fast. Both components of this dish are great examples: the little jacket of tahini painted on top of the fish fillets keeps them moist even under the scorching heat of the broiler, while shredding the Brussels sprouts into a festive heap of green confetti means you can stir-fry them in a flash. You could even use a food processor with a slicing disk to do the work for you.

Heat the broiler with the rack in the top position. Line a baking sheet with aluminum foil.

To make the Brussels sprout slaw, heat the oil in a large skillet over medium-high heat. Add the mustard seeds and cook, stirring frequently, until they begin to pop. Add the shallots, season with salt, and toss to coat. Lower the heat to medium and cook, stirring frequently, until the shallots are lightly browned, about 4 minutes. Add the Brussels sprouts and a pinch of salt and toss to coat. Pour in ⅓ cup water, reduce the heat to medium, and cook until the sprouts are crisp-tender, about 4 minutes. Stir in the lemon juice and toss to coat. Season with more salt, if desired.

To prepare the rockfish, season the fillets with salt. In a small bowl, combine the yogurt, tahini, za'atar, garlic, and a pinch of salt. Stir until smooth, then brush the mixture on top of each fillet.

Transfer the fish to the prepared baking sheet, tahini side up, and drizzle with the oil. Broil until the fish is just opaque all the way through and the tahini mixture on the surface is browned, about 5 minutes.

Serve the fish and slaw topped with the pumpkin seed and cashew crunch.

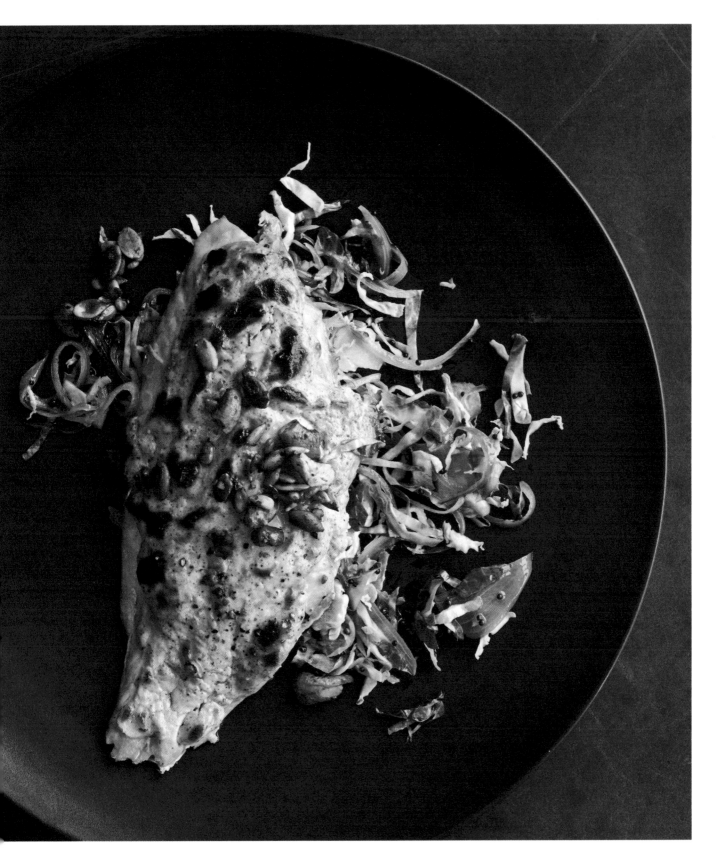

BRAISED CARROTS WITH ZA'ATAR

15 MINUTES	SERVES 4

- 1 pound carrots (8 to 10 medium), cut on the bias into 1-inch pieces
- 2 teaspoons olive oil
- Fine sea salt
- 1 teaspoon za'atar

While most of the ingredients I cook with in winter are seasonally appropriate, I often season them with warmer-climate flavors, like the za'atar here. Za'atar is a Middle Eastern spice blend that typically combines dried herbs—including the namesake za'atar, an oregano cousin—with tart, citrusy sumac and mellow sesame seeds. It gives a sunbaked earthiness and a bit of tang to the food it garnishes, and once you have it in the kitchen, you'll find yourself sprinkling it on yogurt, hummus, and roasted meats. I order mine from worldspice.com, but if you can't find it, don't fret—you could use a pinch of dried thyme and/or dried oregano instead.

Place the carrots in a 3-quart saucepan and add water to cover by 1 inch. Add the oil and salt. Bring to a boil over high heat, then turn the heat down to an easy simmer. Cook the carrots, stirring occasionally, until tender but not mushy, about 12 minutes. Pour off the liquid. Toss the za'atar with the carrots and season with additional salt.

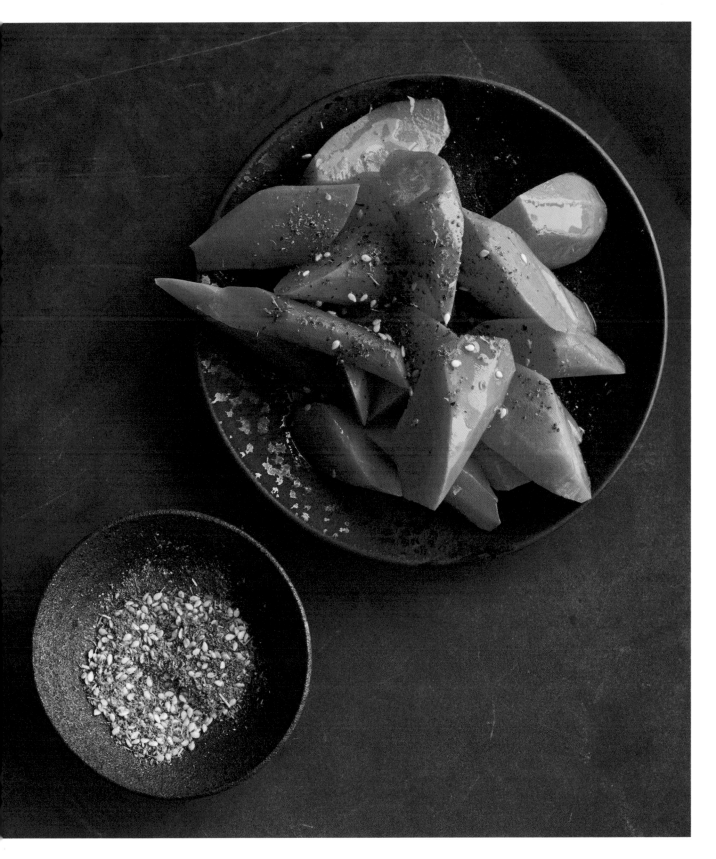

OVEN-ROASTED CHICKEN WITH RADICCHIO AND WALNUT-PARSLEY PESTO

40 TO 50 MINUTES (15 ACTIVE)	4 SERVINGS AND 1 LUNCH THE NEXT DAY

- 3 large skin-on, bone-in chicken breasts
- Fine sea salt and freshly ground black pepper
- 9 fresh sage leaves
- 2 heads radicchio, cut into 8 to 10 wedges, each with some core attached
- 1 tablespoon plus 1 teaspoon olive oil
- 1 tablespoon balsamic or sherry vinegar
- ¼ to ½ cup Walnut-Parsley Pesto (page 264), for serving
- Flaky sea salt to finish

Crimson radicchio is so pretty, but it definitely puts the bitter in bitter greens. One trick is to lace it with some sweetness—such as the balsamic in this recipe. The bitterness is also checked by roasting the radicchio until the edges of the leaves are frilled and caramelized, lending complex notes to a simple weeknight chicken.

Place one rack in the lower third of the oven and one in the upper third. Preheat the oven to 425°F.

Loosen the chicken skin without removing it completely and season the chicken with fine sea salt and pepper above and below the skin. Lay 3 of the sage leaves beneath the skin of each breast and let the chicken sit at room temperature for about 15 minutes before cooking.

Meanwhile, arrange the radicchio on a baking sheet and season with fine sea salt and pepper. Drizzle with 1 tablespoon of the oil, turning once to distribute the oil without breaking apart the radicchio wedges.

Place the sheet on the upper rack and roast until the radicchio is tender and crisp-browned at the edges, about 15 minutes. Remove the radicchio from the oven and spoon the vinegar on top.

Heat the remaining 1 teaspoon oil in a large ovenproof skillet over medium-high heat. Pat the skin side of the chicken breasts with a paper towel to remove any liquid, then place them skin side down in the skillet. Cook, undisturbed, until the skin is golden brown, about 5 minutes. Carefully flip the chicken and place the pan in the oven. Roast until a thermometer registers 165°F at the thickest part of the breast, 15 to 18 minutes. Let the chicken rest for a few minutes, then carve the breasts off the bone and into thick slices.

Place some radicchio on each serving plate and spoon on about 1 tablespoon of the pesto. Serve the chicken on top of the radicchio and sprinkle with flaky sea salt.

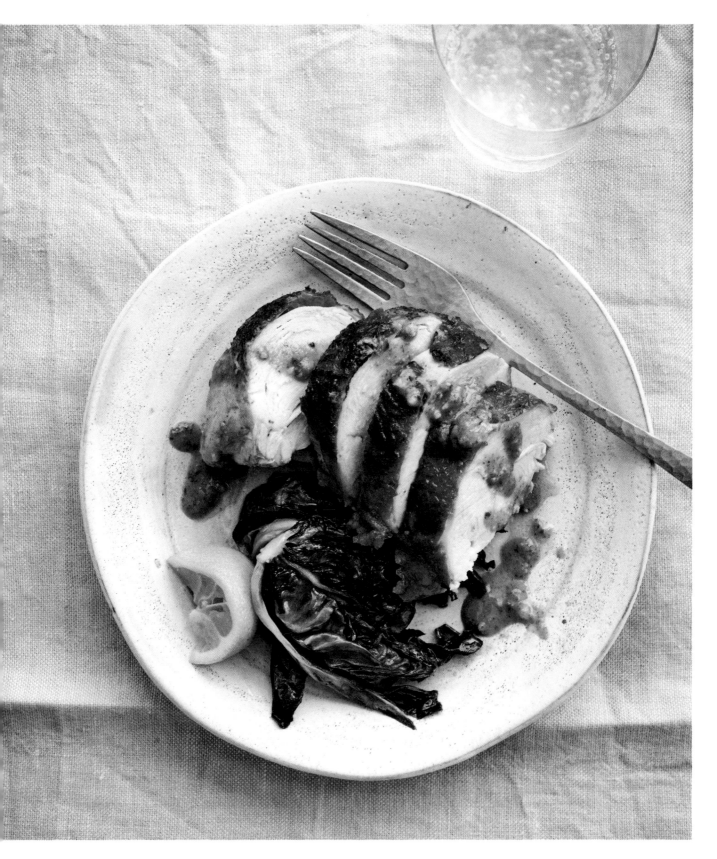

MACKEREL WITH LEMON AND WALNUT-PARSLEY PESTO

15 MINUTES (8 ACTIVE)	4 SERVINGS

- 4 (4-ounce) skin-on Atlantic mackerel (also sold as Boston, Common, Caballa, or Saba mackerel) fillets
- Fine sea salt and freshly ground black pepper to taste
- Neutral oil, such as canola or grapeseed, for the pan
- 2 teaspoons freshly squeezed lemon juice
- 4 tablespoons Walnut-Parsley Pesto (page 264)
- 1 lemon, cut into wedges, for serving

We see a lot of mackerel skies during winters in Seattle, but we don't see so much mackerel on menus—unless, of course, it's a Japanese restaurant, where simply broiled mackerel shows what a delicious fish it can be. Mackerel is full of omega-3s and is a forgiving fish to cook, but you may need to seek it out at an Asian market (or in the freezer at your local fishmonger). Here I use the basic broiler technique, topping the fillets with our trusty walnut-parsley pesto for a nicely browned, crackly topping to the tender-textured fish. If you can't find mackerel, salmon or black cod would work, but they're thicker fillets and will likely need more time to cook. Roast them until almost done in a medium oven (350°F), and then place them just below the broiler to brown.

Score the skin of the mackerel fillets and trim off any remaining belly bones. Season the fillets to taste with salt and pepper. Chill and let rest for 15 minutes before cooking.

Place the oven rack in the top position and heat the broiler. Line a baking sheet with aluminum foil. Rub a very thin layer of oil on the foil. Lay the fillets on the prepared sheet, skin side down, and sprinkle with lemon juice. Spread a thin layer of walnut-parsley pesto on each fillet and broil until the fish is just opaque at the center and the surface is browned, rotating once, about 6 minutes total. Serve with the lemon wedges.

WHITE BEAN SALAD WITH POMEGRANATE AND PARSLEY

If winter food ever feels a bit drab, I reach for pomegranate seeds to bring bracing tartness, bright color, and crunch to a dish (oh, and lots of antioxidants, too). Toss together 1¾ cups cooked, drained cannellini beans (1 [15-ounce] can), ⅓ cup pomegranate seeds, 1 tablespoon fresh lemon juice, 1 tablespoon extra-virgin olive oil, ¼ cup thinly sliced scallions, and 2 tablespoons chopped flat-leaf parsley leaves. Season to taste with fine sea salt and freshly ground black pepper.

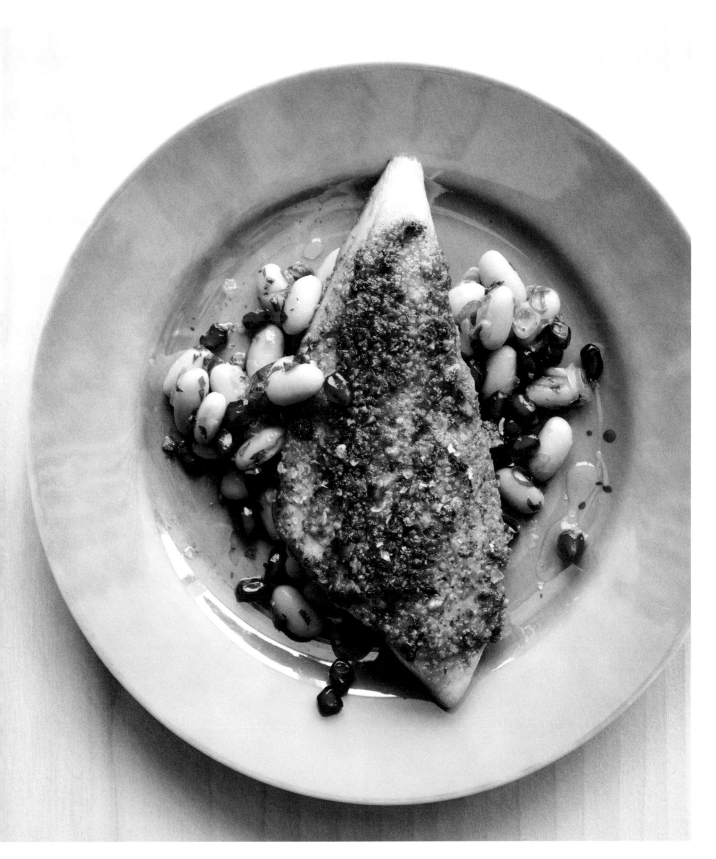

VEGETABLE POT-AU-FEU

30 TO 40 MINUTES	4 SERVINGS AND 1 LUNCH THE NEXT DAY

- 2 large carrots, cut on the bias into 2-inch pieces
- 2 large leeks (white and light green parts, well rinsed), cut on the bias into 2-inch pieces
- 2 large or 3 medium parsnips, peeled, halved lengthwise if large (remove the woody center if needed), and cut on the bias into 2-inch chunks
- ½ medium Savoy cabbage head, cut into 4 wedges, each with some core attached
- 2 fresh flat-leaf parsley sprigs
- 5 cups homemade chicken stock (see page 301) or low-sodium canned
- Fine sea salt and freshly ground black pepper to taste
- 1 tablespoon chopped fresh flat-leaf parsley, for garnish

Pot-au-feu is the name for the long-cooked stew of veggies and tough meat cuts. In theory, the French farmhouse cook would simply throw new bits of meat, produce, and water into the ever-simmering pot to replenish it with each serving.

This is considerably quicker to cook and shows you what a rich meal you can put together with vegetables as the centerpiece. If you want to make the soup totally vegetarian, use homemade vegetable stock (see page 302).

Place the carrots, leeks, parsnips, cabbage, parsley sprigs, and stock in a large heavy pot and bring to a boil over medium-high heat. Reduce the heat to low, cover, and simmer until the vegetables are tender but not falling apart, about 20 minutes.

Season with salt and pepper and top with the chopped parsley.

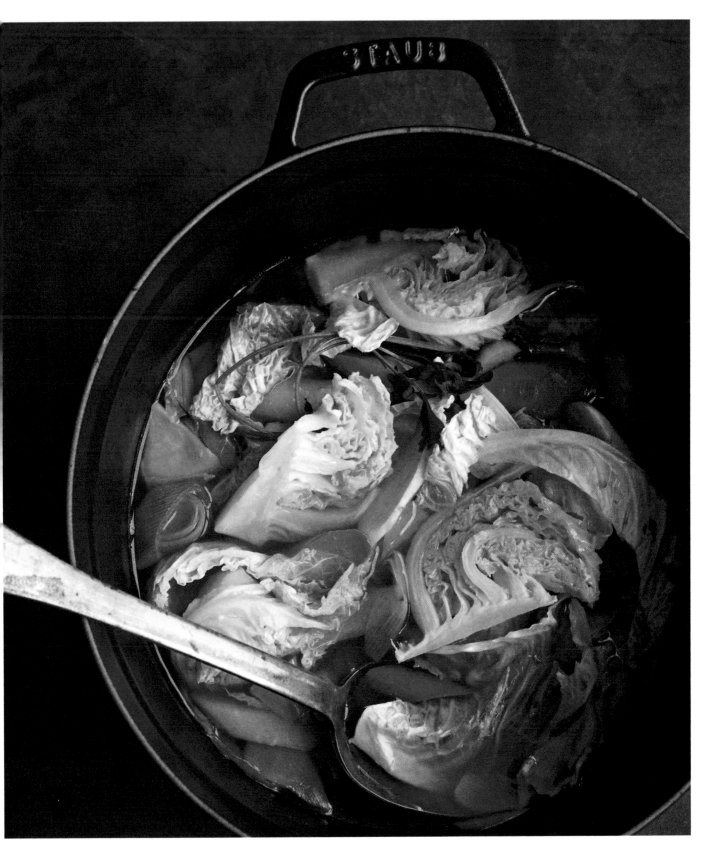

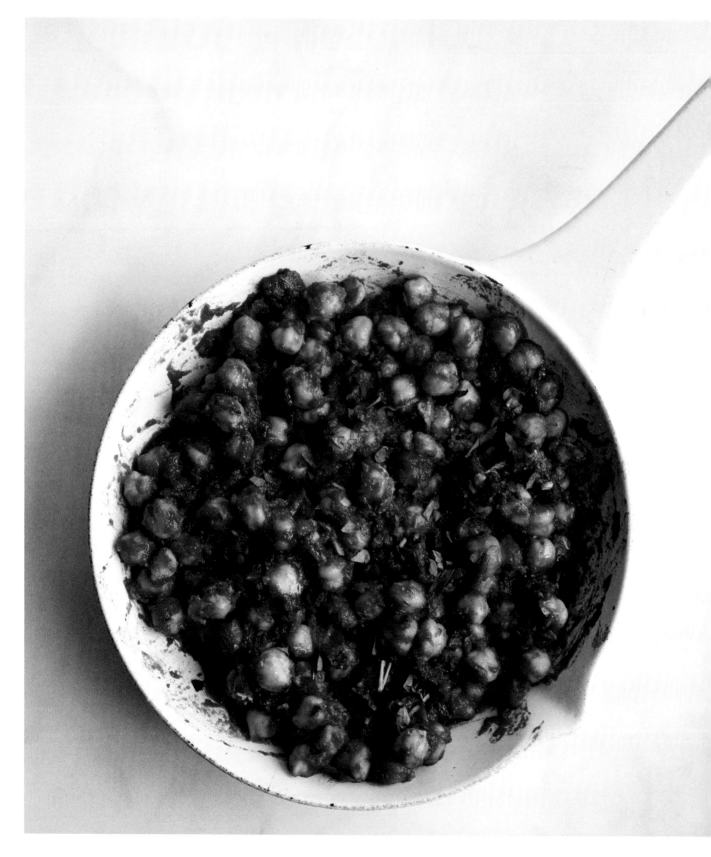

SMOKY SPICED CHICKPEAS

15 MINUTES	4 SERVINGS AND 1 LUNCH THE NEXT DAY

- 2 tablespoons olive oil
- 1 small dried chile, such as chile de arbol or japones
- 1 teaspoon cumin seeds
- 2 garlic cloves, sliced
- 1½ cups tomato puree
- 1 bay leaf
- ½ teaspoon smoked paprika
- 2 (15-ounce) cans chickpeas, drained, or 3 cups cooked chickpeas
- Fine sea salt
- ¼ cup chopped sun-dried tomatoes
- Freshly ground black pepper
- Fresh parsley leaves, for garnish

Some vegetarian entrees are meatier than others, and this one is full of satisfying flavor, with a thick, slightly smoky tomato sauce coating the tender chickpeas. It tastes great beside the Kale Sautéed with Onions, Leeks, and Turmeric on page 255, but it also works well tossed with whole wheat pasta and chopped fresh oregano or topped with a gorgeous fried egg at brunch.

In a large skillet, heat the oil over medium heat. Add the chile and cumin seeds and toast, stirring frequently, until the cumin is fragrant and has darkened a shade, about 1 minute. Add the garlic and stir for 30 seconds. Stir in the tomato puree, bay leaf, paprika, chickpeas, and ½ cup water (use caution, as the tomato may splatter). Season with salt and lower the heat; simmer, stirring occasionally, until the tomato sauce has reduced and coated the chickpeas, about 6 minutes. Stir in the sun-dried tomatoes and adjust the seasoning with additional salt and black pepper to taste. Top with the parsley leaves.

ROASTED CAULIFLOWER WITH THYME AND OLIVES

25 MINUTES	4 SERVINGS AND 1 LUNCH THE NEXT DAY

- 2 tablespoons olive oil
- 1 large cauliflower head, cut into ½-inch-thick pieces
- Fine sea salt to taste
- 1 tablespoon fresh thyme leaves (from 4 to 5 sprigs)
- ¼ cup Kalamata olives, rinsed, drained, pitted, and halved
- 1½ teaspoons finely grated orange zest
- Red pepper flakes, preferably Aleppo or Marash, to taste

If it's dinnertime, more often than not I'm roasting produce on a sheet pan (see more on this on page 302). It's the laziest way I know to get good veggie flavor on my plate, and I love the irregular browned edges that develop in a hot oven.

I chase away monotony by tossing vegetables with something intense and aromatic right when they're piping hot from the oven. The heat will make the fragrance of those last-minute ingredients bloom. It could be a grated garlic clove or a bit of sesame oil or some chopped fresh herbs. But cauliflower puts me in a Mediterranean mood, and so I fold in some grated orange zest, a handful of olives, and a spiky pinch of red pepper flakes. Oh, and if like me you hate scrubbing sheet pans, consider lining the pan first with compostable parchment paper.

Preheat the oven to 425°F.

Spread 1 tablespoon of the oil on a baking sheet and spread the cauliflower pieces in a single layer. Sprinkle with the salt, thyme, and additional oil. Roast the cauliflower, flipping the florets once, until evenly browned, 20 to 25 minutes.

Remove from the heat and gently toss the cauliflower with the olives, orange zest, and red pepper flakes. Taste and add more salt, if desired.

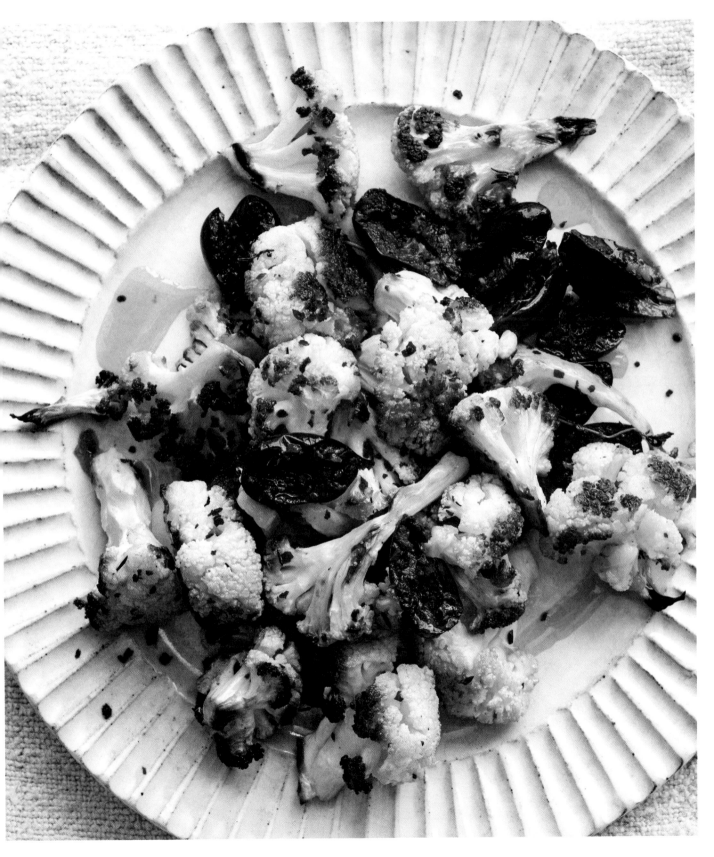

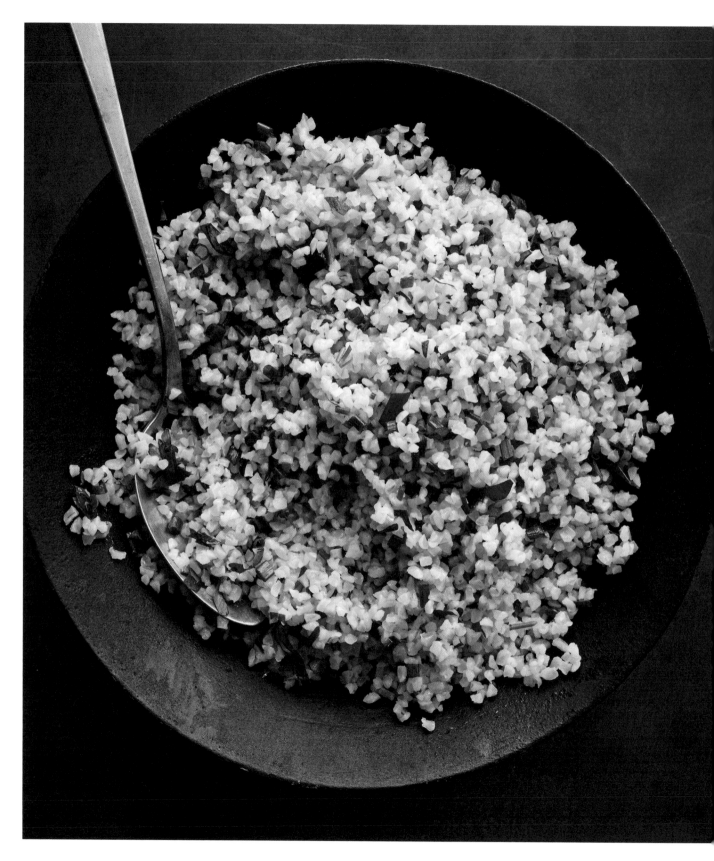

BULGUR WITH PARSLEY AND CHIVES

25 MINUTES (5 ACTIVE)	4 SERVINGS

- 1 lemon
- 1 tablespoon olive oil
- 1 cup medium bulgur wheat
- Fine sea salt to taste
- ½ cup chopped fresh flat-leaf parsley leaves
- ¼ cup chopped fresh chives
- Freshly ground black pepper to taste

My kids are not great whole-grain eaters, but bulgur is part of the transition effort. From white pasta they grew to love *maftoul*, a kind of whole wheat couscous, and from there, tender, nutty bulgur isn't that far away. They like it plain, but I love it with a great big shower of fresh herbs on top. The other handy thing about bulgur is its quick cooking time.

Using a peeler, remove the bright yellow peel of the lemon, leaving behind the white pith. Cut the lemon into wedges and reserve.

Place the lemon peel and oil in a small sauté pan and heat it over medium heat for 1 minute. Turn off the heat and set the pan aside to let the oil infuse with the lemon.

Meanwhile, place the bulgur in a medium saucepan with 2 cups water and salt. Bring the water to a boil over high heat, turn the heat to low, cover, and cook until the bulgur is tender, about 12 minutes.

Pour off any excess water and fluff the bulgur with a fork. Cover and let stand another 5 minutes.

Place the bulgur, parsley, and chives in a large bowl; add the lemon-infused oil and stir. Remove the pieces of lemon peel, taste, and season with salt and pepper.

Serve with the lemon wedges to squeeze over.

MOROCCAN LAMB SHANKS WITH POMEGRANATE

3½ HOURS (20 MINUTES ACTIVE)	4 SERVINGS AND 1 LUNCH THE NEXT DAY

- 1 teaspoon coriander seeds
- ½ teaspoon fennel seeds
- ½ teaspoon cumin seeds
- ¼ teaspoon red pepper flakes, preferably Aleppo or Marash
- Pinch of saffron (optional)
- Kosher salt and freshly ground black pepper to taste
- 2 lamb shanks (about 2½ pounds)
- 1 tablespoon cornstarch
- 1 tablespoon olive oil
- 1 medium red onion, cut into 1-inch wedges
- 2 medium carrots, cut into 2-inch pieces
- 1 large leek (white and light green parts), cut into 2-inch pieces
- 1 cinnamon stick
- 8 fresh thyme sprigs
- 1½ cups pomegranate juice
- 1½ cups homemade chicken stock (see page 301), low-sodium canned, or water
- ¼ cup pomegranate seeds, for garnish
- ¼ cup fresh mint leaves, for garnish
- Flaky sea salt to finish

Sometimes, especially on a weekend, you just need a braise going in the background. Marissa reminded me that it might be nice to include a lamb shank in our winter repertoire, and when she did, I was thrilled. In the cleanse we tend to focus on pretty quick-cooking cuts of meat and seafood, but nothing feels more soul-soothing and wintry than the long-braised, velvety, on-the-bone cut. It's not the leanest cut of meat in the world, but most of its unctuousness comes not from fat but from the connective tissue that weaves through the shank. We've flavored the shank with North African spices and woken up the rich meat and vegetables with a handful of pomegranate seeds and fresh mint leaves sprinkled on just before serving. If you're serving 4 for dinner and want to use lamb leftovers for lunch, you might want to throw an extra shank in the pot for that purpose.

Preheat the oven to 350°F.

Using a spice grinder or mortar and pestle, coarsely grind together the coriander seeds, fennel seeds, cumin seeds, and red pepper flakes. Crumble the saffron into the mixture, if using, and stir in 1 teaspoon kosher salt, plus black pepper to taste.

If there is an opaque white layer enrobing the shanks, remove it by cutting it a bit at the edge and then pulling at the corner: it should come off with a little coaxing. Do not remove the iridescent membrane below, which holds the meat together. Season the shanks with the coriander mixture and let them rest for at least 30 minutes (or chill overnight).

Thirty minutes before you want to cook them, dredge the shanks in the cornstarch, shaking off any excess. In a large heavy braising dish or Dutch oven, heat the oil over medium heat. Add the shanks and brown them on all sides, 10 to 12 minutes. Transfer the shanks to a platter or baking dish and add the onion, carrots, and leek to the pan. Cook, stirring and scraping up any brown bits that have accumulated in the pan. After 1 minute, add the

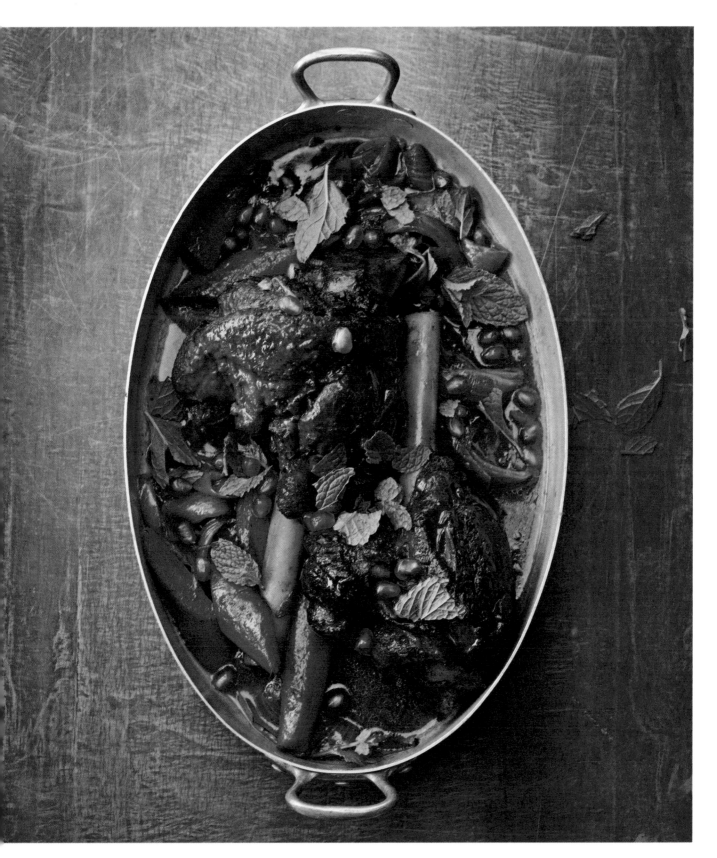

cinnamon and thyme and pour in the pomegranate juice and stock. Scrape the pan bottom again and bring the liquid up to a simmer. Return the shanks to the pan and season again with kosher salt and black pepper.

Cover the pot and transfer it to the oven. Braise for about 1½ hours, then check the liquid level, making sure there is at least 1 inch of stock in the pan. If not, add water or stock to bring it up to that mark, then continue braising until the meat is completely tender and falling off the bone, about 2½ hours.

Using a slotted spoon, remove the meat and large chunks of vegetables from the pot. Discard the thyme and cinnamon stick. Use a spoon to skim off as much fat as possible from the surface; tilting the pan a bit can help with gathering the fat layer. To serve, bring the liquid to a simmer and place the meat and vegetables in the pot to warm up again, if necessary.

Serve the lamb pieces off the bone with some sauce and top with pomegranate seeds, mint leaves, and flaky sea salt.

WALNUT-PARSLEY PESTO

Pictured on page 262

20 MINUTES (5 MINUTES ACTIVE)	MAKES 1½ CUPS

- 2 cups walnut halves
- 1 garlic clove, chopped
- 2 anchovy fillets, roughly chopped
- ½ cup olive oil, plus more as needed
- 1 tablespoon sherry vinegar
- ¼ teaspoon smoked paprika
- ¼ cup roughly chopped fresh flat-leaf parsley leaves
- Fine sea salt and freshly ground black pepper

Sometimes I fall for exotic ingredients, but day in and day out, I lean on the plainest foods. Here's a rich and versatile sauce that summons depth of flavor from the most ordinary of ingredients: parsley and walnuts. One trick is toasting the nuts to fragrant richness, and the other is another easy grocery store find: a couple of anchovy fillets. Don't worry, they don't taste fishy amid all the other ingredients—they just whisper something rich and satisfying from backstage. You can use them to the same subtle effect when braising greens or whisking up a vinaigrette.

Preheat the oven to 300°F. Arrange the walnuts on a baking sheet and toast until golden, about 15 minutes. Let cool.

Pulse the garlic and anchovies in a food processor until combined. Add half the walnuts and process into a paste, about 2 minutes. Add the ½ cup oil, the vinegar, and the paprika and process to combine. Add the remaining walnuts and the parsley and pulse until there are roughly chopped bits of nut within the paste, about 1 minute. Season to taste with salt and pepper; add more olive oil (up to 2 tablespoons) to make a more fluid pesto as desired. Store in an airtight container in the refrigerator for up to 1 week.

ROOT VEGETABLE MINESTRONE

45 MINUTES (15 ACTIVE)	5 TO 6 SERVINGS

- 1 medium onion, chopped
- 1 large carrot, chopped
- 2 tablespoons olive oil
- 1 teaspoon fennel seeds, crushed in a mortar or with the back of a pan
- 2 garlic cloves, peeled and sliced
- 2 tablespoons tomato paste
- 1 large parsnip, peeled and cut into 1-inch pieces
- ½ large celery root, peeled and cut into 1-inch pieces
- 2 medium golden beets, peeled and cut into 1-inch pieces
- 4 fresh marjoram sprigs or ½ teaspoon dried oregano
- ½ cup dry white wine
- Fine sea salt and freshly ground black pepper to taste
- 4 cups chopped cabbage
- 1 (28-ounce) can whole tomatoes, crushed with your fingers
- Parmesan rind (optional)
- 1 (15-ounce) can cannellini beans, drained, or 1¾ cups cooked beans (see page 303)
- 1 bunch kale, well washed, large stems removed, and leaves torn
- Red pepper flakes, preferably Aleppo or Marash, to taste

When I finish my cleanse every year, I use up all the odds and ends in the crisper drawer in something I call aftermath soup. In go the handfuls of spinach and kale left over from lunch salads; in go the half cup of mushrooms and the stray carrots that didn't make it into any meal. It's a delicious way to keep all those good ingredients from going to waste, and it proves that soup can make a noble and satisfying meal. This soup is a more refined version of that kitchen-sink soup; it's full of the earthy-sweet depth of root vegetables, but brightened by tomatoes and chile flakes. And though aged cheese isn't generally part of the cleanse, feel free to throw a Parmesan rind in the pot if you have one. It will share some of its irresistible complexity with the stock, and you wouldn't want it to go to waste, would you?

In a food processor, pulse the onion and carrot until finely chopped, about 2 minutes.

In a large heavy-bottomed soup pot or Dutch oven, heat the oil over medium heat. Add the fennel seeds and toast until fragrant, about 1 minute. Add the garlic, onion, and carrot. Cook, stirring frequently, until any liquid released by the vegetables reduces and the vegetables begin to brown, about 5 minutes. Add the tomato paste, stir until it's well distributed through the vegetables, and cook about 3 minutes. Add the parsnip, celery root, beets, and marjoram or oregano and stir in the white wine, scraping up the browned bits from the bottom of the pan. Cook, stirring frequently, until the wine is almost completely evaporated and the vegetables are coated with the tomato mixture; season with salt and black pepper. Add the cabbage, crushed tomatoes with their juices, 4 cups water, and the Parmesan rind, if using.

Bring the liquid to a boil, then reduce the heat and simmer, stirring occasionally, until the vegetables are tender but not mushy, about 30 minutes. Stir in the beans, kale, red pepper flakes, and ½ cup water if the soup is too thick. Cook for 5 minutes, taste, and add more salt and black pepper as desired.

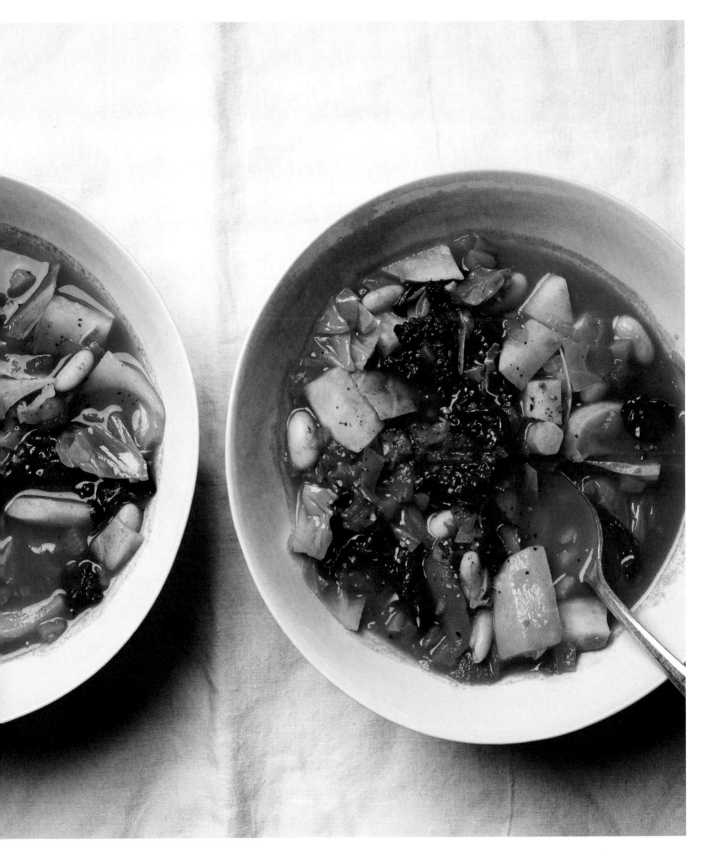

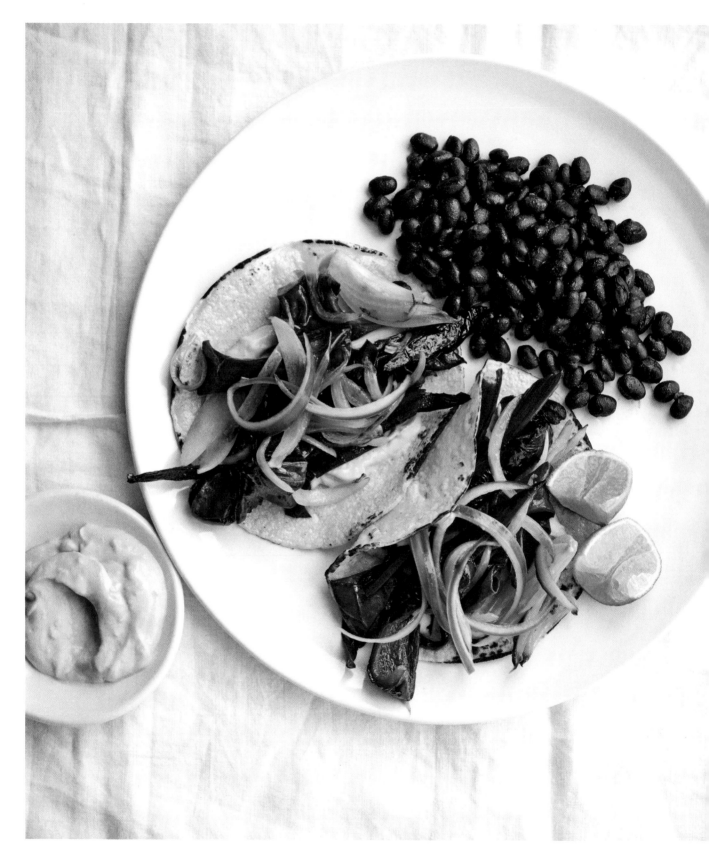

SWISS CHARD AND POBLANO TACOS WITH AVOCADO CREMA

25 MINUTES	4 SERVINGS

Avocado crema

- 1 ripe avocado, pitted and peeled
- 1 tablespoon freshly squeezed lime juice
- ¾ cup plain Greek yogurt
- 1 garlic clove, chopped
- Fine sea salt to taste

Tacos

- 2 tablespoons neutral oil, such as canola or grapeseed
- 2 poblano (pasilla) chiles, cored, seeded, and cut into 1-inch-wide strips
- 2 bunches chard, well washed, large stems removed and cut into 4-inch pieces, leaves sliced into ribbons
- 1 medium onion, sliced
- Fine sea salt
- 1 garlic clove, sliced
- 8 small corn tortillas
- 1 batch Quick Citrus-Pickled Onion (see page 323)

I took an eye-opening trip a few years ago to Mexico City, where the food was extraordinary everywhere from the poshest restaurants to the street-cart snacks. While tacos can certainly be a very meaty affair, there are also traditional vegetable fillings for tortillas, including *acelgas*, or chard. This is my quick-fired none-too-traditional riff on the stewed chard tacos I loved in the Condesa neighborhood. I also took the liberty of adding quick-pickled onions and a creamy little avocado sauce.

To make the crema, in a blender or food processor, blend together the avocado, lime juice, yogurt, garlic, and salt. Place plastic wrap directly on the surface of the puree and chill until serving.

To make the taco filling, in a large covered skillet or braising pot, heat 1 tablespoon of the oil over medium heat. Add in the poblano strips and chard stems and cook, undisturbed, until browned, about 2 minutes. Turn and brown on the other side, about 1 more minute. Remove them from the pan and wipe out the pan.

Heat the remaining 1 tablespoon oil and add the onion and a pinch of salt. Cook, stirring occasionally, until the onion is softened, about 5 minutes. Stir in the garlic and cook for 1 minute. Stir in the chard leaves and another pinch of salt and cook until the greens are wilted and tender, 2 to 3 minutes.

Heat the tortillas one by one in a dry skillet over medium-high heat, about 30 seconds per side (if you have a gas flame, you can do this directly over the flame). Wrap the tortillas in clean dish towels or napkins to keep them warm as you go.

To assemble the tacos, place some avocado crema in a tortilla. Top with the chard stems, poblanos, chard-leaf mixture, and pickled onions.

BRAISED CHICKEN WITH SQUASH AND PRUNES

40 MINUTES	4 SERVINGS AND 1 LUNCH THE NEXT DAY

- ¼ teaspoon ground cumin
- ¼ teaspoon ground cinnamon
- ¼ teaspoon ground cayenne pepper
- 5 chicken thighs on the bone (about 2½ pounds)
- Fine sea salt
- 1 tablespoon olive oil
- 1 small butternut squash (about 2½ pounds), peeled and cut in 4 × ½-inch wedges
- Freshly ground black pepper to taste
- 2 shallots, thinly sliced
- ½ cup halved prunes
- 1 cup homemade chicken stock (see page 301) or low-sodium canned
- 2 tablespoons chopped fresh mint leaves, for garnish
- Flaky sea salt to finish

Prunes are tangy, sweet, and so good to cook with. Give them a shake here, with this warm-spiced chicken stew that nods to Persian squash-and-prune _khoresh_. I use my trusty enameled braising pan for this dish; it's a good 12 inches wide. If you don't have a covered skillet that wide, brown everything in batches, then cook it together with the stock or transfer to a baking dish, cover securely, and bake at 425°F until done.

Mix together the cumin, cinnamon, and cayenne. Season the chicken thighs with the spice mixture and fine sea salt.

Heat the oil in a wide heavy skillet over medium heat. Blot the chicken thighs to dry them, then place them skin side down in the oil. Cook until the skin is browned on the skin side only, 7 to 9 minutes. Transfer the chicken to a plate.

Working in batches if needed, turn the heat to medium-high and place the squash wedges in the pan in a single layer. Season the squash with fine sea salt and pepper. Cook until brown on one side, 4 to 5 minutes. Transfer to the plate with the chicken and repeat with the remaining squash pieces.

Add the shallots and sauté until browned, about 3 minutes. Return the chicken to the pan, skin side up, along with any accumulated juices on the plate. Nestle the prunes around the chicken, followed by the squash. Add the stock, bring the liquid to a boil, reduce the heat, and simmer, covered, until the squash is tender and the chicken is cooked through, 12 to 15 minutes. Uncover and simmer until the liquid is glossy and thick, about 4 more minutes.

Serve the chicken with squash, prunes, and a spoonful of the pan sauce. Top with mint and flaky sea salt.

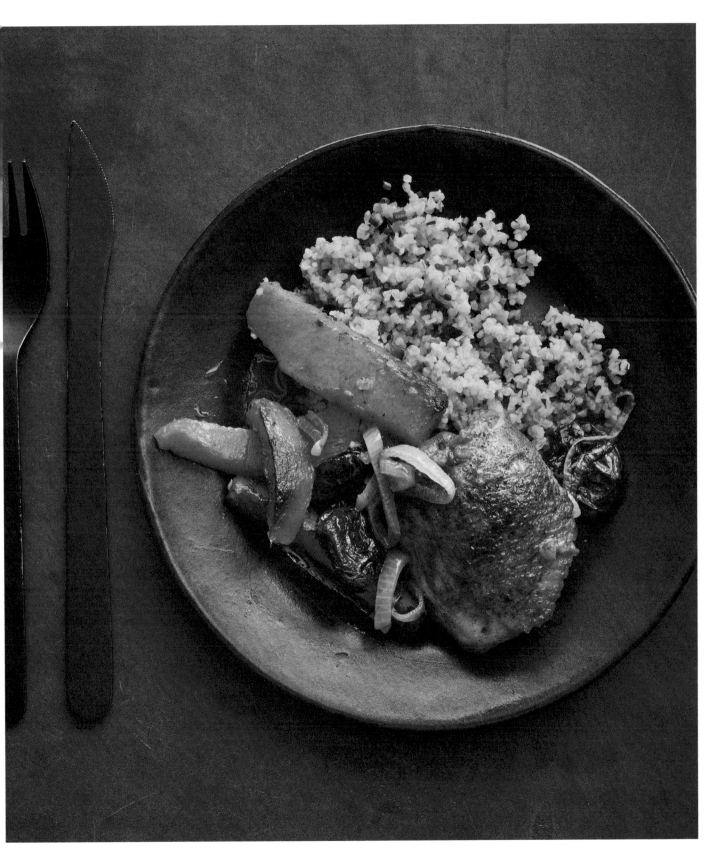

SEA SCALLOPS WITH CELERY ROOT AND MEYER LEMON SALAD

ABOUT 10 MINUTES	4 SERVINGS

- 2 Meyer lemons, plus more for garnish, or 1 tablespoon finely grated conventional lemon zest plus 2 tablespoons lemon juice

- 2 teaspoons Dijon mustard

- 2 tablespoons olive oil

- 1 tablespoon capers, soaked and drained if packed in salt, rinsed if packed in vinegar, chopped

- Fine sea salt and freshly ground black pepper to taste

- 12 large dry-pack sea scallops

- 1 tablespoon neutral oil, such as canola or grapeseed

- 6 cups finely julienned peeled celery root (from about 1 softball-size celery root)

- ¼ cup fresh parsley leaves and tender stems (about ¼ bunch)

- Flaky sea salt to finish

Celery root can look pretty imposing in the market: with bumpy, gnarled skin, it can be anywhere from the size of a tennis ball to that of a bowling ball (a candlepin bowling ball, at least). But the best celery roots aren't too big; the giants tend to have spongy centers. Instead, pick a small to medium root and peel off its hide with a sharp knife. Inside you'll find ivory-green flesh that's crisp, a bit nutty, and utterly delicious in salads. This take on a classic remoulade provides perfect contrast to the silken luxury of seared scallops.

Supreme the lemons, reserving the peel (see page 306). Chop the lemon flesh and transfer it to a small bowl. Very finely chop the peel until you have about 1 tablespoon; add to the bowl with the chopped lemon. Juice the remaining lemon and add 2 tablespoons to the lemon mixture, along with the mustard, oil, and capers. (If you're working with a conventional lemon, stir in the zest and juice here.) Season the mixture with fine sea salt and pepper and more lemon juice, if needed.

Season the sea scallops with fine sea salt and a bit of pepper. Heat the neutral oil in a nonstick pan over medium-high heat. Pat the scallops dry and sear them in the pan, leaving 1 inch of clearance between the scallops (you may need to work in batches). Cook, undisturbed, until the underside is caramel brown, about 1 minute. Turn the scallops and cook until warmed through but still a bit translucent in the center, another minute.

In a medium bowl, toss the celery root with the parsley leaves and stems and dress it with the Meyer lemon mixture. Season with additional fine sea salt and pepper, if desired. Serve the salad with the scallops, finished with flaky sea salt and garnished with Meyer lemon wedges.

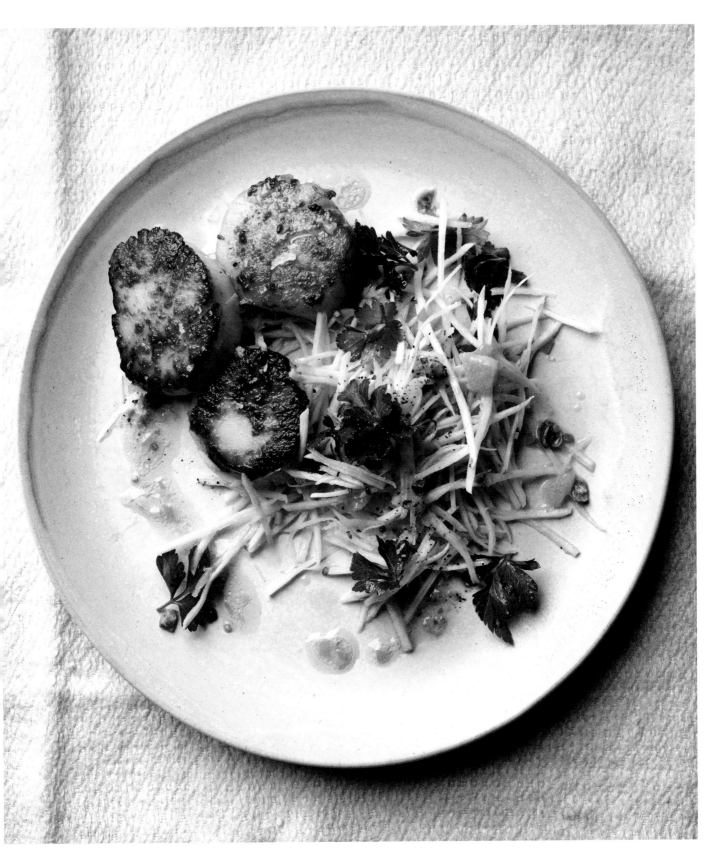

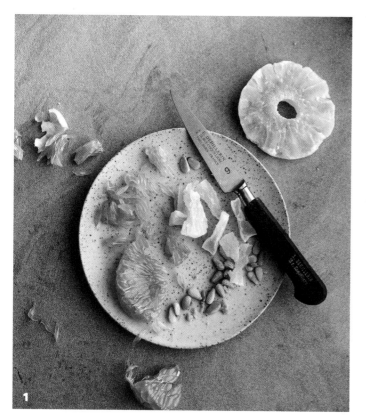

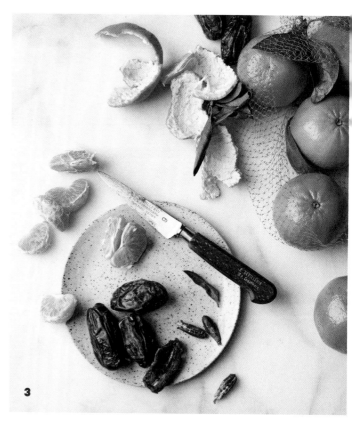

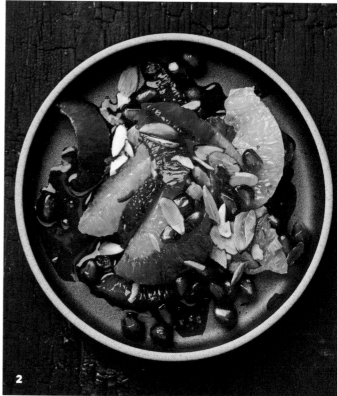

WINTER DESSERT SUGGESTIONS

The suggested portions below are for one person.

1. Pomelo with toasted pine nuts and dried pineapple
½ pomelo, 1 or 2 teaspoons pine nuts, and 1 tablespoon chopped dried pineapple

2. Navel and blood orange supremes with pomegranate seeds and toasted almond flakes
½ blood orange, ½ navel orange, ¼ cup pomegranate seeds, 1 tablespoon almond flakes

3. Tangerine with dates
1 tangerine, 2 dates

4. Mango carpaccio with citrus threads, sea salt, and chile
½ mango, ¼ cup grapefruit or finger lime threads (you can get citrus threads by peeling the membrane off a slice of citrus and teasing apart the juicy fibers inside)

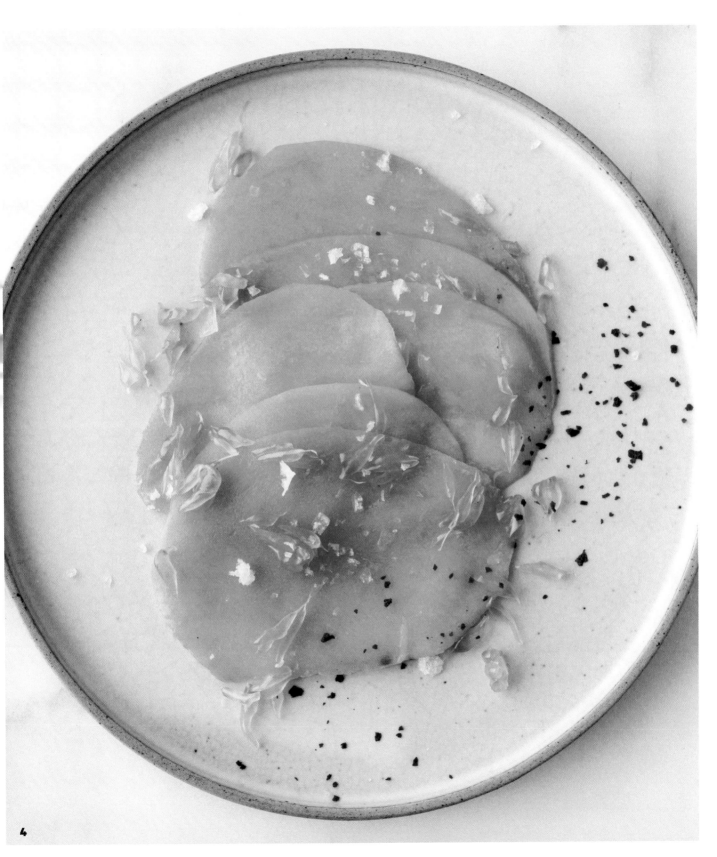

DAY 1

(STARTS WITH DINNER)

DINNER
Pan-Roasted Salmon with
Grapefruit-Cabbage Slaw
(page 251)

Refried Black Beans
(page 252)

DESSERT
Tangerines with dates
(pictured on page 286)

DAY 2

BREAKFAST
Coconut Oatmeal with Cacao
Nibs and Dates (page 233)

LUNCH
Leftover salmon with grated
carrots, celery root, mint,
Belgian endive, and toasted
sesame seeds with Creamy
Tahini Dressing (pictured on
page 214)

SNACK
Plain Greek yogurt with
Spiced Pumpkin Seed and
Cashew Crunch (page 316)

DINNER
Oven-Roasted Chicken
with Radicchio and Walnut-
Parsley Pesto (page 262)

Roasted Cauliflower with
Thyme and Olives
(page 270)

DESSERT
Navel and blood orange
supremes with pomegranate
seeds and toasted almond
flakes (pictured on
page 286)

DAY 3

BREAKFAST
Spiced Pumpkin Steel-Cut
Oats with Pecans (page 236)

LUNCH
Leftover chicken and
cauliflower with apple, red
kale, toasted walnuts, with
Sherry Vinaigrette (pictured
on page 243)

SNACK
Sliced pear with chèvre

DINNER
Tahini-Broiled Rockfish
with Brussels Sprout Slaw
(page 258)

Braised Carrots with Za'atar
(page 260)

DESSERT
Mango carpaccio with citrus
threads, sea salt, and chile
(pictured on page 287)

DAY 4

BREAKFAST
Apples and Pomegranate
with Toasted Quinoa and
Yogurt (page 237)

LUNCH
Leftover rockfish with mint,
lemon zest, and Creamy
Tahini Dressing (dressing
recipe on page 314) with
chickpeas and butter lettuce

SNACK
Hard-boiled egg (see
page 301) with Smoked
Salt Furikake (page 323)

DINNER
Vegetable Pot-au-Feu
(page 266)

Bulgur with Parsley and
Chives (page 273)

DESSERT
Salted Seedy Chocolate Bark:
The Original (page 327)

DAY 5

BREAKFAST
Scrambled Eggs with
Smoked Salmon, Chives, and
Rye Cracker (page 234)

LUNCH
Leftover pot-au-feu
vegetables with bulgur,
mustard greens, and Meyer
Lemon–Shallot Vinaigrette
(pictured on page 242)

SNACK
Roasted Beet and Tahini Dip
(page 318) with crudités

DINNER
Kale Sautéed with Onions,
Leeks, and Turmeric
(page 255)

Smoky Spiced Chickpeas
(page 269)

DESSERT
Pomelo with toasted pine
nuts and dried pineapple
(pictured on page 286)

DAY 6

BREAKFAST
Coconut Oatmeal with Cacao
Nibs and Dates (page 233)

LUNCH
Leftover chickpeas with
hard-boiled egg (see
page 301), side salad
of spinach, pistachios,
dried apricot, and Sherry
Vinaigrette (page 315)

SNACK
Apple with almond butter

DINNER
Miso Flank Steak with
Shiitake–Mustard Green
Escabeche (page 248)

Acorn Squash Puree with
Chili Oil (page 247)

DESSERT
Navel and blood orange
supremes with pomegranate
seeds and toasted almond
flakes (pictured on page 286)

CLEANSE MENU

DAY 7

BREAKFAST
Two-Egg Omelet with
Walnut-Parsley Pesto
(page 239)

LUNCH
Leftover flank steak and
mushrooms, escarole, celery,
toasted sesame seeds,
and Whole-Grain Mustard
Vinaigrette (page 315)

SNACK
Plain Greek yogurt with
Spiced Pumpkin Seed and
Cashew Crunch (page 316)

DINNER
Moroccan Lamb Shanks with
Pomegranate (page 274)

Bulgur with Parsley and
Chives (page 273)

DESSERT
Salted Seedy Chocolate Bark:
The Original (page 327)

DAY 8

BREAKFAST
Spiced Pumpkin Steel-Cut
Oats with Pecans (page 236)

LUNCH
Leftover Moroccan lamb
shanks with shaved fennel,
frisée, pistachios, and Meyer
Lemon–Shallot Vinaigrette
(pictured on page 240)

SNACK
Roasted Beet and Tahini
Dip (page 318) with all-rye
crackers

DINNER
Mackerel with Lemon and
Walnut-Parsley Pesto
(page 264)

White Bean Salad with
Pomegranate and Parsley
(page 264)

DESSERT
Tangerine with dates
(pictured on page 286)

DAY 9

BREAKFAST
Scrambled Eggs with
Smoked Salmon, Chives, and
Rye Cracker (page 234)

LUNCH
Leftover white bean salad,
arugula, roasted Delicata
squash (see page 302),
pumpkin seeds, and Whole-
Grain Mustard Vinaigrette
(page 315)

SNACK
Sliced pear with chèvre

DINNER
Root Vegetable Minestrone
(page 278)

DESSERT
Navel and blood orange
supremes with pomegranate
seeds and toasted almond
flakes (pictured on page 286)

DAY 10

BREAKFAST
Apples and Pomegranate
with Toasted Quinoa and
Yogurt (page 237)

LUNCH
1 cup minestrone, with side
salad spinach and orange
sections with Whole-Grain
Mustard Vinaigrette
(page 315)

SNACK
Roasted Beet and Tahini
Dip (page 318) with all-rye
crackers

DINNER
Tunisian-Style Poached
Eggs in Red Pepper Sauce
(page 244)

Barley Pilaf with Spinach and
Pine Nuts (page 246)

DESSERT
Pomelo with chopped dried
pineapple (pictured on
page 286)

DAY 11

BREAKFAST
Two-Egg Omelet with
Walnut-Parsley Pesto
(page 239)

LUNCH
Canned albacore tuna
with leftover barley, pine
nuts, and tatsoi with Whole-
Grain Mustard Vinaigrette
(page 315)

SNACK
Apple with almond butter

DINNER
Swiss Chard and Poblano
Tacos with Avocado Crema
(page 281)

Quick Citrus-Pickled Onion
(page 323)

Refried Black Beans
(page 252)

DESSERT
Mango carpaccio with citrus
threads, sea salt, and chile
(pictured on page 287)

DAY 12

BREAKFAST
Coconut Oatmeal with Cacao
Nibs and Dates (page 233)

LUNCH
Leftover chard with hard-
boiled egg (see page 301)
alongside shaved vegetable
salad with cauliflower, carrot,
and sauerkraut and Whole-
Grain Mustard Vinaigrette
(page 315)

SNACK
Leftover avocado crema with
crudités

DINNER
Braised Chicken with Squash
and Prunes (page 282)

Bulgur with Parsley and
Chives (page 273)

DESSERT
Salted Seedy Chocolate Bark:
The Original (page 327)

DAY 13

BREAKFAST
Apples and Pomegranate
with Toasted Quinoa and
Yogurt (page 237)

LUNCH
Leftover chicken, roasted
Delicata squash (see
page 302), Spiced Pumpkin
Seed and Cashew Crunch
(page 316), frisée, Creamy
Tahini Dressing (page 314)

SNACK
Sliced pear with chèvre

DINNER
Sea Scallops with Celery
Root and Meyer Lemon Salad
(page 284)

Barley Pilaf with Spinach and
Pine Nuts (page 246)

DESSERT
Tangerine with dates
(pictured on page 286)

DAY 14

BREAKFAST
Spiced Pumpkin Steel-Cut
Oats with Pecans (page 236)

LUNCH
Leftover barley, served with
shredded carrots, olives, and
arugula with Creamy Tahini
Dressing (page 314)

SNACK
Hard-boiled egg (see
page 301) with Smoked Salt
Furikake (page 323)

DINNER
Curried Pork with Garnet
Yams and Green Beans
(page 256)

Braised kale with Spiced
Pumpkin Seed and Cashew
Crunch (page 316)

DESSERT
Mango carpaccio with citrus
threads, sea salt, and chile
(pictured on page 287)

SHOPPING LIST

We've put together a shopping list for you following the number of servings in our recipes; that means dinner recipes are for four people, but breakfasts, lunches, snacks, and desserts are portioned for one person. Please adjust according to your needs!

PANTRY

CANNED AND DRIED GOODS
- albacore tuna, 3- to 4-ounce can
- almond butter
- anchovy fillets
- black beans, 4 (15-ounce) cans
- bonito flakes
- cannellini beans, 2 (15-ounce) cans, or 3½ cups cooked
- capers
- chicken stock, homemade or low-sodium canned, 11½ cups
- chickpeas, 3 (15-ounce) cans
- coconut milk, 2 cans
- cornstarch, 1 tablespoon
- curry paste, Thai, yellow
- nonstick oil spray
- olives, Kalamata, ½ cup
- pumpkin puree, 2 cans
- sun-dried tomatoes, ¼ cup
- tahini
- tomato paste
- tomato puree
- whole tomatoes, 28-ounce can

CONDIMENTS
- Chinese chili oil
- Dijon mustard
- harissa
- miso, white
- nori
- soy sauce, light
- whole-grain mustard

DRIED FRUIT
- dried apricots, ¼ cup
- dried pineapple, ¼ cup
- prunes, ½ cup
- unsweetened coconut flakes, ¼ cup

GRAINS
- all-rye crackers
- barley, semi-pearled, 2½ cups
- bulgur, medium grind, 3 cups
- quinoa, ½ cup
- steel-cut oats, 1½ cups

NUTS AND SEEDS
- cacao nibs, ½ cup
- cashews, ¼ cup
- hemp seeds, 2 tablespoons
- pecans, ¼ cup
- pepitas (pumpkin seeds), ¾ cup
- pine nuts, ¾ cup
- pistachios, 2 tablespoons
- sesame seeds, 6 tablespoons
- sliced almonds, ¼ cup
- sunflower seeds, shelled, ¼ cup
- walnuts, 4 cups

OILS AND VINEGARS
- balsamic vinegar
- canola, grapeseed, or vegetable oil
- olive oil, at least a quart
- rice wine vinegar
- sherry vinegar
- toasted sesame oil
- walnut oil (okay to substitute neutral oil)
- white wine vinegar

SPICES
- kosher salt (can use fine sea salt)
- ancho chile powder, ½ teaspoon
- bay leaf, 1
- black peppercorns
- cayenne pepper, ground, 1 teaspoon
- cinnamon stick, 1
- cinnamon, ground, 1 teaspoon
- cloves, ground, pinch (optional)
- coriander seeds, 1 teaspoon
- cumin seeds, 2 teaspoons
- cumin, ground, 1½ teaspoons
- dried oregano, ½ teaspoon
- fennel seeds, 1½ teaspoons
- fine sea salt, 1 container, typically 26 ounces
- five-spice powder, ½ teaspoon
- flaky sea salt, small container
- garam masala (can use Madras curry powder), 1 teaspoon
- mustard seeds, 2 tablespoons
- red pepper flakes, preferably Aleppo or Marash, ¼ cup
- saffron, pinch (optional)
- small dried chiles, such as chile de arbol, 4
- smoked paprika, 1 teaspoon
- smoked sea salt, 1 tablespoon
- za'atar, 2 teaspoons (can substitute dried oregano or thyme)

SWEET ITEMS
- agave syrup
- bittersweet chocolate, 8 ounces
- honey
- pure maple syrup

WINE
- white wine, ½ cup

SHOPPING LIST

DAIRY AND OTHER REFRIGERATED ITEMS

- chèvre, 1 (4- or 5-ounce) package
- eggs, large, 1 dozen
- plain Greek yogurt, 1 quart
- pomegranate juice, 16-ounce bottle
- sheep's milk yogurt, ½ cup (can substitute plain Greek yogurt)

MEAT AND SEAFOOD

- chicken breasts, skin on, bone in, 3 large pieces
- flank steak, preferably grass-finished (1¼ pounds)
- lamb shanks, 2 (or 3, if planning on leftovers)
- rockfish or snapper fillets, skinless, 1½ pounds
- salmon, preferably wild, 5 (4-ounce) fillets
- hot smoked salmon (can also use canned sardines), 1½ ounces

PRODUCE

- acorn squash, 2 medium
- apple, Opal or other yellow-skinned variety, 1
- apple, Braeburn or Honeycrisp, 2
- avocado, 1
- beets, 1 pound
- Belgian endive, 1 head
- blood oranges, 2
- Brussels sprouts, 1½ pounds
- butter lettuce, 1 small head
- cabbage, Savoy, 1 medium head
- carrots, 14 medium, 2 large
- cauliflower, 1 large head
- celery root, 1 small
- celery, 1 heart
- chile, Fresno or jalapeño, 1
- chives, 1 bunch
- cilantro leaves, 1 bunch
- dates, Medjool, 6
- escarole, 1 small head
- garlic, 1 head
- ginger, 1 medium piece
- grapefruit, pink, 1 large
- kale, 4 bunches, preferably a mix of curly and lacinato
- leeks, 4 large
- lemons, 7
- lemons, Meyer, 2
- mango, 1 medium
- mint, 1 bunch
- mushrooms, shiitake, 8 ounces
- mustard greens, 2 bunches
- onions, 2 medium
- onions, red, 2 medium
- oranges, 2
- parsley, flat-leaf, 2 bunches
- parsnips, 2 large
- pear, 1
- pomegranate, 1 large
- pomelo or pink grapefruit, 2
- radicchio, 2 heads
- radish, 1 small bunch
- sage, 1 small bunch
- shallots, 5
- spinach, 2 to 3 cups
- tangerines, 1
- thyme, 1 bunch
- turmeric root, 1 small (okay to substitute ground)

SHOPPING LIST

Do a quick inventory before heading out shopping for your second week—some of your dairy, produce, and sauces may be in fine shape for a second week!

DAIRY AND OTHER REFRIGERATED ITEMS

- chèvre, 1 (4- or 5-ounce) package
- corn tortillas, 8 small
- eggs, large, 1 dozen
- yogurt, plain Greek, 1 cup
- yogurt, sheep's milk, 1 cup (can substitute plain Greek)
- sauerkraut, 1 cup

MEAT AND SEAFOOD

- chicken thighs, on bone, 5 pieces (2½ pounds)
- trimmed pork shoulder, 1 pound
- hot smoked salmon (can also use canned sardines), 1½ ounces
- mackerel, Atlantic, 4 (4-ounce) skin-on fillets (also sold as Boston, Common, Caballa, or Saba mackerel)
- sea scallops, 12 large

PRODUCE

- apples, preferably Opal or other yellow-skinned variety, 2
- apple, Honeycrisp or Braeburn, 1
- arugula, 6 to 8 cups (2 bunches)
- avocado, 1
- baby spinach, 30 ounces
- beets, 2 large
- blood orange, 1
- butternut squash, 1 small (about 2½ pounds)
- cabbage, 1 small head
- carrots, 3 medium and 1 large
- cauliflower, 1 small head
- celery root, 2 large
- celery, 1 heart
- chard, 2 bunches
- chile, Fresno or jalapeño, 1
- chiles, poblano (pasilla), 2 fresh
- chives, 1 bunch
- cilantro sprigs, 1 small bunch
- dates, Medjool, 6
- Delicata squash, 2 small
- fennel, 1 large bulb
- frisée, 2 small heads
- garlic, 1 head
- garnet yams or other sweet potato, 1 pound
- ginger, 1 small piece
- golden beets, 2
- haricots verts or other green beans, 4 ounces
- kale, 4 bunches, preferably a mix of curly and lacinato
- leeks, 3 large
- lemons, 6
- lemons, Meyer, 2
- lime leaves (optional), 2
- limes, 4
- mangoes, 2
- marjoram, 4 sprigs (okay to use oregano)
- mint, 1 small bunch
- onions, 4 medium
- onions, red, 2 medium
- oranges, 3
- parsley, flat-leaf, 2 bunches
- parsnip, 1 large
- pears, 2
- pomegranate, 1 large
- pomelo or pink grapefruit, 2
- radishes, 1 small bunch
- red bell peppers, 4
- scallions, 1 bunch
- shallots, 4
- tangerines, 2
- tatsoi or salad mix, 3 to 4 cups
- tomato, 1 large
- turmeric root, 1 small (okay to substitute ground)

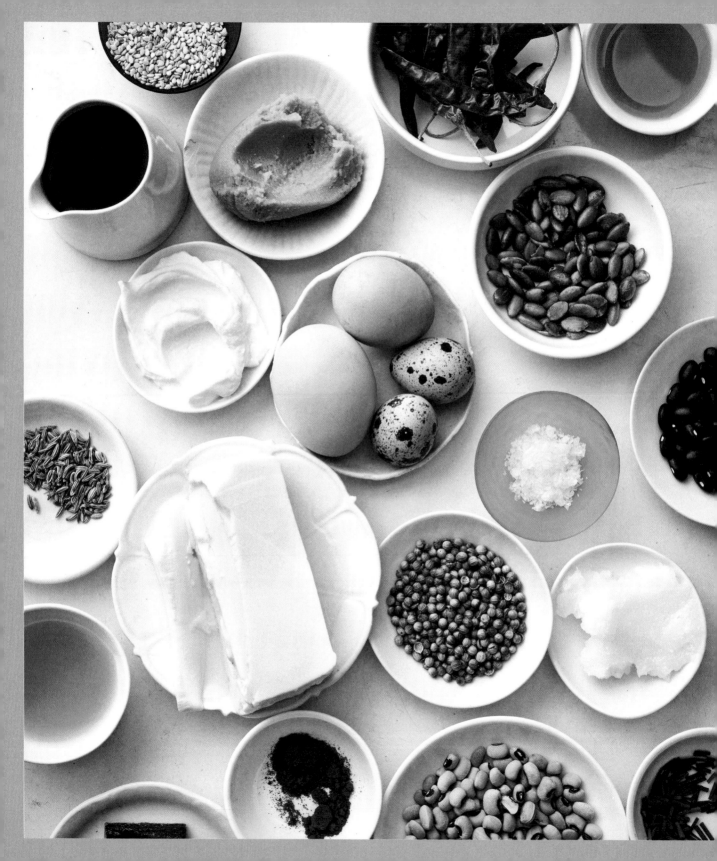

THE FOOD LOVER'S CLEANSE PANTRY

Welcome to the pantry! When I lead the online cleanse, I encourage readers to prepare some recipes that can work in several different meals. Here's a cache of recipes that can be helpful throughout the year: vinaigrettes to dress those lunchtime salads, condiments to add a bit of thrill to the simplest vegetables and meats, and colorful dips to chase away your late-afternoon munchies. I've also included basic methods that you can use to prep your food in advance and take some of the pressure off your day-to-day cooking. And finally, you'll also find a few notes on ingredients: where to find them and what to look for in the market as you're choosing them.

PANTRY NOTES

You've seen some ingredients popping up throughout the book: the staples of my everyday kitchen. Here are a few sourcing notes on those foundations.

SALT

I used to be a kosher salt fan, and I still like it for even seasoning of large cuts of meat, but I've come to appreciate the more direct salinity and finer texture of fine sea salt, so we call for fine sea salt as the basic seasoning. My current favorite is the slightly speckled sugar-textured salt from the Utah salt flats called Real Salt (you can find it on Amazon). No matter what salt you use, remember to salt as you go along, not just at the beginning or the end of cooking. Use a little at a time and adjust with more salt if it's necessary.

For finishing, we often call for flaky sea salt, which gives crunchy bursts of salinity and texture wherever it lands. I love the delicate pyramidal crystals of Maldon salt, and for a little variety the elegantly smoked version of Maldon salt.

BLACK PEPPER

Salt and pepper are an automatic reflex, and you'll find freshly ground black pepper called for throughout the book. That said, I often find that dishes are better with just a touch of the pungent stuff (or none at all). Even more than with other seasonings, make sure to start with just a touch of pepper and increase to taste.

RED PEPPER FLAKES

In my home cooking I use red pepper just as much as or more than ground black pepper. You'll notice we call for medium-hot Mediterranean red pepper flakes, such as Aleppo or Marash. That's because generic red pepper flakes are so hot you can't really get any flavor along with the chile heat. Peppers like Aleppo pepper (originally from Syria), Marash (my favorite, available from zingermans.com), Urfa Biber (Turkey), and piment d'Espelette (the Basque regions of Spain and France) all deliver distinctly fruity and/or smoky notes along with a bit of heat. Since they aren't too hot, you can use enough of them to really taste their impact on the food. And that little bit of heat may give your metabolism a little boost along with your taste buds.

I do use small whole chile peppers, usually chiles de arbol or chiles japones, in longer-cooked dishes. They add distinctive heat and flavor and are easy to fish out when the cooking is done.

SPICES

I lean heavily on spices to give my food flavor without piling on extra calories. In big cities, it's easy to get a huge variety of spices and blends at groceries, health food stores, and Asian specialty stores. If you don't have a great selection in your town, however, the Internet is a great place to turn to for spices. World Spice (worldspice.com) is my hometown favorite, and New York's Kalustyan's (kalustyans.com) has just about every spice imaginable.

MISO

Miso is a paste of legumes that has been combined with cultured rice or barley to produce a thick fermented paste. Because it's a live cultured product, it can serve as a probiotic (as long as you don't kill the microflora with high-heat cooking). But most of all, it adds a wonderful richness to the dressings, marinades, and soups we use it for. In this book, we call for white (or shiro) miso, the gentlest, sweetest variety. From there you might delve into the funkier flavors of barley, chickpea, and red misos. Among other brands, I like South River Miso, made in Massachusetts from traditional Japanese methods.

OLIVE OIL

I love olive oil for its flavor and its lushness, but I don't make too big a deal about it: I tend to rely on well-priced extra-virgin oil from Crete, which is green and assertive enough to remind you it's not canola oil but not too aggressively peppery. You can save your very fancy small bottles of olive oil for finishing dishes.

COCONUT OIL

Coconut oil is a solid at room temperature, and it's become a favorite for sautéing and stir-frying when the flavors are skewing Indian, Caribbean, or Southeast Asian. Keep it out of the direct heat of the sun or your stove, and make sure to keep an extra jar around as a skin-soothing salve.

TOFU

Even though it's been the butt of countless jokes, tofu takes on great flavor and texture if you handle it well. It's important to find very fresh tofu and to get the right texture for your needs. For creamy sauces such as Chipotle Mayonnaise (page 123), you'll want extra-soft silken tofu, while for roasting and stir-fries, you want to seek out extra-firm or firm tofu packed in water. To maximize crispness, it's best to press the excess water from the tofu following the method in the recipes.

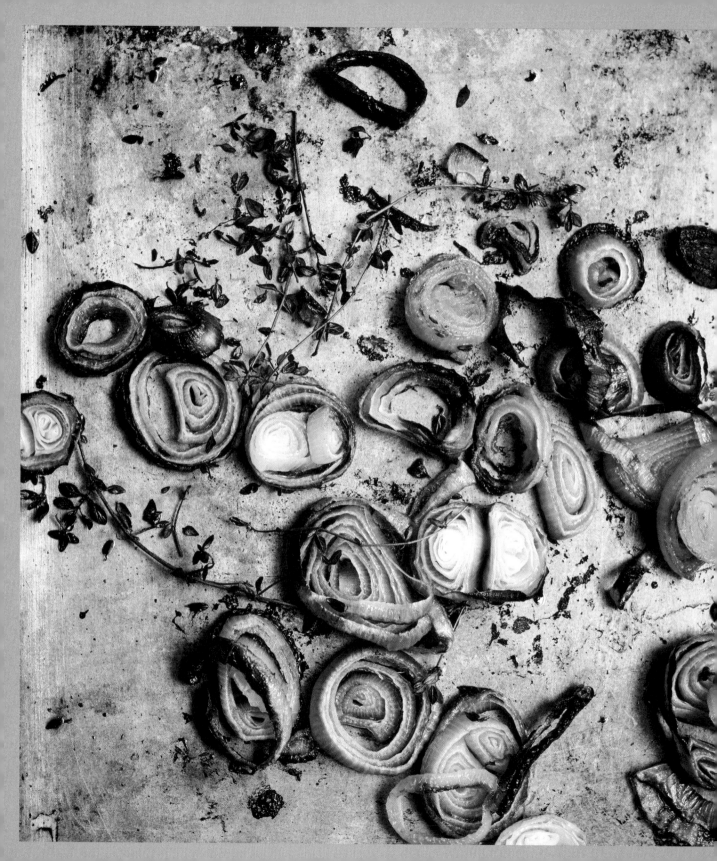

PANTRY METHODS

As you go through the cleanse, there are certain key methods and ingredients that come up again and again, so here are the basics to make them easier and better. They're also the building blocks to improvising your own cleanse-style menus.

HOW TO MAKE A BIG BATCH OF STEEL-CUT OATS

The key to actually eating longer-cooking whole-grain porridge in the morning is to have it ready to go. Here's a method to make scrumptious steel-cut oats in bulk so that you can just heat and go when you're sleepy:

Bring 4 cups of water to a boil for every 1 cup of oats being cooked. Add a pinch of salt and stir in the oats. Reduce heat to a low simmer and cook, stirring occasionally, to the desired texture (20 minutes will give you a pretty creamy result). For later use, let cool to room temperature and store in the refrigerator for up to 5 days. To serve, warm the oats in a small saucepan over medium heat or in the microwave. Either way, stir in ¼ cup water or almond milk to keep it from scalding.

Note: You can reduce the cooking time even further by pouring the same amount of boiling water over the oats at night and letting sit at room temperature until the morning. When ready to cook, proceed as above.

HOW TO BOIL AN EGG

I love a hard-boiled egg, one of the most reliable snacks around, though in truth I like them softish rather than completely firm. Place the egg(s) in a small saucepan and cover with water by 1½ inches. Bring to a boil over medium-high heat, then turn the heat off. Let the eggs stand 9 minutes for an egg that's still a tad runny in the middle, or 10 for one that's firm but fudgy in texture. Place the boiled egg(s) in a bowl of ice water to stop the cooking, and after a few minutes of cooling, peel them in the water to rinse off any bits of shell.

HOW TO MAKE CHICKEN STOCK

I can be extravagant with my groceries, but I like to get the most out of them, which is why I like to make stock with leftover bones and meat scraps. I do use commercial chicken stock sometimes, but I'm much happier when I brew my own: home-cooked chicken stock tastes both mellower and richer than the canned stuff. I tend to save chicken carcasses in the freezer as my family and I make our way through a few roast chicken meals and then use them for a big batch. If I don't have any around, I pick up some very inexpensive chicken backs at the store and use them as the basis for my stock. The aromatic elements can vary from batch to batch, but here's the basic setup:

- Place 2 chicken carcasses, cleaved in half if possible, or 2 pounds chicken backs, wings, or feet in a large stockpot. Cover with water by about 3 inches, and then add vegetables and aromatics, including, ideally, 1 leek, cleaned and halved; 1 carrot; 1 medium onion, halved; 1 bay leaf; 1 garlic head with its upper third sliced off horizontally to expose the cloves below; 4 parsley sprigs; 4 thyme sprigs; 8 peppercorns; and 2 or 3 dried shiitakes. Don't fret if you don't have every last ingredient: it will taste nice anyway.

- Bring the water to a boil over medium-high heat, then turn the heat down to a lazy simmer. Skim off any unsightly froth and/or fat at the top of the stock, but unless you're working in a French restaurant, you don't need to be too fastidious. Simmer the stock for 3 to 8 hours, making sure the chicken is always covered with water. The shorter time is good for most applications, but if you want a very rich concentrated stock for sauces, go ahead and cook longer.

- Carefully strain through a fine mesh-strainer, pushing on the solids to extract flavor. Discard the solids. If you're not using it right away, place the hot stock in its container into another bowl or pot of ice water. Stir the stock to chill to room temperature right away.

- Chill the stock completely in the refrigerator; when it's cold, scrape the congealed fat off the surface. Keep chilled for up to 5 days, or divide into small containers and freeze for up to 3 months. (It freezes well in ice cube trays.)

HOW TO MAKE VEGETABLE STOCK

I really dislike commercial vegetable stock; it has a weird yeasty flavor that reminds me of no vegetable in particular. Since the cleanse tends to generate a lot of vegetable scraps, I try to get a couple of batches of infinitely better homemade vegetable stock going instead. Here's a rough formula, but please feel free to play around with whatever tasty vegetable leavings you have on hand.

- In a large pot, place 2 leek tops, rinsed and cut into large pieces; 2 carrots, cut into large pieces; 1 cup mushrooms or mushroom stems; 1 onion, cut into 2-inch wedges; 1 parsnip, peeled and cut into large chunks; the fronds and outer layer of a fennel bulb; 4 parsley sprigs; 4 thyme sprigs;

2 tablespoons tomato paste; 1 whole chile de arbol or japones; 1 teaspoon fennel seeds and 1 teaspoon peppercorns.

- Cover with water by 2 inches. Bring the water to a boil over medium-high heat, then turn the heat down and simmer for 25 to 35 minutes.

- Strain the liquid (discard the solids) and cool it to room temperature. Store it in small containers and use it within 5 days or freeze it for up to 3 months. (It freezes well in ice cube trays.)

HOW TO ROAST VEGETABLES

I'm a huge sheet pan cook. Roasting vegetables on sheet pans means that I can focus on some more fiddly part of a meal (or help my kids with piano practice) at the same time. Veggies emerge toasty brown and tender, and they're great to keep around to add texture and flavor to the next day's lunch salad. Though you'll find a few variations elsewhere in the book, here's the basic method for roasting veggies of all sorts.

- Preheat the oven to 425°F.

- Cut the vegetables either into 1-inch pieces (best for carrots, parsnips, celery root, beets, and large squashes) or ½-inch cross-section slices (best for Delicata squash, fennel, zucchini, and sunchokes).

- Figure about 1 cup raw veggies per person and about 1½ teaspoons olive oil per person. Toss the veggies with oil, salt, and pepper, keeping individual veggies separate from one another.

- If you have it, line the baking sheet(s) with compostable parchment paper (this will save you a little dishwashing work).

- Spread the vegetables out on a single layer on the baking sheet with about ½ inch of space between each piece, using more than one tray if necessary.

- Roast the vegetables in the oven, tossing once during cooking, until they're tender and browned in spots. The time depends on the vegetable and the chunk size, but figure 15 to 30 minutes. If you have more than one pan, rotate the pans once during the roasting.

For a burst of extra flavor, toss the veggies with something aromatic: 1 grated garlic clove, a teaspoon of finely grated citrus zest, lemon juice, chopped herbs, sesame oil and green onions, and/or hot sauce. Taste and add more salt if necessary.

HOW TO COOK DRIED BEANS

Cooking your own dried beans takes a bit more planning than using canned, but the effort adds so much character to your legume dishes. Here's the gist, using white beans as a model. You can use this same method for any number of dried beans: pinto, black, flageolet, garbanzos, or gigantes, keeping in mind that cooking times vary considerably.

- Soak 2 cups dried white beans in at least two times their volume of water overnight in the refrigerator.

- Drain the soaked beans and place them in a large pot with any or all of the following aromatic ingredients: 1 peeled carrot; 4 thyme sprigs; 1 leek, rinsed and trimmed; 1 garlic head with its top sliced off to reveal the cloves; 1 small peeled onion; 1 or 2 small dried chiles; 1 teaspoon fennel seeds and/or a bay leaf. Fill the pot with cold water that extends 2 inches above the beans.

- Bring to a boil, skim off the residue that collects at the surface of the water. Turn heat down to a simmer and stir in 2 tablespoons olive oil and about 1½ teaspoons sea salt per quart of water. Cook gently until the beans are tender to their centers, about 35 to 45 minutes.

- Taste beans and add red pepper flakes, additional salt and/or fennel to taste. Let the beans cool in their cooking water. Before serving, drain them and remove the aromatic vegetables.

HOW TO STEAM-ROAST BEETS

Whether you're making a batch of Roasted Beet and Tahini Dip (page 318) or just looking for some hefty vegetable flavor for your lunchtime salads, roasted beets are easy to make ahead of time.

- Preheat the oven to 425°F. Scrub some beets and make sure they're more or less the same size; cut any gargantuan ones in half. Place them in a single layer in a baking dish or pan with sides at least 2 inches high. Season with salt and pepper, slosh in 1 or 2 tablespoons olive oil, and toss in any herbs (thyme, rosemary, parsley) that you might have on hand. Pour in ¼ cup of water to create steam. Cover the dish securely with aluminum foil and roast until a knife slips into the beets easily, which can take from around 45 minutes to 70 minutes, depending on the size of the beets.

- Cover again tightly as the beets cool to room temperature, so they're easier to peel. You can peel them by rubbing with a clean kitchen towel (it won't be clean for long . . .) or with a paring knife. Store in the refrigerator in an airtight container for up to 5 days.

HOW TO BRAISE GREENS

Braised greens are just the thing when you've run out of ideas for a side dish, and they're also a great component to a brown-bag office lunch. The best greens to braise have a little structure, such as chard, kale, cabbage, or escarole. Spinach is absolutely delicious, too, of course, but it will wilt down to almost nothing, so be sure to use enough to make it worth your while, or mix it in with something else. Very broadly speaking, 1 bunch spinach will serve 2 people.

- Wash the greens: Cut the greens off any sturdy stems. Immerse the greens in a large bowl of water and swish them around. Keep them in the bowl until you start cooking. If you're working with chard, chop the stems into small pieces and include them with the leaves.

- In a large skillet with a cover, over medium heat, heat 1 tablespoon of olive oil per bunch of greens. Slip a sliced garlic clove and a pinch of red pepper flakes (preferably a medium-hot Mediterranean chile, such as Aleppo or Marash). Stir, then pull the leaves up out of their washing water and place them in the skillet. Cover and cook until the leaves have wilted a bit and are easy to stir with tongs. Season them with salt and stir well. Cook until tender; spinach will cook the quickest, then chard, kale, escarole, and cabbage. Remove the greens and season with salt to taste.

- For extra flavor, stir in any of the following: lemon juice; fresh herbs, such as dill, cilantro, mint, and/or basil; toasted nuts or seeds; a teaspoon of sesame oil; or the hot sauce of your choice.

HOW TO BLANCH VEGETABLES

Blanching vegetables means cooking them briefly in boiling water; it's a great way to have some nonraw vegetables around for snacking or tossing in a grain salad. When I'm doing a cleanse, it's a great way to prepare for both lunch salads and snacks, when I might want a little textural variation from raw veggies alone.

- Set a big pot of salted water over medium-high heat and trim and cut the vegetables to the desired size.

- When the water comes to a boil, add the vegetables in separate batches. Leafy greens take 15 seconds to 2 minutes, depending on their heartiness. Green beans and asparagus take 1 or 2 minutes to get to a crisp-tender state. Root vegetables and crucifers like broccoli and cauliflower take longer, though if you want them to finish quickly, simply cut them in smaller pieces.

- Use a slotted spoon or spider to fish your blanched veggies out of the water. If you're trying to maximize crispness, you can remove them from a pot to a bowlful of ice water. Once they're cool, drain, then lay them in a single layer on a baking sheet covered with a towel or paper towel so they dry further.

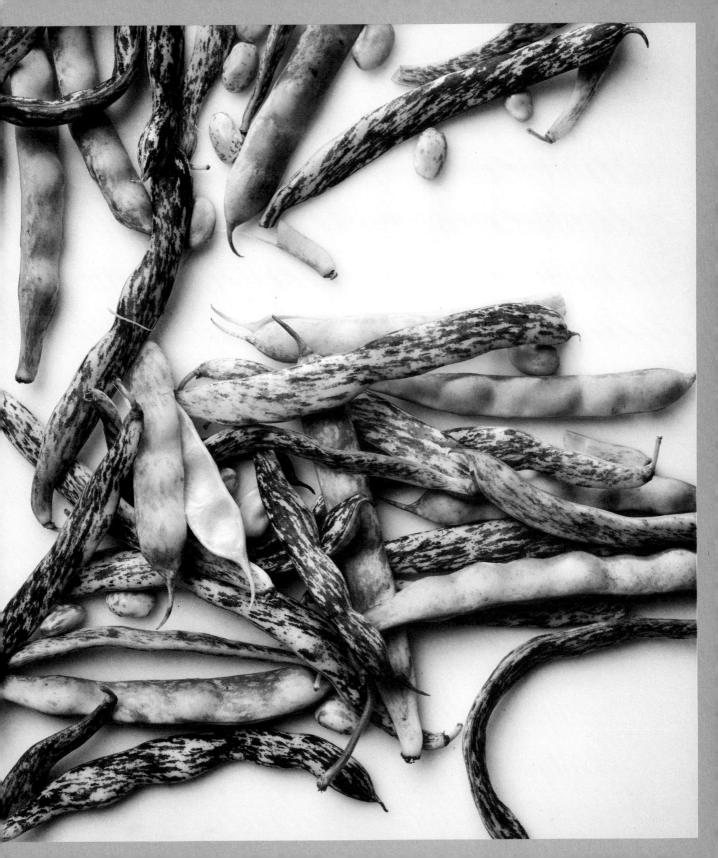

HOW TO TOAST NUTS AND SEEDS

Nuts and seeds taste better when they're toasted, and since they're a big part of the cleanse, it's a worthy step. One good thing is that you can store cooled, toasted nuts and seeds in an airtight container for 3 to 5 days before using, so they're ready to go when a recipe calls.

Small nuts and seeds, such as slivered almonds, pine nuts, amaranth, flaxseeds, pumpkin seeds, sesame seeds, sunflower seeds, chia seeds, and whole spices, are best toasted in a pan (you can use the same method for unsweetened coconut flakes, as well). Place the nuts or seeds in a dry skillet over medium heat (only one kind at a time! Nuts and seeds toast at different rates). Stir the nuts or seeds as they cook. Some seeds, such as amaranth, pumpkin seeds, and flaxseeds, will helpfully let you know when they're done by popping and snapping vigorously. Others, particularly higher-oil ones, such as pine nuts, hempseeds, and sesame, will not give such audible cues; just look for a slight golden shift in color, and don't step away until they're done: these are the easiest to burn. Place the toasted seeds on a cool plate to cool; otherwise, they may overcook from the residual heat in the pan.

Larger nuts, such as pecans, hazelnuts, pistachios, walnuts, cashews, and almonds, do best toasting in the oven. Preheat the oven to 300°F and have a rimmed baking sheet ready for each variety you're toasting. Spread the nuts in an uncrowded layer on the baking sheet and toast them in the oven until they're fragrant and slightly golden at their centers; from 6 minutes to 15 minutes depending on the nut. Pecans and pistachios are the quickest; other nuts can take considerably longer.

HOW TO REST MEATS

Letting meat rest for a while before carving or serving allows juices to be more thoroughly reabsorbed by the meat. Slice too early, and a lot of the moisture in your lamb or your chicken will end up on the cutting board, but if you wait a bit, say 10 minutes, you'll find that most of the juices will stay where you want them. It's also a good idea to rest your meat because when you remove meat from the oven the temperature will continue to rise for a bit before cooling off. Throughout the book we give you a few target temperatures for roasting meats and poultry to doneness. Those are final temperatures. So if you want your lamb or your flank steak medium-rare, remove it from the oven around 125°F to 128°F for a final resting temperature closer to medium-rare's 130°F (see page 58). Also remember that this effect is more significant in larger cuts of meat; a chicken cutlet will not increase in heat as much as a big roast beef.

HOW TO SUPREME CITRUS FRUIT

Here's how to make neat, membraneless segments, or supremes, of lemons, oranges, or grapefruit:

- Cut a ½-inch slice off the top and bottom of one fruit and place it with the flat side down. Using a sharp knife in a curving downward motion, slice off a band of the skin, pith, and a thin layer of flesh from the fruit. Rotate and repeat until the fruit is completely skinned. Holding the fruit in hand, cut a V shape parallel to the membranes of each section to release the crescent of citrus flesh. Repeat with the remaining sections of the fruit.

- If you need juice from the fruit, once you've cut all the sections, squeeze the membrane to extract the juice.

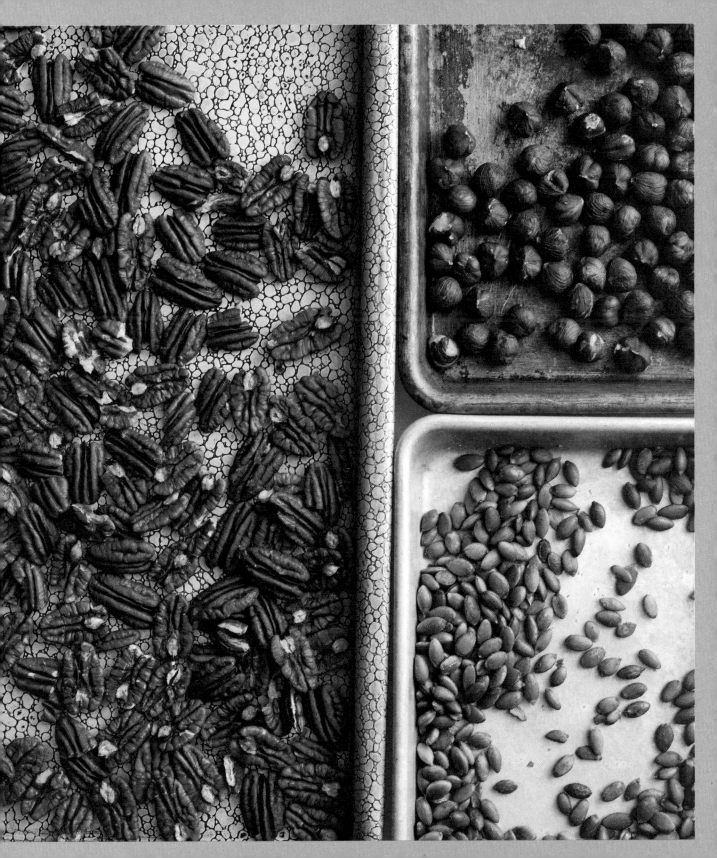

HOW TO COOK WHOLE GRAINS AND OTHER SIDES

Healthier eating can come with small switches: even if you're not doing the whole cleanse, try switching whole grains for white pasta or rice a couple days a week. Cracked bulgur, millet, and quinoa are the fastest to cook, in about 15 minutes, with no previous soaking. They're the speed grains, and good to keep in mind if you're pressed for time.

Most often, I recommend cooking whole grains like pasta in a large quantity of salted water, just like pasta. I bring the water to a rolling boil, add the grains, and then reduce the heat so they cook at a steady simmer. Simply drain the grains before including them in a pilaf or salad. I use this method for farro, barley, millet, and quinoa.

The exceptions to the pasta-style rule are cracked grains, such as bulgur and cracked freekeh, and whole-grain rices, which I cook like, well, rice. It seems to keep them fluffier than the other style. Place these in a pot with the correct amount of water and a pinch of salt. Bring to a boil, then reduce the heat and cover. Simmer until the water is fully absorbed and the grains are fluffy (see the approximate cooking times in the chart). Stir, then turn off the heat, cover the pan again, and let steam for 5 minutes. They may still need a little draining at this point.

SOAKING

You can soak long-cooking grains before cooking to cut back significantly on the cooking time. I recommend doing this especially with farro, unhulled barley, wheat berries, whole freekeh, and rye berries. When you're ready to cook, drain and use fresh water to cook the grains with the pasta method.

COOKING AHEAD

Whole grains generally store really well; in fact, you may find they hydrate more fully if you cook them and then store them at least overnight in an airtight container in the refrigerator. Once you've cooked them, toss them with a small bit of olive or neutral oil and spread them out on a sheet pan to cool until room temperature, then place them in an airtight container and chill until ready to use. It's best to use refrigerated grains within 5 days of cooking.

If you need to make the grains further ahead, cool them fully and then freeze them in an airtight container. To thaw, place the quantity you need to cook in a strainer and run cool water over the grains, breaking up chunks with your hands.

Reheating: I usually reheat refrigerated or thawed grains in a small saucepan over medium heat with ¼ cup water or stock. You can also place them in a microwave-safe container, sprinkle with a couple of tablespoons of liquid, cover, and microwave until warm.

COOKING WHOLE GRAINS AND OTHER SIDES

CRACKED FREEKEH	• Rice method	• 2 cups water to 1 cup freekeh	• 20 minutes	• Tender
QUINOA	• Pasta method	• Large pot of boiling water	• 10 to 12 minutes	• Crisp-tender, visible endosperm
BULGUR	• Rice method	• 2 cups water to 1 cup bulgur	• 12 to 14 minutes	• Tender
BARLEY (PEARL)	• Pasta method, presoaking recommended	• Large pot boiling water	• 40 to 50 minutes without soaking	• Chewy-tender
BHUTANESE RED RICE	• Rice method	• 1¾ cups water to 1 cup red rice	• 25 to 30 minutes	• Tender
BLACK (FORBIDDEN RICE)	• Rice method, presoaking recommended	• 1¾ cups water to 1 cup black rice	• 30 to 35 minutes, presoaking recommended	• Tender
FARRO	• Pasta method, presoaking recommended	• Large pot boiling water	• 30 to 40 minutes without soaking	• Chewy-tender
BROWN BASMATI RICE	• Rice method	• 2½ cups water to 1 cup brown basmati	• 45 to 55 minutes	• Tender
MILLET	• Pasta method	• Large pot boiling water	• 15 to 18 minutes	• Tender but not clumpy
BUCKWHEAT GROATS	• Rice method	• 2 cups water to 1 cup buckwheat	• 12 to 15 minutes	• Tender

DRESSINGS AND VINAIGRETTES

BUTTERMILK DRESSING

TOTAL TIME: 5 MINUTES
MAKES 1¼ CUPS (UP TO 2 TABLESPOONS PER SERVING)

I have a pet buttermilk culture that I need to refresh a couple of times a week, so I'm always pleased when I come up with another good use for the gently soured milk. My live-culture buttermilk slips into smoothies, and of course when I'm not doing the cleanse, it makes pancakes taste great. This recipe is one of my favorite uses: it's reminiscent of ranch dressing, but with a lighter, cooler touch. It pairs beautifully with tender herbs, such as chives, parsley, tarragon, and mint, but I don't mix those in until I assemble the salad, since they don't keep as well as the dressing will on its own.

- ¾ cup buttermilk
- 2 tablespoons extra-virgin olive oil
- 2 tablespoons canola oil
- 1 tablespoon lemon juice
- Pinch of freshly ground black pepper
- 1 teaspoon fine sea salt
- 1 teaspoon rice vinegar
- 1 tablespoon lemon zest

Combine all the ingredients in a small mixing bowl and whisk to incorporate. Taste and season with more salt if necessary.

Do ahead: The dressing will keep 3 to 5 days in the refrigerator. If it loses some zing during storage, add a bit more lemon juice to brighten it up.

SESAME-MISO VINAIGRETTE

TOTAL TIME: 5 MINUTES
MAKES ⅔ CUP (ABOUT 2 TABLESPOONS PER SERVING)

Miso gives vinaigrettes an almost buttery richness and a satisfying creamy texture (and introduces some healthy microflora to your food, too). White miso is the mellowest variety, and you can find it at Asian groceries and health food stores alike. From there, you may want to experiment with other varieties of miso—I love barley and chickpea misos, and they work equally well in soups.

- 1 Fresno chile, with seeds, finely chopped
- ¼ cup vegetable oil
- 2 tablespoons fresh lime juice
- 2 tablespoons white miso
- 1 tablespoon unseasoned rice vinegar
- 1 teaspoon toasted sesame oil
- 1 teaspoon toasted sesame seeds (see page 306)
- ½ teaspoon grated peeled fresh ginger

Whisk together all the ingredients in a small bowl.

Do ahead: The dressing will keep 1 week in the refrigerator. If it loses some zing during storage, add a bit more lime juice or vinegar to brighten it up.

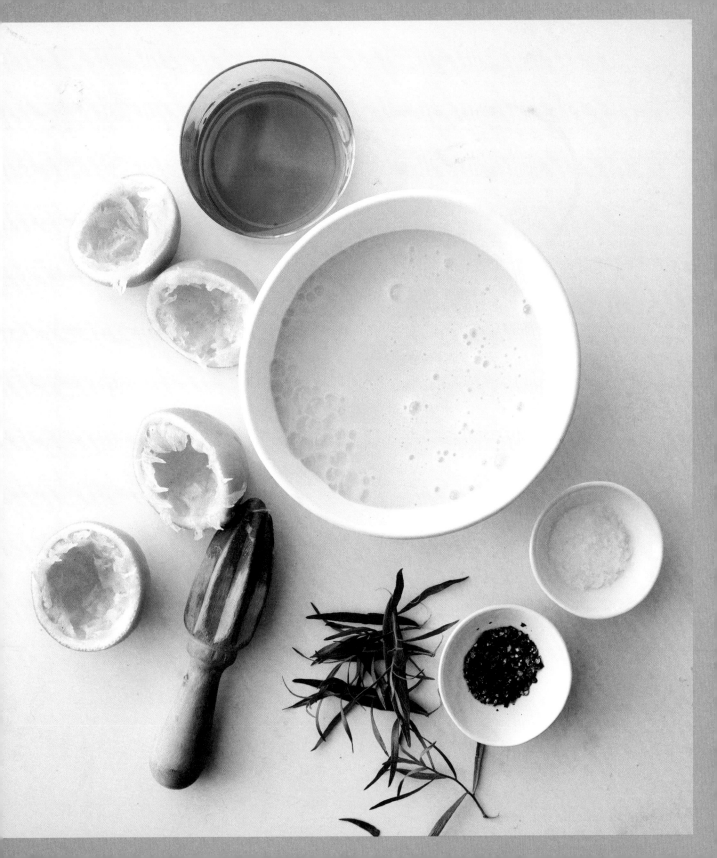

BROKEN OLIVE VINAIGRETTE

TOTAL TIME: 5 MINUTES
MAKES ABOUT ⅔ CUP (UP TO 2 TABLESPOONS PER SERVING)

Chopped and loosely structured, this rusticated vinaigrette can swerve from sauce to salad dressing, depending on the moment. It goes great with grilled meats (such as the pork skewers it's served with on page 156), but it can also be tossed with tomatoes, cucumbers, or sturdy lettuces for a lovely lunch salad. I like to use a mix of green and black olives for depth of flavor and color.

- ¼ cup extra-virgin olive oil
- 6 tablespoons roughly chopped green and black olives
- 1 teaspoon finely grated lemon zest
- 1 tablespoon freshly squeezed lemon juice, plus more to taste
- ½ teaspoon fennel seeds, crushed
- Fine sea salt and freshly ground black pepper to taste

Whisk together all the ingredients. Taste and add more lemon juice, if desired.

Do ahead: The dressing will keep 1 week in the refrigerator. If it loses some zing during storage, add a bit more lemon juice to brighten it up.

HONEY-CHAMOMILE DRESSING

TOTAL TIME: 5 MINUTES
MAKES ABOUT ½ CUP (ABOUT 1 TABLESPOON PER SERVING)

To make a piece of fruit seem a little more, well, dessertlike, it pays to frame it well. Slice your apples elegantly, or place your berries in a beautiful bowl. Grate a bit of citrus zest on top or add a pinch of flaky Maldon sea salt. And give your fruit a lovely accent such as this soft floral sauce. A bit of steeped chamomile adds a sunny floral flavor to this sweetened dressing, which elevates the best fruit of any season. If you can locate fresh chamomile flowers or whole dried ones—which are commonly available in the bulk section of the natural foods store—you can sprinkle a few on your fruit along with the dressing for a bit of extra loveliness. If not, you can steep chamomile tea bags instead.

- 2 tablespoons dried chamomile or about 6 tea bags
- ½ cup boiling water
- 2 teaspoons honey
- ½ cup sheep's milk yogurt or other plain yogurt
- Additional chamomile blossoms (dried or fresh), for garnish (optional)

Place the chamomile in a mug or small bowl. Pour in the boiling water and let it infuse for 5 minutes. Strain and measure 2 tablespoons of the chamomile infusion into a medium bowl. Stir the honey into the warm infusion, then the yogurt. Sprinkle with the chamomile blossoms, if using, and serve with fruit.

Do ahead: The dressing will keep 1 week in the refrigerator; stir before serving to reemulsify.

MEYER LEMON–SHALLOT VINAIGRETTE

TOTAL TIME: 5 MINUTES
MAKES ABOUT 1 CUP (ABOUT 2 TABLESPOONS PER SERVING)

Back in the nineties, when I first read Annie Somerville's ahead-of-its-time *Fields of Greens* cookbook, I couldn't understand why Meyer lemons kept popping up everywhere. Growing up on the East Coast, I'd never seen one before and felt slightly annoyed by the specificity. Lemons were lemons, weren't they? When I moved to California and got my hands on some, I finally understood: Meyer lemons are a delicate-skinned hybrid of lemon and mandarin orange, and everything about them is tasty—skin, flesh, even pith. They give recipes a distinctive tangy floral flavor. When I worked for a short while at Chez Panisse, we would add minced lemon skin, pith, and zest to many of our vinaigrettes, and to this day I do the same in the winter and spring, when Meyer lemons are plentiful. If you cannot get Meyer lemons in your grocery, you can use 2 teaspoons of the finely grated skin of a conventional lemon instead, but just the bright yellow skin; conventional lemons have a bitter pith.

- 2 Meyer lemons, washed well
- 2 tablespoons finely minced shallot
- 1 tablespoon white wine or champagne vinegar
- ¼ cup plus 3 tablespoons extra-virgin olive oil
- Fine sea salt and freshly ground black pepper to taste

Cut the pointed ends off 1 lemon and stand it vertically. Using fluid, curved, downward knife strokes, slice off a swath of skin, pith, and about ⅛ inch of the interior flesh of the lemon. Repeat until all the skin is removed. Finely chop the fleshy skin to make 2 tablespoons total and add it to a medium bowl with the shallot.

Squeeze the interior flesh of the peeled lemon to gather any juice, and if necessary, juice the remaining lemon to make a total of 2 tablespoons juice. Whisk the juice into the shallot mixture and stir in the vinegar. Let sit for at least 10 minutes.

Gradually whisk in the oil and season to taste with salt and pepper.

Do ahead: The dressing will keep 3 to 5 days in the refrigerator. If it loses some zing during storage, add a bit more lemon juice or vinegar to brighten it up.

CAESAR-STYLE VINAIGRETTE WITH FIGS

TOTAL TIME: 15 MINUTES
MAKES 1 CUP (ABOUT 2 TABLESPOONS PER SERVING)

This is an adaptation of a dressing I made at my first restaurant job, in the kitchen of Campanile in L.A. The dressing gets a creamy richness and a touch of sweetness by whizzing some dried figs into the mix.

- ¼ cup boiling water
- 2 dried figs, stemmed and chopped
- 1 garlic clove
- 1 small anchovy fillet, chopped
- Fine sea salt
- 3 tablespoons red wine vinegar
- ¼ cup plus 3 tablespoons olive oil
- Freshly squeezed lemon juice to taste
- Freshly ground black pepper to taste

Pour the boiling water over the chopped figs and let sit for 10 minutes to soften.

If using a mortar and pestle, smash the garlic and the anchovy fillet with a pinch of salt and grind to a smooth paste. Drain the excess water from the figs (reserving for later) and add the figs to the mortar. Smash to form a thick paste. Whisk in the vinegar and the fig-soaking water, followed by the oil. Working ½ teaspoon at a time, add lemon juice to taste, then season with salt and a generous crack of pepper.

If using a blender or a hand blender, mince the garlic and anchovy and add them to the blender. Pour in the vinegar and fig-soaking water, followed by the oil. Blend until smooth and season with lemon juice, salt, and pepper as above.

Do ahead: The dressing will keep 1 week in the refrigerator. If it loses some zing during storage, add a bit more lemon juice or vinegar to brighten it up.

CREAMY TAHINI DRESSING

TOTAL TIME: 5 MINUTES
MAKES 1⅓ CUPS (UP TO 2 TABLESPOONS PER SERVING)

Tahini sneaks into so many of my dishes because it adds creaminess with just a bit of bitter edge to keep things from getting cloying. This is tahini at its most basic: thinned with water, accented with garlic, and smoothed out with a touch of yogurt and agave syrup. You could use it just as easily as a chicken or fish marinade as you can a salad dressing. Add a bit more water if you need to thin it out once it has lived in the fridge for a few hours.

- ½ cup tahini
- ½ cup boiling water
- 1 garlic clove, grated
- 2 tablespoons plain yogurt
- 1 tablespoon toasted sesame oil
- 1 teaspoon agave syrup
- 2 tablespoons lemon juice, plus more to taste
- Fine sea salt and freshly ground black pepper to taste

Whisk or blend the tahini with the boiling water to create a smooth puree. Stir in the garlic, yogurt, oil, agave syrup, and lemon juice. Season with salt and pepper and additional lemon juice to taste.

Do ahead: The dressing will keep 1 week in the refrigerator. If it loses some zing during storage, add a bit more lemon juice to brighten it up.

WHOLE-GRAIN MUSTARD VINAIGRETTE

TOTAL TIME: 5 MINUTES
MAKES ABOUT 1 CUP (UP TO 2 TABLESPOONS PER SERVING)

Whole-grain mustard adds body and texture to a vinaigrette, and it works especially well on heartier greens such as escarole, frisée, and cabbage. Do look for a whole-grain mustard that isn't honey-sweetened; you can better adjust the sweetness of the vinaigrette with agave syrup or honey added when you mix it up.

- ½ cup olive oil
- ½ cup walnut or neutral oil, such as canola or grapeseed
- ¼ cup white or red wine vinegar
- ¼ cup whole-grain mustard
- 2 teaspoons agave syrup or honey
- ½ teaspoon fine sea salt, plus more to taste
- ½ teaspoon freshly ground black pepper

Whisk together all the ingredients in a small bowl or shake, covered, in a jar. Taste for seasoning and add more salt, if desired.

Do ahead: This can be made ahead and kept for up to 5 days in the refrigerator. As you go through the week, shake again to recombine the ingredients. If it loses some zing during storage, add a bit more mustard or vinegar to brighten it up.

SHERRY VINAIGRETTE

TOTAL TIME: 5 MINUTES
MAKES ¾ CUP (UP TO 2 TABLESPOONS PER SERVING)

This is my most basic go-to vinaigrette. If you haven't introduced yourself to sherry vinegar, please do; good vinegar makes a salad almost as much as the greens. Sherry vinegar strikes a happy medium between the astringency of wine vinegars and the sugary tones of balsamic. The best ones come directly from Jerez, the sherry-producing region of Andalucía, Spain, and they're worth a little splurge.

- 1 medium shallot, minced
- 2 tablespoons sherry vinegar
- 1 tablespoon fresh lemon juice
- 1 teaspoon Dijon mustard
- ¼ cup plus 3 tablespoons extra-virgin olive oil
- Fine sea salt and freshly ground black pepper to taste

Whisk together the shallot, vinegar, lemon juice, and mustard in a small bowl and let the shallot macerate for at least 15 minutes. Gradually whisk in the oil. Season with salt and pepper.

Do ahead: The dressing will keep 1 week in the refrigerator. If it loses some zing during storage, add a bit more lemon juice or vinegar to brighten it up.

SPREADS AND SNACKS

WHITE BEAN DIP

TOTAL TIME: ABOUT 5 MINUTES
MAKES 3½ CUPS (¼ CUP PER SERVING)

White bean dip is a great wholesome party option when you're working your way through the cleanse. The smooth white dip is a great canvas for color: sprinkle with some chopped herbs and serve it up with a beautiful riot of crudités: endive, carrots of all colors, florets of Romanesco or cauliflower, cherry tomatoes, and quickly blanched green beans or asparagus (see page 304). If you're making it your afternoon snack, simplify and serve with a cup of one or two kinds of raw vegetables.

- 2½ cups cooked white beans (see page 303), drained and cooking water reserved
- Cooked leeks and garlic cloves from cooking the beans
- 1 teaspoon chopped fresh sage leaves, plus more to taste
- 2 tablespoons lemon juice, plus more to taste
- ¼ cup extra-virgin olive oil
- Fine sea salt and freshly ground black pepper to taste
- Red pepper flakes, such as Aleppo or Marash, to taste

In a food processor, puree the beans, leeks, and garlic. Add the sage and lemon juice. While the motor is running, pour the oil into the bean mixture. If the texture is too thick for a dip, add some cooking water to smooth it out. Add salt, pepper, and red pepper flakes to taste, as well as more sage and/or lemon juice, if desired. Cool and store in an airtight container in the refrigerator for up to 5 days.

SPICED PUMPKIN SEED AND CASHEW CRUNCH

TOTAL TIME: 30 MINUTES (5 MINUTES ACTIVE)
MAKES ABOUT 1 CUP (1 TO 2 TABLESPOONS PER SERVING)

For a salty, savory, crunchy boost, sprinkle this on roasted vegetables, soups, and hot cereal. Garam masala, the peppery northern Indian spice blend, is available at many groceries, as well as health food and Asian specialty stores.

- Nonstick vegetable oil spray
- 1 large egg white
- 1 teaspoon light agave syrup
- ½ teaspoon garam masala or curry powder
- ½ teaspoon kosher salt
- ⅛ teaspoon ground cayenne pepper
- ¼ cup coarsely chopped raw cashews
- ¼ cup shelled pepitas (pumpkin seeds)
- ¼ cup shelled sunflower seeds

Preheat the oven to 300°F. Coat a rimmed baking sheet with nonstick spray. Whisk together the egg white, agave syrup, garam masala, salt, and cayenne in a medium bowl. Add the nuts and seeds and toss to coat. Using a slotted spoon, transfer the mixture to a baking sheet, letting the excess egg drip back into the bowl.

Bake, tossing once, until the mixture is golden brown, 20 to 25 minutes. Let it cool on the baking sheet.

Do ahead: The crunch can be made up to 10 days ahead. Store airtight at room temperature.

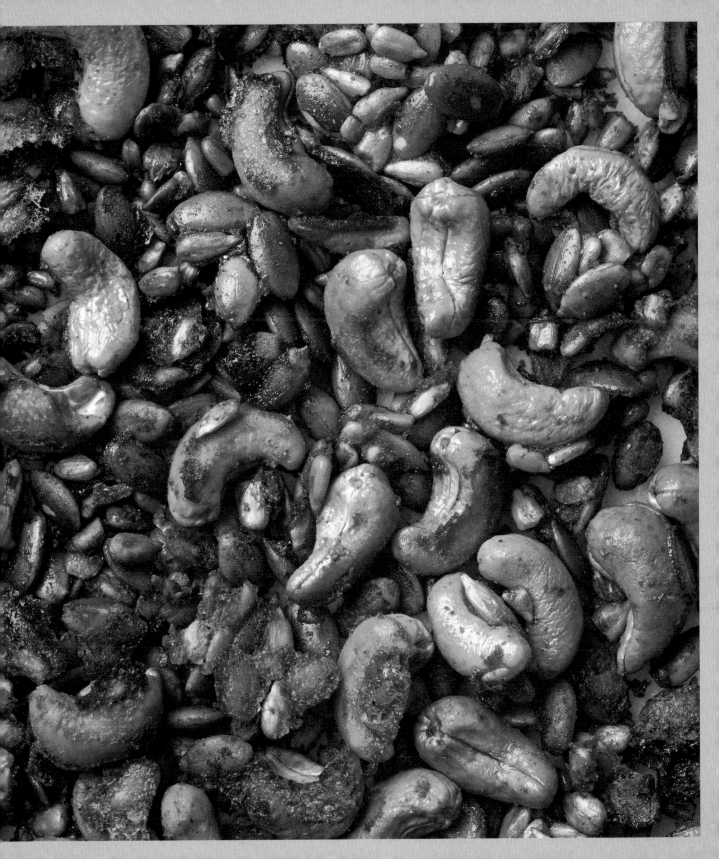

ROASTED BEET AND TAHINI DIP

TOTAL TIME: 10 MINUTES
MAKES 1½ CUPS (2 TABLESPOONS PER SERVING)

I love the flavor of beets, but I won't lie; sometimes it's all about the color for me. When you grate them up and mix them with garlicky tahini, you get a vivid dip that makes a healthier party dip or afternoon snack seem all the more fun. This recipe calls for roasted beets; see my method for steam-roasting beets on page 303 (and roast a couple of extras while you're at it, as a backup side dish or a garnish for a lunchtime salad).

A serving of this dip is perfect with 1 cup raw vegetables or 3 or 4 thin all-rye crackers.

- 1 tablespoon tahini
- 1 tablespoon very hot water
- 1 garlic clove, grated
- 2 tablespoons lemon juice, plus more to taste
- 1 tablespoon extra-virgin olive oil
- ⅛ teaspoon smoked paprika
- 2 large roasted beets, peeled and grated
- Fine sea salt and freshly ground black pepper to taste

In a large bowl, mix together the tahini and hot water until the paste is pale and pliable. Whisk in the garlic, lemon juice, oil, and paprika to form a smooth mixture. Fold in the grated beets and season to taste with the salt and pepper and more lemon juice, if desired. Store chilled in an airtight container for up to a week.

SPICY CARROT DIP

TOTAL TIME: ABOUT 20 MINUTES
MAKES 2 CUPS (¼ CUP PER PERSON)

Carrots are so simple, but they can deliver voluptuous flavor when they're simply stewed and then pureed into a golden dip that's great for crudités (and when you're not cleansing, pita bread).

A serving of this dip is perfect with 1 cup raw vegetables or 3 or 4 thin all-rye crackers.

- ¼ cup plus 1 tablespoon olive oil
- 2 garlic cloves, sliced thinly
- 1½ pounds carrots (about 12 medium), cut into ½-inch pieces
- Fine sea salt to taste
- 2 tablespoons lemon juice
- ½ teaspoon ground cumin
- ¼ teaspoon red pepper flakes, such as Aleppo or Marash pepper, plus more to taste
- Freshly ground black pepper to taste

In a large skillet with a lid, heat 1 tablespoon of the oil over medium heat. Add the garlic and cook until fragrant, then add in the carrots and a pinch of salt. Pour in 1 cup of water, bring to a boil, turn the heat to low, and cover. Cook until the carrots are tender, about 15 minutes. Drain the liquid and return the skillet to the heat to cook off any remaining liquid and let the carrots develop an amber glaze, about 5 minutes.

Place the carrots in a food processor or blender and puree with the remaining ¼ cup oil, the lemon juice, cumin, and red pepper flakes until very smooth. Taste and add more salt, red pepper flakes, and black pepper to taste. Store chilled in an airtight container for up to a week.

GRILLED CAPONATA RELISH

TOTAL TIME: 25 MINUTES
MAKES 1¾ CUPS (2 TO 3 TABLESPOONS PER SERVING)

After I've cooked a dinner on the grill, I often try to make a little something extra using the last heat of the coals. Here's a special relish that you can make in the evening and keep around to serve with morning eggs, mix into salads, or use as the basis for midafternoon snacks throughout your cleanse (serve it with a crumble of chèvre). Fragrant with mint and dappled with capers, this caponata is based on the classic Sicilian relish, but it gets smoky flair from a bit of charring on the grill.

- 1 pound (about 4 small) Japanese or Chinese eggplant, stemmed and cut lengthwise into ½-inch wedges
- 3 tablespoons extra-virgin olive oil
- Fine sea salt to taste
- 1 large sweet onion
- 2 celery stalks, trimmed
- Canola oil, for the grill
- 1 tablespoon honey
- 2 tablespoons red wine vinegar
- 1 tablespoon capers, soaked and drained if packed in salt, rinsed if packed in vinegar
- 1 garlic clove, minced
- 12 cherry tomatoes, halved
- Fresh mint leaves from 2 to 3 sprigs, roughly torn
- Flaky sea salt and freshly ground black pepper to taste

Build a charcoal fire or preheat the grill to medium-high.

Toss the eggplant with 1 tablespoon of the olive oil and season with fine sea salt.

Cut the onion crosswise into ½-inch slices, keeping the concentric rings together in each slice (if you have skewers handy, stick a skewer through the rings to hold them together). Lay the slices on a large plate and drizzle with 1 tablespoon of the olive oil. Season with fine sea salt.

Rub the celery stalks with the extra oil on the onion plate.

Scrape the grill well with a brush and, using tongs, rub the grate with a paper towel coated with canola oil.

Lay the eggplant wedges, onion rings, and celery stalks on the grill. Grill the onion rings until they're browned with slightly charred grill marks, about 6 minutes. Using a spatula or tongs, turn them over carefully, keeping the concentric rings together. Grill until browned on the other side, about 4 minutes. Remove the skewers, if using, and roughly chop.

Grill the eggplant wedges until browned on one side, about 5 minutes. Turn the slices over and grill until the eggplant has browned and softened, about 5 minutes. Remove from the heat and roughly chop.

Cook the celery, rotating frequently, until crisp grill marks develop and the celery is cooked but still crisp, about 6 minutes total. Roughly chop and set aside.

In a large bowl, whisk together the honey, vinegar, capers, garlic, and the remaining 1 tablespoon olive oil. Stir in the chopped celery, onion, and eggplant and then the cherry tomatoes and mint. Stir well and season with flaky sea salt and pepper.

PRESERVED LEMON HARISSA

TOTAL TIME: ABOUT 20 MINUTES
MAKES ABOUT 1 CUP (1 TABLESPOON PER SERVING)

For recipes such as Tunisian-Style Poached Eggs in Red Pepper Sauce (page 244), you can easily get harissa at Whole Foods or from online retailers such as chefshop.com. But along the way, I decided to take harissa into my own hands to deliver an earthy chile sauce that's just the right blend of heat and warm spices. This version is accented with the funky taste of preserved lemons.

- 1 cup boiling water
- 2 pasilla chiles negro, stemmed and seeded
- 1 tablespoon coriander seeds
- 1½ teaspoons cumin seeds
- 1½ teaspoons fennel seeds
- 1 teaspoon caraway seeds
- ½ teaspoon ground cinnamon
- 1 teaspoon sweet paprika (not smoked)
- ½ teaspoon red pepper flakes, preferably Aleppo or Marash, plus more to taste
- 1 red bell pepper, roasted, peeled, cored, and seeded*
- 1 teaspoon wine vinegar (red, white, or sherry)
- 1 garlic clove, minced
- 2 tablespoons minced preserved lemon peel (flesh scooped out and discarded)
- 2 tablespoons olive oil
- Fine sea salt to taste

To roast a red pepper, place the oven rack about 6 inches from the broiler element. Lightly rub the red pepper with olive oil and place it on a baking sheet on the oven rack. Cook, using tongs to turn occasionally, until all sides of the pepper are blistered (about 15 minutes total). Place in a bowl, cover the bowl with a plate, and let the pepper steam. When cool enough to handle, peel off the skin and remove the stem and seeds.

Pour the boiling water over the pasilla chiles negro and cover with a piece of plastic wrap directly on the surface. Let the peppers soak until soft, about 15 minutes.

Meanwhile, in a dry skillet, combine the coriander, cumin, fennel, and caraway seeds. Cook over medium heat, stirring frequently, until the spices are aromatic and lightly toasted, 3 to 4 minutes. Let cool. In a small food processor, spice grinder, or mortar and pestle, combine the coriander mixture with the cinnamon, paprika, and red pepper flakes and grind to a powder.

Drain the pasilla chiles negro, reserving the soaking water. Place the chiles, roasted bell pepper, coriander mixture, vinegar, garlic, preserved lemon peel, and oil in a food processor. Process into a coarse puree; if it needs a bit more liquid, add some pepper soaking water, 1 tablespoon at a time. Taste and add salt and more pepper flakes to taste. Store in the refrigerator in an airtight container for up to two weeks.

HERBED YOGURT SPREAD

TOTAL TIME: 5 MINUTES
MAKES ABOUT 1 CUP (2 TO 3 TABLESPOONS PER SERVING)

This bright dip brings some green goddess deliciousness to your afternoon snacks and a little voluptuous pleasure to your eggs in the morning. Don't drive yourself crazy over the herbs: use a mixture of whatever tender herbs—like dill, chervil, basil—you can easily gather together. Heartier thyme leaves might also work (go easier on the thyme, though—it's more pungent).

A serving of this dip is perfect with 1 cup raw vegetables or 3 or 4 thin all-rye crackers.

- 1 cup plain Greek yogurt
- 1 tablespoon olive oil
- 1 tablespoon finely minced shallot
- 2 teaspoons red wine vinegar, white wine vinegar, or sherry vinegar
- 2 tablespoons chopped fresh tarragon leaves
- ¼ cup chopped fresh mint leaves
- 2 tablespoons chopped fresh flat-leaf parsley leaves
- 2 tablespoons chopped fresh chives
- Fine sea salt and freshly ground black pepper

Line a sieve with 2 coffee filters (if using the cone kind, open them up at the seams first). Scoop the yogurt into the lined sieve and suspend it over a deep bowl. Let the yogurt drip for at least 15 minutes to thicken (the longer the better).

Scoop the thickened yogurt into a medium bowl. Whisk in the oil, shallot, and vinegar. Stir in the tarragon, mint, parsley, and chives. Season with salt and pepper. Store in an airtight container in the refrigerator for up to 5 days.

SMOKED TROUT SPREAD

TOTAL TIME: ABOUT 10 MINUTES
MAKES 1 CUP (2 TO 3 TABLESPOONS PER SERVING)

I'm a huge whitefish salad fan, and this easy-to-make recipe keeps a little of the delicious deli essence, but instead of mayonnaise and sour cream, it's bound with Greek yogurt and olive oil. Serve it on thin rye crackers or fill celery stalks or piquillo peppers with the spread.

- 1 Meyer lemon or zest and juice from 1 large conventional lemon
- 2 smoked trout fillets, preferably refrigerated rather than canned, skinned, deboned, and crumbled
- 4 teaspoons chopped fresh dill
- 2 tablespoons plain Greek yogurt
- 2 tablespoons olive oil
- Fine sea salt and freshly ground black pepper to taste

If using the Meyer lemon, cut the pointed ends off the lemon and stand it vertically. Using fluid, curved, downward knife strokes, slice off a swath of skin, pith, and about ⅛ inch of the interior flesh of the lemon. Continue until all the skin is removed. Finely chop enough of the skin strips to make 1 tablespoon and place it in a medium bowl.

Squeeze the remaining lemon flesh and measure out 1½ tablespoons of lemon juice; add it to the bowl. (If using conventional lemon, place zest and 1½ tablespoons juice in the bowl.) Stir in the trout, dill, yogurt, and oil and use a wooden spoon to mash the fish mixture into a chunky but spreadable paste. Add more lemon juice, if desired, and season with salt and pepper to taste.

CHICKPEA AND HAZELNUT DUKKAH

TOTAL TIME: ABOUT 12 MINUTES
MAKES 1¾ CUPS (1 TABLESPOON PER SERVING)

Dukkah is a dry dip that comes originally from Egypt, and it got very trendy in Australia a few years ago before making waves here. I'm totally smitten with the combination of toasted nuts and seeds. You can use it as a dip (a little olive oil helps glue the mixture to your carrots or radishes), or you can sprinkle it on salads and stews for a last-minute burst of texture and flavor. Roasted chickpeas (ceci) are available at a lot of Mediterranean import stores and at nuts.com. If you can't locate them, feel free to substitute ¼ cup more hazelnuts.

- ½ cup hazelnuts
- ¼ cup sesame seeds
- 2 tablespoons coriander seeds
- 2 tablespoons cumin seeds
- 1 teaspoon caraway seeds
- 1½ teaspoons fennel seeds
- ¼ cup roasted chickpeas or a combination of chickpeas and favas
- ½ teaspoon ground cinnamon
- ¼ teaspoon red pepper flakes, preferably Aleppo or Marash
- 1 teaspoon salt

To toast the hazelnuts, preheat the oven to 300°F. Spread the hazelnuts on a sheet pan and toast until the nuts are light golden brown at their centers, 8 to 10 minutes. Let cool, then rub the nuts vigorously with a clean kitchen towel to remove most of the skins. Lift the nuts free of the skins.

To toast the sesame seeds, heat the seeds in a dry skillet over medium heat. Stir and shake until the seeds are pale golden brown, about 2 minutes. Remove from the pan and set aside to cool.

Combine the coriander, cumin, caraway, and fennel seeds in the same skillet over medium heat and cook, stirring frequently, until lightly toasted, about 2 minutes. Remove from the pan and set aside to cool.

Place the hazelnuts, sesame seeds, coriander mixture, chickpeas, cinnamon, red pepper flakes, and salt in a food processor (or you can work in batches with a spice grinder). Pulse until coarsely chopped.

Serve as a topping for salads, yogurt, or stews, or use as a dip with crudités.

Do ahead: The dukkah can be made up to 10 days ahead. Store airtight at room temperature.

SMOKED SALT FURIKAKE

TOTAL TIME: 10 MINUTES
MAKES ABOUT ⅓ CUP

Furikake, a classic Japanese rice seasoning, gives you a couple of key flavors all at once: there's salt, of course, in this case smoky salt, and then there's the flavor-doubling effect of umami, which is present in both the seaweed and the bonito. I sprinkle it on eggs, on rice, and on seafood of all sorts.

- 2 tablespoons sesame seeds
- 1 sheet toasted nori, torn into small pieces
- 2 tablespoons bonito flakes (available at most Asian groceries or health food stores)
- 1 tablespoon smoked sea salt

Toast the sesame seeds in a dry skillet over medium heat. Stir frequently and remove when pale golden brown, about 2 minutes. Let cool.

In a small food processor, spice grinder, or mortar and pestle, grind the nori, bonito, and ½ tablespoon of the salt into a fine powder. Mix the powder with the cooled toasted sesame seeds and the remaining ½ tablespoon salt. Store in an airtight container for up to a month.

QUICK CITRUS-PICKLED ONION

TOTAL TIME: 32 MINUTES (2 MINUTES ACTIVE)
MAKES ¾ CUP

If you keep a batch of this on hand, you can instantly up your salad game at lunch. It's also great atop grilled or braised meats, on your midafternoon egg snack, or with smoked fish at breakfast time.

- ½ large red onion, thinly sliced (¾ cup)
- ¼ cup lime juice (from about 2 limes)
- 2 tablespoons orange juice
- ½ teaspoon dried oregano
- Fine sea salt to taste

In a medium bowl, toss the onion with the lime and orange juices, oregano, and a solid pinch of salt. Place in the refrigerator and let sit at least 30 minutes; if you want to make this ahead of time, it'll keep for 2 days in the refrigerator.

DESSERTS
SEASONAL CHOCOLATE BARK VARIATIONS

I don't do well with "healthy" desserts. A lower-fat, higher-fiber cookie is still a cookie, and I'm likely to eat too many. But from the first cleanse on, Marissa and I wanted to incorporate a minidessert that offers a sense of celebration and sweetness at the end of a day of discipline. Dark chocolate, which has relatively little sugar, balanced out by lots of flavor and antioxidants, seemed the way to go. A little bit goes a long way, and I thought it would be even more compelling if topped with seriously textured garnishes. The first time out, I scattered melted chocolate to make the original Salted Seedy Chocolate Bark. The barks have changed with subsequent years, and for the book, I thought it would be great to have one for each season.

SPRING

RASPBERRY-PISTACHIO CHOCOLATE BARK

TOTAL TIME: 2 HOURS 5 MINUTES (5 MINUTES ACTIVE)
MAKES 8 SERVINGS

- 8 ounces bittersweet chocolate with at least 70% cacao content, chopped
- ¼ cup chopped pistachios
- ¼ teaspoon flaky sea salt or kosher salt
- ¼ cup crumbled freeze-dried raspberries

Line a baking sheet with a silicone mat or a sheet of parchment paper.

Place the chocolate in a microwave-safe bowl. Microwave at 50% power for 1 minute. Stir and continue cooking in 30-second bursts, stirring after each one, until the chocolate is melted.

Pour the chocolate onto the prepared baking sheet and smooth it out into an even layer (it will not cover the entire pan). Evenly sprinkle the pistachios over the chocolate and season with the salt. Sprinkle the crumbled berries over the chocolate and let it cool for 2 hours or more.

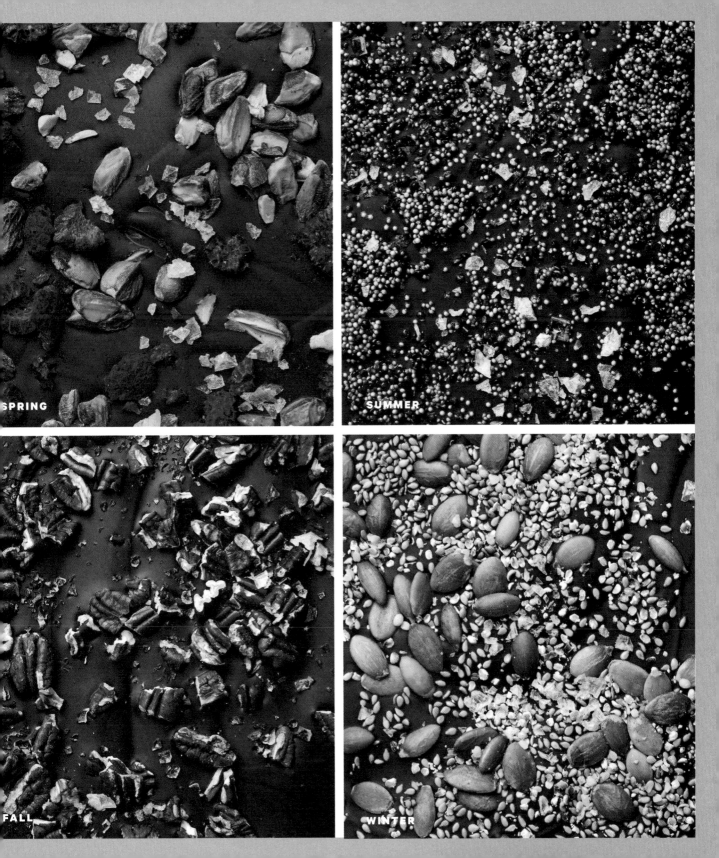

SPRING

SUMMER

FALL

WINTER

SUMMER

HONEY-TOASTED QUINOA AND AMARANTH BARK

TOTAL TIME: 2 HOURS 5 MINUTES (5 MINUTES ACTIVE)
MAKES 8 SERVINGS

- 8 ounces bittersweet chocolate with at least 70% cacao content, chopped
- ½ teaspoon ground cinnamon
- Small pinch of ground cayenne pepper (optional)
- 2 tablespoons red or black quinoa
- 2 tablespoons amaranth seeds
- 1 teaspoon honey
- Flaky sea salt or kosher salt to taste

Line a baking sheet with a silicone mat or a sheet of parchment paper.

Place the chocolate in a microwave-safe bowl. Microwave at 50% power for 1 minute. Stir and continue cooking in 30-second bursts, stirring after each one, until the chocolate is melted. Stir in the cinnamon and, if using, the cayenne.

In a dry skillet, heat the quinoa over medium heat, stirring and shaking frequently; once the quinoa starts popping vigorously (about 1 minute), cook 10 more seconds and remove the quinoa to a plate. Place the amaranth seeds in the pan and cook until they're vigorously popping, about 1 minute. Return the quinoa to the pan, stir, and turn off the heat. Drizzle in the honey and stir vigorously until the seeds gather in crisp clusters.

Pour the chocolate onto the prepared baking sheet and smooth it out into an even layer (it will not cover the entire pan). Evenly sprinkle the amaranth-quinoa combination over the chocolate, then sprinkle with salt to taste. Let cool for 2 hours or more.

FALL

PECAN-GINGER BARK

TOTAL TIME: 2 HOURS 5 MINUTES (5 MINUTES ACTIVE)
MAKES 8 SERVINGS

- ½ cup pecans
- 8 ounces bittersweet chocolate with at least 70% cacao content, chopped
- 1½ teaspoons grated peeled fresh ginger
- ¼ teaspoon flaky sea salt or kosher salt

Preheat the oven to 300°F and spread the pecans on a baking sheet. Cook until the nuts are warmed through and fragrant, 6 to 8 minutes. Let cool, then chop.

Line the baking sheet with a silicone mat or a sheet of parchment paper.

Place the chocolate in a microwave-safe bowl. Microwave at 50% power for 1 minute. Stir and continue cooking in 30-second bursts, stirring after each one, until the chocolate is melted. Stir in the ginger (the chocolate will look a bit lumpy after this addition).

Pour the chocolate onto the prepared baking sheet and smooth it out into an even layer (it will not cover the entire pan). Evenly sprinkle the pecans over the chocolate, then sprinkle with the salt. Let cool for 2 hours or more.

SALTED SEEDY CHOCOLATE BARK: THE ORIGINAL

TOTAL TIME: 2 HOURS 5 MINUTES (5 MINUTES ACTIVE)
MAKES 8 SERVINGS

- ¼ cup raw shelled pepitas (pumpkin seeds)
- 2 tablespoons hemp seeds
- 2 tablespoons sesame seeds
- ¼ teaspoon flaky sea salt or kosher salt
- 8 ounces bittersweet chocolate with at least 70% cacao content, chopped

Line a baking sheet with a silicone mat or a sheet of parchment paper.

Heat a dry skillet over medium-high heat and add the pumpkin seeds. Toast, stirring occasionally, until the seeds first start to pop, about 1 minute. Pour the seeds into a bowl. Add the hemp seeds to the same skillet and toast, stirring frequently, until the seeds are fragrant and just starting to turn a pale straw gold, about 45 seconds. Add them to the bowl with the pumpkin seeds. Toast the sesame seeds in the same skillet over medium-high heat until fragrant and just starting to turn golden, about 45 seconds. Add them to the bowl with other seeds. Add the salt and toss to combine.

Place the chocolate in a microwave-safe bowl. Microwave at 50% power for 1 minute. Stir and continue cooking in 30-second bursts, stirring after each one, until the chocolate is melted.

Pour the chocolate onto the prepared baking sheet and smooth it out into an even layer (it will not cover the entire pan). Sprinkle the seed mixture evenly over the chocolate. Let it stand at room temperature for at least 2 hours.

TO SERVE CHOCOLATE BARK

Break it into 8 pieces (the chocolate may be a bit soft, depending on the brand) and store them in an airtight container in the refrigerator. If desired, let the chocolate stand at room temperature for 10 minutes before eating.

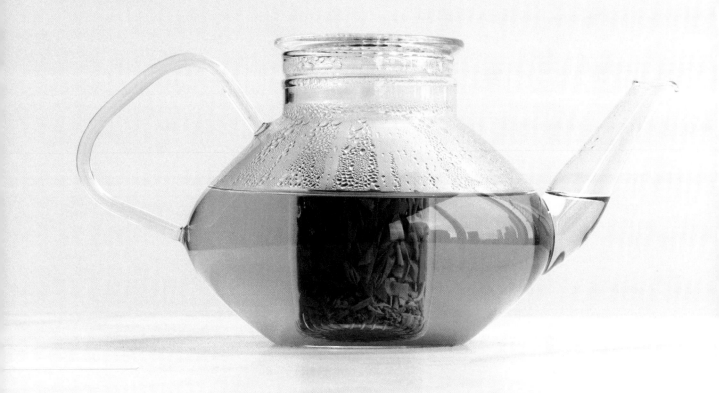

ACKNOWLEDGMENTS

My first thank-you is to the community of people who have participated in The Food Lover's Cleanse online. You were my sounding board, my (constructive) critics, and my dedicated audience, who made me feel as if we were really onto something. It's been to a wonderful thing to cook and eat with you.

Thank you to everyone who built the Food Lover's Cleanse on bonappetit.com. Marissa Lippert, my nutritional guru and friend—your enthusiasm for good food made it possible to plan a wholesome eating plan focused on delightful flavor and the joys of market-fresh eating. Thanks for being there all this time. Emily Fleischaker got the snowball rolling; who knew it would roll so fast and get so big? Thanks also to editors Julia Bainbridge, Matt Gross, and Carey Polis, who shaped the plan in subsequent years. Thanks to the sharp eyes and creative minds in the *Bon Appétit* test kitchen who made the recipes bulletproof, including Dawn Perry, Janet McCracken, and Allie Lewis Clapp. Thanks to the photographers who have made the web cleanse look so good over the years, including Kimberly Hasselbrink and Danny Kim. Thanks too to Danielle Walsh and Laura Loesch-Quintin, who helped me connect more directly with our wonderful readers.

In making this book, I've been incredibly grateful to the *Bon Appétit* staff, who have contributed their (strong) opinions, style, and belief in this project. I know it was a lot of work, and I'm so glad you found time for it. Thanks to Adam Rapoport, Carla Lalli Music, Alex Pollack, Alex Grossman, Stacey Rivera, and Meryl Rothstein. And to Greg Ferro, thanks

for your calm manner and kindness as we juggled so many elements in putting this together.

Michael Graydon and Nikole Herriott's images made this book the beautiful object it is. Thank you to the entire photography team, who crafted these breathtaking images at a hurricane pace: food stylist Rebecca Jurkevich; prop stylists Amy Wilson and Nina Lalli; photo assistants Jon Vachon and Andrew Katzowitz; food styling assistants Sue Li, Drew Salvatore, Misha Spivack, and Elizabeth Jaime; and Julia Callon, who kept the whole operation moving forward from Times Square all the way to Lower Manhattan. Thanks to Sarah Gephart and Olivia de Salve Villedieu at MGMT. design for pulling all this material into a beautiful form.

Yewande Komolafe diligently tested all these recipes and always knew how to gracefully perfect a recipe. Thanks for rallying around this complicated project.

Thank you to my editor, Cassie Jones, for believing in this project and for asking all the right questions.

Kim Witherspoon, my agent, called me almost ten years ago to see what I might like to develop into a book. It took me a while to decide, but when I did, I knew it was right. Thanks for waiting for me.

Here in Seattle, I know I got a little tightly wound as I developed these recipes and eating plans. Thanks to Sam Dickerman, Leah Dickerman, Teri Gelber, Curtis Vredenburg, Brad Hinckley, Hanouf Grandinetti, and Sarah Flotard for keeping me calmish. And most of all, thanks to my beautiful family for reminding me that eating well is all about who you're eating with: I love you, Andrew, Gus, and Adele.

UNIVERSAL CONVERSION CHART

OVEN TEMPERATURE EQUIVALENTS

250-120°F = 120°C
275°F = 135°C
300°F = 150°C
325°F = 160°C
350°F = 180°C
375°F = 190°C
400°F = 200°C
425°F = 220°C
450°F = 230°C
475°F = 240°C
500°F = 260°C

MEASUREMENT EQUIVALENTS

Measurements should always be level unless directed otherwise.

⅛ teaspoon = 0.5 mL
¼ teaspoon = 1 mL
½ teaspoon = 2 mL
1 teaspoon = 5 mL
1 tablespoon = 3 teaspoons = ½ fluid ounce = 15 mL
2 tablespoons = ⅛ cup = 1 fluid ounce = 30 mL
4 tablespoons = ¼ cup = 2 fluid ounces = 60 mL
5⅓ tablespoons = ⅓ cup = 3 fluid ounces = 80 mL
8 tablespoons = ½ cup = 4 fluid ounces = 120 mL
10 tablespoons = ⅔ cup = 5 fluid ounces = 160 mL
12 tablespoons = ¾ cup = 6 fluid ounces = 180 mL
16 tablespoons = 1 cup = 8 fluid ounces = 240 mL

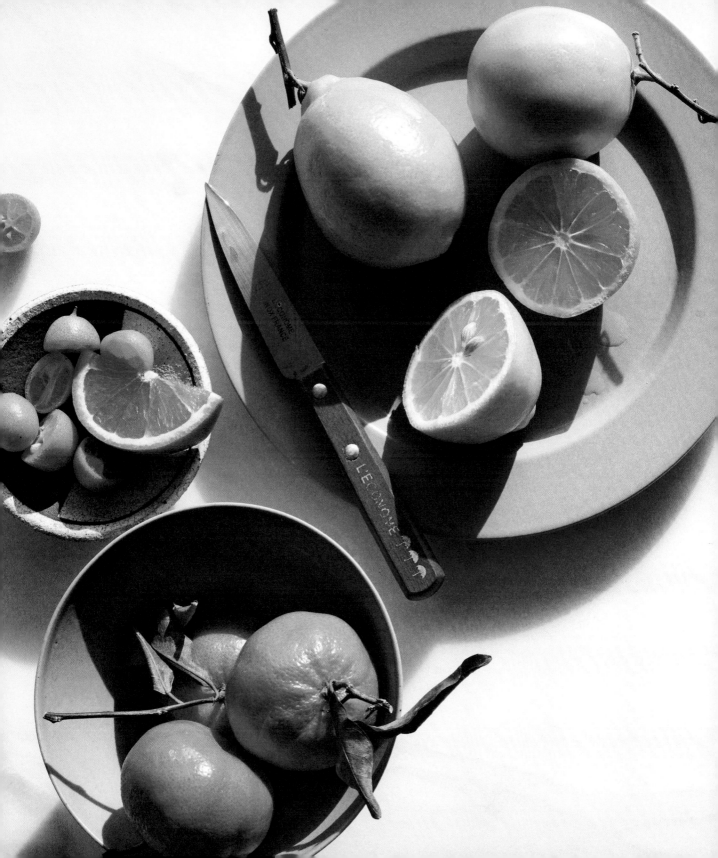

INDEX

Note: Page references in *italics* indicate photographs.

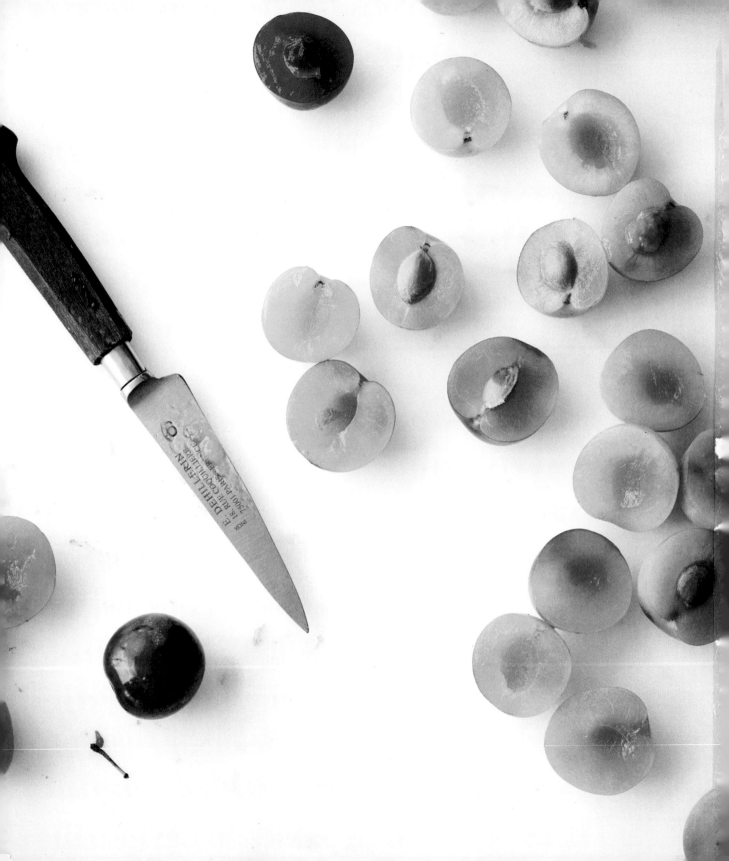